Core Review for Critical Care Nursing

Second Edition

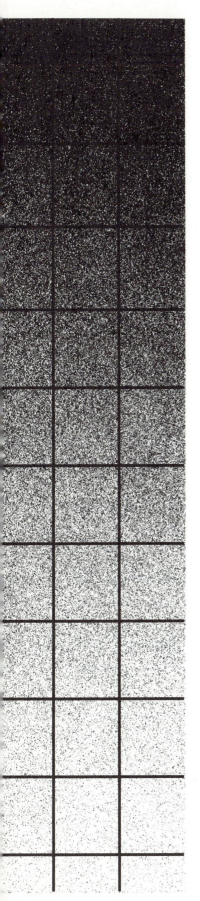

Core
Review
for
Critical Care
Nursing
Second Edition

JoAnn Grif Alspach, RN, MSN, EdD, Editor
Nursing Education Consultant, Critical Care,
Editor, *Critical Care Nurse*
Annapolis, Maryland

1991
W.B. SAUNDERS COMPANY
Harcourt Brace Jovanovich, Inc.
Philadelphia   London   Toronto   Montreal   Sydney   Tokyo

W. B. SAUNDERS COMPANY
Harcourt Brace Jovanovich, Inc.

The Curtis Center
Independence Square West
Philadelphia, PA 19106

Library of Congress Cataloging-in-Publication Data

Core review for critical care nursing/editor, JoAnn Grif Alspach.—
2nd ed.

p. cm.

Includes bibliographical references.

ISBN 0–7216–3228–9

1. Intensive care nursing—Examinations, questions, etc. [DNLM:
   1. Critical Care—examination questions. 2. Critical Care—nurses'
   instruction.   WY 18 C7975]

RT120.I5C67   1991

610.73'61—dc20   91-10415

Editor: Thomas Eoyang
Designer: Joan Wendt
Production Manager: Peter Faber
Manuscript Editor: Karen Okie
Illustration Coordinator: Brett MacNaughton
Cover Designer: Ellen M. Bodner

Core Review for Critical Care Nursing, 2nd Edition   ISBN   0–7216–3228–9

Printed in the United States of America.

Last digit is the print number: 9   8   7   6   5   4   3   2   1

Contributors

Kathleen E. Ellstrom, R.N., M.S., CCRN, CS
Clinical Nurse Specialist—Medical ICU and Research Nurse, Division of Pulmonary and Critical Care Medicine, University of California–Irvine Medical Center, Orange, California
Pulmonary

Karen L. Cooper, R.N., M.S.N., CCRN, CEN, CNA
Director of Nursing Education, STAT Nursing Services; Staff Nurse, PACU, UCSF Medical Center; Staff Nurse, ICU and Emergency Room, Mt. Zion Medical Center, San Francisco, California
Cardiovascular

Randy M. Caine, R.N., Ed.D., CS, CCRN
Associate Professor of Nursing, Director—Trauma/Emergency; Clinical Nurse Specialist Program, California State University, Long Beach, California
Neurologic

Janice P. Fracassi, R.N., M.S.N., CCRN, CNA
Director of Nursing, Critical Care and Emergency Services, Community Medical Center, Toms River, New Jersey
Renal

Jill A. Gershan, R.N., M.S.N., CCRN
Graduate Student, Marquette University, Milwaukee, Wisconsin
Endocrine

Martha A. Dickerson, R.N., M.S., CCRN
Manager, Clinical Staff Development, Michael Reese Health Plan, Chicago, Illinois
Hematologic

Barbara C. Opperwall, R.N., M.S.N., CS, CCRN
Clinical Nurse Specialist, Sinai Hospital of Detroit, Detroit, Michigan
Gastrointestinal

Patricia G. Rienzo, R.N., B.S.N., CCRN, M.S.
Community Educator, New London Hospital, New London, New Hampshire
Legal/Ethical

Reviewers

1. Pulmonary

   Jenny Hamner, R.N., M.S.N., CCRN
   Assistant Professor, School of Nursing, Auburn University,
   Auburn, Alabama

2. Cardiovascular

   Mary Abraham, R.N., M.A., CCRN
   Head Nurse, Surgical ICU, M. D. Anderson Cancer Center,
   Houston, Texas

3. Neurologic

   Jacqueline Sullivan, R.N., M.S.N., CCRN, CNRN
   Clinical Nurse Specialist, Neurosurgical ICU, Clinical Assistant
   Professor, Thomas Jefferson University, Philadelphia,
   Pennsylvania

4. Renal

   M. Lynn Rodgers, R.N., M.S.N., CCRN
   Critical Care Educator, Deaconess Hospital, Evansville, Indiana

5. Endocrine

   Mary Beth Harrington, R.N., M.S.N., CCRN
   Staff Nurse, Lahey Clinic Medical Center, Burlington,
   Massachusetts

6. Hematology

   Ann S. Bines, R.N., M.S., CCRN
   Clinical Nurse Manager, Post-Anesthesia Recovery Room, Olson
   Pavilion, Northwestern Memorial Hospital, Chicago, Illinois

7. Gastrointestinal

   Joyce Wolf Roth, R.N., M.S.N., CCRN
   Coordinator Nursing Education, Critical Care and Women's and
   Children's Health, New York Hospital–Cornell Medical Center,
   New York, New York

8. Legal/Ethical

Margo Halm, R.N., M.A., CCRN
Clinical Nurse Specialist II, Critical Care Nursing Division,
University of Iowa Hospitals and Clinics, Iowa City, Iowa

Preface

Quality of care of the critically ill patient requires that nurses be competent in critical care nursing practice and be able to provide care by effectively using the nursing process. The AACN *Core Curriculum for Critical Care Nursing* provides a framework for the universe of knowledge involved in critical care nursing practice. The *Core Review for Critical Care Nursing* is designed as a study guide to assess mastery of the content of the *Core Curriculum*.

This second edition of the *Core Review* retains many of the first edition's useful features. It continues to cover all topics contained in the most recent *Core Curriculum for Critical Care Nursing*, blending core content with the five steps of the nursing process. The 600 test items continue to evaluate a nurse's ability to assess, diagnose, plan, implement, and evaluate nursing care for patients with life-threatening health problems. The test items still comprise four-option multiple choice questions with explanations of correct and incorrect answers. References for each answer and annotated bibliographies are again provided to help users identify relevant references.

This second edition covers new topics included in the revised (1991) fourth edition of the *Core Curriculum* and introduces several new features as well. Among the new topics added to the *Core* are vascular surgery, immunosuppression and AIDS, neurosurgery, arteriovenous malformations, gastrointestinal surgery and trauma, bowel infarction and obstruction, and legal and ethical aspects of critical care nursing.

Most of the new features in this edition were introduced in order to more thoroughly emphasize a nursing orientation rather than a disease or medical model of care. These new features include the following:

—Greater use of case studies to demonstrate application of the nursing process.

—Inclusion of nursing diagnosis into the sample tests.

—Inclusion of various content areas in each test to approximate their proportional coverage in the CCRN examination blueprint.

—Location of answers at the end of each test so that test completion is not disrupted and more closely resembles completion of the CCRN examination.

—Use of a range of cognitive levels (i.e., knowledge-comprehension, application-analysis, and synthesis-evaluation) in the sample test items consistent with their distribution in the CCRN examination.

Inasmuch as the *Core Curriculum* is built around the CCRN examination blueprint, the sample tests in this book may be useful study guides for the CCRN examination. These tests are intended to simulate the general types of questions included in the CCRN examination, although none of the questions were or will be actual examination items. Because the CCRN examination is continually updated, candidates preparing for the exam are encouraged to request a copy of the most current blueprint from the AACN Certification Corporation.

The contributors to this book have made every attempt to provide a study guide that is helpful in validating a nurse's ability to apply the content of the *Core Curriculum* to critical care nursing practice. We welcome your comments on how well we have achieved our objectives.

JoAnn Grif Alspach
Editor

Instructions

Each of the three review tests in this book consists of 200 four-option multiple choice questions. To simulate taking a CCRN examination, mark your answer to each question for that test and allow a maximum of four hours to complete each test. After you have completed each test, compare your answers with those that appear in the answer key that follows that test.

A list of additional study references is provided for you in the annotated bibliographies for each content area of the CCRN examination. These bibliographies are located after the last of the three tests.

Table of Contents

CORE REVIEW TEST

1

1–1. The level of the mean arterial pressure (MAP) is a function of the cardiac output and

    A. Systemic vascular resistance.
    B. Pulse pressure.
    C. Myocardial contractility.
    D. Left ventricular stroke work.

1–2. The most abundant intracellular cation is

    A. Sodium.
    B. Potassium.
    C. Calcium.
    D. Magnesium.

1–3. Physiologic actions of glucocorticoids include

    A. Increased glycogenolysis.
    B. Decreased gluconeogenesis.
    C. Decreased cardiac contractility.
    D. Increased lysosomal membrane fragility.

1–4. Which of the following is a correct statement regarding the pia mater?

    A. It contains the larger blood vessels of the brain.
    B. It consists of two layers of tough, fibrous tissue.
    C. It contains channels that reabsorb cerebrospinal fluid (CSF).
    D. It contains blood vessels that form the choroid plexus.

1–5. Gas exchange occurs

    A. Down a pressure gradient.
    B. Through active transport.
    C. By bulk flow.
    D. By laminar flow.

1–6. Internal respiration occurs

    A. In the alveolus.
    B. Across the alveolar-capillary membrane.
    C. In the mitochondria.
    D. By diaphragmatic contraction.

1–7. The standards of care to which a nurse certified in critical care (CCRN) is held accountable are

A. Determined by hospital policy.
B. The same standards any RN must uphold.
C. The standards of the American Association of Critical-Care Nurses (AACN).
D. More advanced than the standards applied to an RN not certified in critical care.

1–8. Factors that accelerate gastric emptying include

A. Insulin and a large volume of liquids.
B. Starchy meals and Vitamin B_{12}.
C. Secretin and protein.
D. Fats and pepsinogen.

1–9. A patient received incompatible blood and developed a hemolytic transfusion reaction. The patient may develop which of the following signs and symptoms?

A. Pain at the intravenous (IV) site, hives, palpitations.
B. Dysphagia, diplopia, myoglobinuria.
C. Hypertension, hypothermia, confusion.
D. Severe back pain, hypotension, hematuria.

1–10. An obese patient with primary hypertension complains to you that he must not be sleeping well because he feels tired all of the time. Review of the night nurses' notes shows that the patient received a backrub at 2200 hours and was snoring loudly at 2400. From 0200 until 0500 the patient was noted to be asleep, but had occasional premature ventricular contractions (PVCs) on the cardiac monitor. The patient's blood pressure upon admission was 240/140 mm Hg and is currently 170/100 mm Hg.
Which of the following interventions would be most appropriate for this patient?

A. Obtain an order for a long-acting sedative so the patient sleeps deeply through the night.
B. Tell the patient that most people have difficulty sleeping at night in the hospital.
C. Tell the patient that with weight loss and blood pressure control his sleeping pattern will improve.
D. Tell the patient that many persons feel tired when they start taking blood pressure medications.

1–11. Cerebral vasospasm

A. Occurs as a result of dilation of cerebral arteries.
B. Is frequently a complication of subarachnoid hemorrhage.
C. Is preceded by a decreased blood pressure.
D. Is characterized by decreased cerebral vascular resistance.

1–12. In a patient experiencing vasospasm, the critical care nurse anticipates the use of

A. Hypervolemic therapy to increase cerebral perfusion pressure (CPP).
B. Hypovolemic therapy to reduce the risk of cerebral edema.
C. Antihypertensive therapy to decrease intracranial pressure.
D. Aggressive diuresis to decrease CPP.

1-13. Factors that can induce a hypoglycemic event include all *except*

A. Prolonged ethanol consumption.
B. Administration of exogenous insulin.
C. Chlorpropamide (Diabinese) ingestion.
D. Hydrocortisone (Solu-Cortef) injection.

1-14. A patient has been stable in the ICU with a pulmonary artery catheter in place for 6 days. His central venous pressure has ranged from 2 to 5 mm Hg and his pulmonary artery diastolic pressures have ranged from 6 to 10 mm Hg. The pulmonary capillary wedge pressure has been 6 mm Hg for 3 days. Over the last 2 hours his pulmonary artery diastolic pressure has risen to 25 mm Hg. No other hemodynamic parameters have changed. His heart rate is 80 beats per minute. What should be the suggested therapy for this condition?

A. Place the patient on oxygen by mask at 40% FI_{O_2}.
B. Remove the pulmonary artery catheter.
C. Give sublingual nitroglycerin, 1/150 grain.
D. Pull back the pulmonary artery catheter 1 cm.

1-15. During insertion of a pulmonary artery (Swan-Ganz) catheter, the balloon is first inflated while the tip of the catheter is in which of the following areas?

A. In the superior vena cava.
B. During passage through the tricuspid valve.
C. In the right ventricle.
D. In the pulmonary artery.

Questions 1–16 and 1–17 refer to the following situation.

The following laboratory results are obtained on a patient with long-standing congestive heart failure (CHF):

Serum Na	149	mEq/l
Serum K	2.7	mEq/l
Serum Cl	98	mEq/l
Serum CO_2	42	mEq/l

1-16. The most likely cause of this patient's potassium imbalance is

A. Metabolic alkalosis.
B. Diuretic therapy.
C. Excessive renin production.
D. Fluid overload.

1-17. In planning nursing interventions for this patient's serum potassium level, the nurse should be aware that

A. ECG changes will be the best indication of the effectiveness of treatment.
B. Immediate correction of any acidotic state is necessary for the treatment to be effective.
C. In cases where large doses of potassium fail to correct hypokalemia, concurrent hypomagnesemia should be suspected.
D. Potassium should always be diluted in dextrose solutions.

1-18. Electrolytes are most rapidly absorbed in the

A. Proximal portion of the large bowel.
B. Distal portion of the large bowel.
C. Proximal portion of the small bowel.
D. Distal portion of the small bowel.

1–19. Patients with chronic obstructive pulmonary disease frequently use pursed-lip breathing, especially when they are dyspneic. This breathing technique

A. Promotes a forceful cough.
B. Decreases need for oxygen.
C. Improves gas distribution.
D. Decreases bronchospasm.

1–20. Obstructive pulmonary disease is characterized by the following pulmonary function test results:

A. Decreased FRC and RV, increased FEV.
B. Increased FVC and FEV.
C. Decreased compliance, increased FEV.
D. Increased FRC, RV, and TLC; decreased FEV.

1–21. Septic shock is most frequently caused by

A. Clostridia.
B. *Escherichia coli.*
C. *Staphylococcus epidermidis.*
D. *Streptococcus pneumoniae.*

1–22. The early stages of septic shock are characterized by

A. Vasoconstriction with the release of histamine.
B. Increased cardiac output with peripheral vasoconstriction.
C. Vasodilation with fluid loss and the release of leukocytes.
D. Increased cardiac output with decreased vascular resistance.

1–23. The oculocephalic or doll's eye reflex causes the patient's eyes to

A. Move in the same direction of passive head movement.
B. Move in the opposite direction of passive head movement.
C. Move upward during head flexion.
D. Move downward during head extension.

1–24. When attempting to elicit the doll's eye response, the critical care nurse must remember that

A. Patients must be able to follow commands.
B. The pupils will accommodate but not react.
C. Cervical spine injury in the patient is a contraindication to performing this test.
D. This test must always be done in conjunction with the oculovestibular test.

Questions 1–25 through 1–28 refer to the following situation.

A patient admitted to the intensive care unit is disoriented and complaining of weakness, leg cramps, and polyuria. He is lethargic with dry, cracked lips; poor skin turgor; a weak rapid pulse; decreased bowel sounds; and rapid, deep respirations.

Laboratory and physical assessment findings are:

Vital Signs		Serum Laboratory	
T	97° F	HCT	47%
BP	70/60 mm Hg	pH	7.29
HR	135/min	K^+	5.1 mEq/l
RR	22/min	Na^+	132 mEq/l
		Osmolality	310 mOsm/l
		Glucose	400 mg/dl
		Cl^-	95 mEq/l
		HCO_3^-	15 mEq/l
		WBC	9,000/mm³
		Neutrophils	50%
		Band cells	3%

Urine nitroprusside test (Acetest)
Negative

1–25. The most likely precipitating cause for this patient developing diabetic ketoacidosis (DKA) is

A. Acute infection.
B. Failure to administer insulin.
C. A stress-mediated release of insulin.
D. Decreased level of circulating catecholamines.

1–26. Considering the given data, another physical finding that you would anticipate in this patient is (are)

A. Jaundice.
B. Pulmonary crackles.
C. Periorbital edema.
D. Fruity breath odor.

1–27. The patient's anion gap is

A. 22 mEq/l.
B. 17 mEq/l.
C. 13 mEq/l.
D. 11 mEq/l.

1–28. This anion gap is most likely to be due to the presence of

A. Lactate.
B. Pyruvate.
C. Phosphate.
D. 3-Hydroxybutyrate.

1–29. Twenty-four hours after a temporary pacemaker insertion, the nurse caring for the patient notes incomplete capture during continuous ECG monitoring. The pacemaker rate is set at 60 beats per minute, demand mode, set at 7 mA. Approximately one pacemaker spike out of 10 is not followed immediately by a ventricular complex. The nurse should first

A. Turn up the sensitivity of the pacemaker.
B. Turn up the mA of the pacemaker.
C. Have the patient lie on his left side.
D. Turn the pacemaker off by decreasing the rate slowly.

1–30. A 68-year-old male is admitted to the intensive care unit because of syncope and cardiac dysrhythmias. On physical assessment, the nurse notes petechiae on his trunk and excessive bruising on his limbs. His gums are moist, spongy, and bleeding easily. The nurse suspects a deficiency in

A. Iodine.
B. Iron.
C. Vitamin C.
D. Vitamin A.

1–31. A 26-year-old male is a member of an ethnic minority who was admitted to the critical care unit with a diagnosis of acquired immune deficiency syndrome (AIDS). He is a homosexual and an intravenous drug user. The nurse assigned to care for this patient asks to be removed from his case. Which of the following reasons for this request would be consistent with the American Nurses Association (ANA) Code for Nurses?

A. The nurse is prejudiced against the minority group to which the patient belongs.
B. The nurse finds the patient's lifestyle morally objectionable.
C. The nurse lacks the necessary knowledge and skill to adequately care for an AIDS patient.
D. The nurse does not want to be exposed to a life-threatening, communicable disease.

1–32. Acute respiratory failure is defined as

A. $Pa_{O_2} > 60$ mm Hg, $Pa_{CO_2} > 50$ mm Hg.
B. $Pa_{O_2} < 60$ mm Hg, $Pa_{CO_2} > 50$ mm Hg.
C. $Pa_{O_2} > 60$ mm Hg, $Pa_{CO_2} < 50$ mm Hg.
D. $Pa_{O_2} < 60$ mm Hg, $Pa_{CO_2} < 50$ mm Hg.

1–33. Patients in acute respiratory failure need to be positioned upright in order to

A. Increase vital capacity.
B. Prevent aspiration.
C. Increase oxygen delivery.
D. Decrease the work of breathing.

1–34. A 39-year-old male has just learned he has leukemia. You have noticed that he does not discuss his diagnosis when his wife comes to visit. He stares at the television and does not talk to her. He also says he's more tired than usual and sleeps much of the time. His wife comes to you expressing her concern about the diagnosis and her husband's reaction. Your plan of care will include which of the following nursing diagnoses?

    I. Powerlessness.
    II. Impaired verbal communication.
    III. Hopelessness.
    IV. Decisional conflict.

    A. I and II only.
    B. II and IV only.
    C. I and III only.
    D. III and IV only.

1–35. A patient in the intensive care unit has a serum phosphorus level of 0.4 mg/dl. This could be a result of any of the following *except*

    A. Hyperalimentation.
    B. Hypoparathyroid state.
    C. Chronic alcoholism.
    D. Diabetic ketoacidosis.

1–36. The following lead II rhythm strip demonstrates

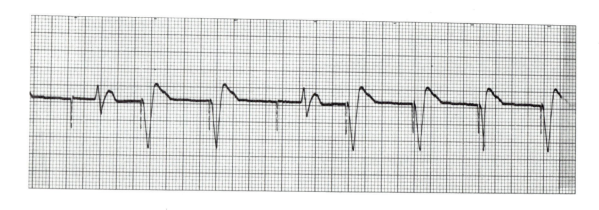

    A. Competition.
    B. Inappropriate sensing.
    C. Incomplete capture.
    D. Failure to pace.

1–37. Which of the following conditions decreases myocardial contractility?

    A. Hypernatremia.
    B. Oxygen saturation of 80%.
    C. Hypocalcemia.
    D. Hypokalemia.

Questions 1–38 and 1–39 refer to the following situation.

A 22-year-old female is admitted through the emergency department after an intentional acetaminophen overdose. It is estimated that she ingested at least 50 325-mg tablets 3 to 4 hours ago. Gastric aspiration was negative for the drug.

1–38. The nurse should anticipate the immediate administration of

    A. Sodium bicarbonate.
    B. Ipecac syrup.
    C. Saline cathartics.
    D. Acetylcysteine.

1–39. This patient is at high risk for development of

    A. Hepatic failure.
    B. Acid-base imbalances.
    C. Agranulocytosis.
    D. Oxyhemoglobinemia.

1–40. A basic neurologic examination includes

    A. Level of consciousness, cranial nerves, vital signs.
    B. Level of consciousness, motor function, cranial nerves.
    C. Motor function, sensory function, vital signs.
    D. Level of consciousness, motor function, vital signs.

1–41. A fixed, dilated, or "blown" pupil noted on assessment usually indicates

    A. Central herniation.
    B. Uncal herniation.
    C. Overdosage of medication.
    D. A subacute disorder.

1–42. Q waves and ST elevations in leads V_2 through V_4 of a 12-lead ECG indicate

    A. Inferior wall myocardial infarction.
    B. Lateral wall myocardial infarction.
    C. Posterior wall myocardial infarction.
    D. Anterior wall myocardial infarction.

1–43. Which of the following complications is most likely to occur in acute inferior wall myocardial infarction?

    A. Mobitz type I heart block (Wenckebach).
    B. Paroxysmal atrial tachycardia (PAT).
    C. Right bundle branch block (RBBB).
    D. Cardiogenic shock.

1–44. For the nursing diagnosis "Decreased myocardial tissue perfusion related to myocardial infarction," the most appropriate expected outcome *upon admission* would be

    A. Patient denies chest pain.
    B. Patient reports chest pain at onset.
    C. Patient and family are able to describe the symptoms of myocardial infarction.
    D. Normal sinus rhythm without ST elevation is demonstrated on the cardiac monitor.

1–45. A patient admitted to the coronary care unit has become angry at the limitations imposed upon him. He is refusing to wear his ECG monitoring electrodes. The most appropriate action for the nurse at this time would be to

    A. Acknowledge the patient's anger.
    B. Tell the patient he is acting unacceptably.
    C. Reason with the patient.
    D. Obtain an order for diazepam (Valium).

1–46. An advantage of continuous arteriovenous hemofiltration (CAVH) over hemodialysis or peritoneal dialysis is that CAVH provides

    A. A rapid and efficient method of fluid and solute removal.
    B. Controlled regulation of fluid balance.
    C. Treatment without use of anticoagulation.
    D. Removal of large amounts of protein components from the blood.

Questions 1–47 to 1–49 refer to the following situation.

A 60-year-old female was admitted to the ICU with a diagnosis of thyroid storm and complaining of dyspnea, nausea, and vomiting. She had a history of angina and hyperthyroidism and underwent cardiac catheterization 3 weeks ago. The family stated that she had become increasingly agitated and inattentive in the last few weeks. She was restless, tremulous, and diaphoretic with flushed skin and had bibasilar crackles. Her heart rate was 150 beats per minute and her ECG showed normal sinus rhythm with an occasional PVC.

Vital signs and laboratory data:

BP	170/80 mm Hg
T	104° F
RR	32/min
Cardiac index	4.7 l/min/m²
Serum glucose	320 mg/dl
WBC	6,000/mm³
Neutrophils	50%
Band cells	3%

1–47. Serum laboratory results consistent with the diagnosis of thyroid storm include

	T_4	T_3	Thyroid Stimulating Hormone (TSH)
A.	increased	increased	decreased
B.	decreased	increased	increased
C.	increased	decreased	decreased
D.	decreased	decreased	increased

1–48. The drug of choice to treat this patient's hyperadrenergic state is

A. Propranolol (Inderal).
B. Nifedipine (Procardia).
C. Verapamil (Calan, Isoptin).
D. Quinidine (Quinidex, Quinora).

1–49. An appropriate nursing diagnosis for this patient is

A. Potential for fluid volume excess related to aldosterone-mediated fluid retention.
B. Potential for decreased cardiac index related to increased myocardial oxygen consumption.
C. Potential for hypothermia related to aggressive cooling measures.
D. Potential for altered swallowing related to thyroid goiter.

1–50. A 22-year-old female with a history of impaired gas exchange related to asthma is admitted to the intensive care unit in acute respiratory distress. Upon examination, she is found to be upright in bed, using accessory muscles for breathing, with decreased chest wall excursion, a fixed costal angle, and distant breath sounds without adventitious sounds. Arterial blood gases on 4 l oxygen per minute by nasal cannula are: pH 7.36, Pa_{CO_2} 45 mm Hg, HCO_3 18 mEq/l, Pa_{O_2} 74 mm Hg, Sa_{O_2} 92%. The appropriate action to take would be

A. Provide emotional support.
B. Set up for intubation.
C. Administer bronchodilator therapy.
D. Draw an aminophylline level.

1–51. The therapeutic range for aminophylline (Theophylline) is

A. 5 to 15 μg/ml.
B. 10 to 20 μg/ml.
C. 15 to 20 μg/ml.
D. 20 to 30 μg/ml.

1–52. B cells are responsible for

A. Humoral immunity.
B. Cellular immunity.
C. Type I hypersensitivity reactions.
D. Cell-mediated hypersensitivity.

1–53. T cells

    A. Are produced by lymphokines.
    B. Secrete mediators for anaphylaxis.
    C. Are programmed to recognize the individual's own tissue.
    D. Are responsible for type II hypersensitivity reactions.

1–54. Evaluation of motor ability in acute spinal cord injury includes assessment of superficial and deep tendon reflexes. This permits assessment for which of the following?

    A. Complete lesions of the spinal cord.
    B. Meningeal irritation.
    C. Progressive edema causing small vessel compression.
    D. Decreased tissue oxygen levels.

1–55. The nursing diagnosis "alteration in temperature" in the acute spinal cord injured patient is the result of

    A. Spinal shock.
    B. Cerebral edema.
    C. Autonomic dysreflexia.
    D. Poikilothermia.

1–56. An 18-year-old female is admitted to your unit with a diagnosis of Brown-Séquard syndrome. As the nurse caring for her, you know that this means that the patient has

    A. Contralateral loss of pain.
    B. Contralateral loss of motor function.
    C. Ipsilateral loss of temperature sensation.
    D. Contralateral loss of vibratory sensation.

1–57. Two days ago, a 20-year-old male sustained blunt head trauma and a knife wound to the abdomen. He had an emergency temporary colostomy and subdural hematoma has been ruled out. Which of the following would be a normal assessment finding for this patient?

    A. Absent bowel sounds.
    B. Bright red blood in the stool.
    C. Dark purple coloration in the stoma.
    D. Abdominal tenderness.

1–58. The anemia of chronic renal failure may be the result of all of the following *except*

    A. Increased erythropoietin production.
    B. Acceleration of red blood cell (RBC) destruction.
    C. Blood loss.
    D. Deficiencies of iron and folic acid.

1–59. The calcium imbalance associated with chronic renal failure is partially a result of

    A. Decreased plasma phosphates.
    B. Decreased intestinal calcium absorption.
    C. Increased parathormone production.
    D. Increased alkalosis.

1–60. A life-threatening complication of intubation is

    A. Rupture of the innominate artery.
    B. Tracheoesophageal fistula.
    C. Granulomata.
    D. Tracheal stenosis.

1–61. A patient on intra-aortic balloon counterpulsation is weaned from 1:2 to 1:4 augmentation. Which of the following findings on 1:4 augmentation indicates intra-aortic balloon dependence?

    A. Systolic blood pressure is 90 mm Hg.
    B. Pulmonary artery diastolic blood pressure is 22 mm Hg.
    C. Heart rate is 100 beats per minute.
    D. The patient complains of chest pain relieved by sublingual nitroglycerin.

1–62. The time is 2200 hours. A patient who had been unstable in the cardiac care unit on an intra-aortic balloon pump (IABP) has a cardiac arrest and dies. The patient in the cubicle across from him, also on IABP therapy, complains of chest pain and requests morphine. The 12-lead ECG shows no changes from the morning ECG and the patient refuses nitroglycerin. The nurse should

A. Offer to give the patient the sleep medication he has ordered and tell the patient to put the light on if he wishes to talk.
B. Give the patient 2 mg of morphine IV and sit with the patient until he falls asleep.
C. Tell the patient he is not as sick as the patient who expired and that he shouldn't worry; that will not happen to him.
D. Tell the patient that it is difficult on all the patients when another patient dies, and focus on the difference in the situations. Encourage the patient to talk with the nurse before deciding which medication to take.

1–63. You receive the following results from the laboratory:

RBC	5.0×10 million/μl
WBC	6,200/μl
Hgb	7.2 gm/dl
Hct	28%
Platelets	200,000/μl

Which of the following laboratory test results is abnormal?

A. RBC.
B. Platelets.
C. Hemoglobin.
D. WBC.

Questions 1–64 through 1–69 refer to the following situation.

An 18-year-old male was admitted with head trauma following an automobile accident. A computed tomography (CT) scan shows evidence of an intracerebral hemorrhage with compensatory volume displacement. Intracranial hypertension is suspected.

1–64. The most likely cause for this patient's intracranial hypertension is

A. Subarachnoid hemorrhage.
B. Brain herniation and intracranial bleeding.
C. Brain swelling and intracranial bleeding.
D. Meningitis.

1–65. The first intervention the nurse should perform to assess this patient's neurologic status is to

A. Take his vital signs.
B. Assess for consensual pupil response.
C. Check his pupils for accommodation.
D. Determine his level of consciousness.

1–66. An immediate priority in the first 15 minutes of intervention for this patient includes

A. Calculating cerebral perfusion pressure (CPP).
B. Determining the scope and extent of his injury.
C. A secondary neurologic examination.
D. Respiratory assessment.

1–67. This patient's Glasgow Coma Score is 3—3—4. The nurse interprets this to mean that the patient

A. Makes no attempt to remove the noxious stimulus used to arouse him.
B. Makes no attempt to vocalize.
C. Opens his eyes when spoken to.
D. Follows simple commands.

1-68. The patient demonstrates a decerebrate posture. The nurse expects to find which of the following?

   A. Flexion of both upper and lower extremities.
   B. Extension of elbows and knees, plantar flexion of feet, and flexion of the wrists.
   C. Flexion of elbows, extension of the knees, and plantar flexion of the feet.
   D. Extension of upper extremities, flexion of lower extremities.

1-69. If this patient were to demonstrate decorticate posturing, the critical care nurse would expect to observe

   A. Flexion of both upper and lower extremities.
   B. Extension of elbows and knees, plantar flexion of feet, and flexion of the wrists.
   C. Flexion of elbows, extension of the knees, and plantar flexion of the feet.
   D. Extension of upper extremities, flexion of lower extremities.

1-70. The most common cause of hypermagnesemia is

   A. Addison's disease.
   B. Severe renal failure.
   C. Hyperthyroidism.
   D. Myxedema.

1-71. The most definitive test for pulmonary embolus is a (an)

   A. Arterial blood gas.
   B. Ventilation/perfusion scan.
   C. Chest x-ray.
   D. Pulmonary angiogram.

1-72. The hypoxia resulting from a pulmonary embolus is a result of

   A. Hypoventilation.
   B. Ventilation/perfusion mismatch.
   C. Right-to-left shunt.
   D. Diffusion defect.

1-73. Treatment for an acute thrombotic pulmonary embolus may include all of the following *except*

   A. Urokinase.
   B. Oxygen.
   C. Embolectomy.
   D. Steroids.

1-74. Cushing's ulcers occur in patients who have

   A. Intracranial injury.
   B. Severe burns.
   C. Chronic drug ingestion.
   D. Bacterial sepsis.

1-75. Which of the following causes a false negative result in the Hemoccult-type slide guaiac test?

   A. Iron supplements.
   B. Ascorbic acid.
   C. Iodine.
   D. Aspirin.

1-76. Which of the following antiarrhythmic medications is a possible cause of torsades de pointes?

   A. Quinidine.
   B. Propranolol.
   C. Digoxin.
   D. Verapamil.

1-77. Which of the following medications is used in the treatment of torsades de pointes?

   A. Quinidine.
   B. Propranolol.
   C. Isoproterenol.
   D. Procainamide.

Questions 1–78 and 1–79 refer to the following situation.

A 47-year-old critical care patient with acute renal failure has just started on hemodialysis treatments. During dialysis he complains of a severe headache that worsens as the treatment progresses. He becomes restless, confused, and nauseous. While his blood pressure is being checked, the patient has a grand mal seizure that lasts approximately 30 seconds.

1–78. The most likely cause of this patient's clinical findings would be

    A. Hypovolemia.
    B. Hypokalemia.
    C. Malignant hypertension.
    D. Cerebral edema.

1–79. Treatment and prevention of a recurrence of these symptoms include

    A. Decreasing blood flow rate through the dialyzer.
    B. Use of a larger dialyzer with a greater surface area.
    C. Lengthening of the dialysis treatment.
    D. Administration of saline IV.

1–80. Brain tumors are classified by

    A. Clinical significance.
    B. Histologic features and grade of malignancy.
    C. Density and location.
    D. Location and accessibility of the tumor.

Questions 1–81 through 1–83 refer to the following situation.

A 24-year-old male has been in the intensive care unit for 3 days following a motorcycle accident that caused a fractured femur, rib fractures, and multiple lacerations. His condition is stable, and he is to be transferred to the floor tomorrow. During the night, he becomes restless, anxious, and confused, with increasing dyspnea, and he is coughing up pink frothy sputum. Vital signs are: pulse 120 beats per minute, BP 126/80 mm Hg, respirations 32 per minute, temperature 37.8° C. Chest x-ray shows a white-out bilaterally in the lungs. Arterial blood gases (ABGs) are drawn on room air and are: pH 7.54, Pa_{CO_2} 30 mm Hg, HCO_3 19 mEq/l, Pa_{O_2} 49 mm Hg, Sa_{O_2} 78%, Ca_{O_2} 15.2 ml/dl.

1–81. The most likely cause of his distress and symptoms is

    A. Fat embolus.
    B. Adult respiratory distress syndrome (ARDS).
    C. Congestive heart failure (CHF).
    D. Pleural effusion.

1–82. By the next day, he is intubated and on a ventilator at settings of FI_{O_2} 0.8, V_T 800, rate 16 per minute assist/control, peak flow rate of 80 l/minute. His ABGs are: pH 7.38, Pa_{CO_2} 45 mm Hg, HCO_3 18 mEq/l, Pa_{O_2} 62 mm Hg, Sa_{O_2} 89%, Ca_{O_2} 16.3 ml/dl, shunt 15%, lung compliance 32 cm H_2O.

    The primary problem his ABGs show is

    A. Respiratory acidosis.
    B. Metabolic alkalosis.
    C. Respiratory alkalosis.
    D. Refractory hypoxemia.

1–83. The treatment of choice for this problem, as indicated by his ABGs, would be

    A. Institute hyperbaric oxygen.
    B. Institute positive end-expiratory pressure (PEEP).
    C. Increase FI_{O_2} to 100% oxygen.
    D. Increase tidal volume.

1–84. Which of the following are necessary elements of negligence?

    I. The provider must have had a duty to provide care.
    II. The provider must have omitted required care.
    III. The patient must have sustained some type of harm.
    IV. A causal relationship must be established between care omitted and harm to the patient.

    A. I and II.
    B. I, II, and IV.
    C. II, III, and IV.
    D. I, II, III, and IV.

1–85. A patient postoperative from mitral valve replacement develops the dysrhythmia shown below 24 hours after surgery. The patient has received 1.0 mg of digoxin during this time as a digitalizing dose. Current hemodynamic values for this patient include a BP of 114/63 mm Hg and pulmonary capillary wedge pressure of 15 mm Hg.
    Which of the following is the most appropriate treatment?

    A. Synchronized cardioversion with 50 joules.
    B. Administer 0.125 mg digoxin by slow IV push.
    C. Perform unilateral carotid massage.
    D. Administer propranolol 1 mg IV at intervals of 5 minutes to a maximum of 10 mg/kg.

1–86. Class I antiarrhythmic medications such as flecainide act on the cell membrane by
    A. Sodium channel blockade.
    B. Potassium channel blockade.
    C. Beta-adrenergic blockade.
    D. Calcium channel blockade.

1–87. A patient is admitted to the intensive care unit following a motor vehicle accident. The patient is to receive two units of packed red blood cells. The patient has cold agglutinins present. Your care for this patient will include

    A. Keeping the patient warm during the transfusion.
    B. Warming the blood during administration.
    C. Administering the blood without a filter.
    D. Transfusing cold blood to the patient.

1–88. A patient with an epidural hematoma usually has

    A. A long period of unconsciousness followed by complete lucidity.
    B. A short period of unconsciousness followed by a lucid period followed by rapid deterioration.
    C. Slowly developing signs of increasing intracranial pressure.
    D. Slow deterioration in CPP.

1–89. A 51-year-old female is admitted with acute pancreatitis. Her BP is 86/40 mm Hg, apical pulse is 110 beats per minute, and rectal temperature is 38.6° C. She is complaining of severe flank pain. Which of the following therapies would most likely be initiated?

    A. 10% dextrose and phenanthrene.
    B. Lactated Ringer's solution and meperidine.
    C. Dobutamine and morphine.
    D. Dopamine and oxycodone.

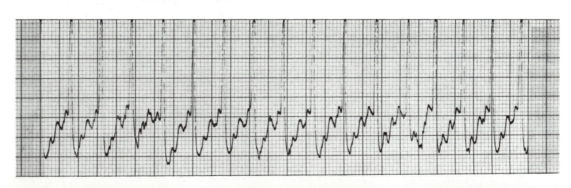

A 27-year-old male has been in the intensive care unit for several days following a severe motor vehicle accident in which he sustained multiple fractures and crush injuries to his lower extremities. His urine output has now decreased and the nurse notes edema of his ankles, feet, back, sacrum, and periorbital areas. On auscultation of lung fields, crackles are heard in both bases. Urinalysis results include

Specific gravity	1.010
Osmolarity	250 mOsm/l
Urea	300 mg/dl
Creatinine	60 mg/dl
Potassium	21 mEq/24 hr

1–90. The most likely cause of this patient's status change is

A. Hypovolemia.
B. Acute tubular necrosis.
C. Glomerulonephritis.
D. Congestive heart failure.

1–91. Inflammation of lung parenchyma associated with alveolar filling by exudate is a description of

A. ARDS.
B. Pneumonia.
C. Pulmonary edema.
D. Chronic bronchitis.

1–92. A patient on a ventilator should be routinely repositioned to

A. Maintain muscle tone.
B. Prevent pressure sores.
C. Keep the body in alignment.
D. Mobilize secretions.

1–93. The portion of the cardiac conduction system that transmits impulses into the subendocardial layers of both ventricles is the

A. Purkinje system.
B. Bundle of His.
C. Bachmann's bundle.
D. Internodal pathway.

1–94. A patient in a junctional (nodal) rhythm has a heart rate of 80 beats per minute. This would be described as

A. A junctional escape rhythm.
B. An accelerated junctional rhythm.
C. A junctional tachycardia.
D. An accelerated junctional tachycardia.

1–95. With a diagnosis of acute bacterial meningitis, it is likely that the laboratory data of the CSF will reveal

A. Protein	450 mg/dl.
B. Glucose	70 mg/dl.
C. WBCs	4 cells/mm^3.
D. Specific gravity	1.007.

1–96. Renin is secreted into the blood by the kidney structure known as the

A. Distal convoluted tubule.
B. Juxtaglomerular apparatus.
C. Loop of Henle.
D. Proximal convoluted tubule.

1–97. Cimetidine and ranitidine inhibit the metabolism of all of the following *except:*

A. Gentamicin.
B. Theophylline.
C. Lidocaine HCl.
D. Procainamide.

1–98. A patient postoperative from coronary artery bypass surgery is on continuous SV_{O_2} monitoring, with values of 96% to 98% on a 50% FI_{O_2} face mask on her second postoperative day. One-half hour later she is changed to a 3 l/min nasal cannula so that she can eat. The SV_{O_2} drops to 87%. The nurse should

A. Place the patient back on the 50% mask as soon as possible.
B. Increase the nasal oxygen delivery to 5 l/min and see if the SV_{O_2} improves.
C. Continue to monitor changes in the SV_{O_2} on a 3 l/min nasal cannula.
D. Medicate the patient for pain and reassess the need to increase oxygen delivery.

1–99. A wide arteriovenous oxygen difference (a-vD$_{O_2}$) of greater than 5.5 volume% indicates

    A. A high cardiac output state.
    B. A low cardiac output state.
    C. High venous oxygen saturation.
    D. Low arterial oxygen saturation.

1–100. A cancer patient with a new permanent tracheostomy refuses to acknowledge or discuss the surgery. The nurse diagnoses the patient's response to the tracheostomy as "Disturbance in self concept: body image." An appropriate response by the nurse might be to

    A. Ignore the patient's response for now.
    B. Advise the family to ignore the tracheostomy.
    C. Encourage the patient to verbalize her concerns.
    D. Force the patient to look at the stoma.

Questions 1–101 and 1–102 refer to the following situation.

A patient is admitted to the intensive care unit following the delivery of her third child. She has hematuria and tachycardia. Her admission laboratory values include:

Na	148 mEq/l
K	4.7 mEq/l
Cl	102 mEq/l
BUN	20 mg/dl
Creatinine	0.9 mg/dl
Hct	12.2 gm/dl
Hgb	32.1%
Platelets	150,000/μl
Fibrinogen	150 mg/dl
Fibrin split products	75 μg/ml
WBC	7,200/μl

1–101. Based on the assessment and laboratory information, you anticipate that the patient is probably developing

    A. An infection.
    B. A coagulopathy.
    C. Anemia.
    D. Uremia.

1–102. The patient is very anxious about her baby's condition. You know that the baby is healthy following delivery. Your response to the patient will be

    A. "Please try to get some rest. Everything will be better in the morning."
    B. "If you had taken better care of yourself, this never would have happened."
    C. "I'll have the pediatrician come to talk to you. He knows more about your baby's condition."
    D. "You seem very worried about your baby's condition. Tell me what concerns you have so I can know how best to help you."

1–103. Which of the following characterizes status epilepticus?

    A. Tonic-clonic movements.
    B. Brief loss of contact with the environment.
    C. Akinetic movements.
    D. Myoclonic movements.

1–104. A 36-year-old female patient is lying in bed, and the padded siderails are raised. The nurse adjusting the patient's IV sees that she suddenly has a seizure. Which of the following is the priority intervention?

    A. Pry open clenched jaws and insert an airway.
    B. Use soft restraints to control violent movements.
    C. Place the call light in the patient's dominant hand and run quickly to the nurse's station for help.
    D. Protect the patient from injury.

1–105. The drug of choice to treat diabetes insipidus is

    A. Mannitol (Osmitrol).
    B. Desmopressin (dDAVP).
    C. Phenytoin (Dilantin).
    D. Oxytocin (Pitocin).

Questions 1–106 to 1–108 refer to the following situation.

A female patient with renal failure has been started on hemodialysis. She tells the triage nurse that she has "fluid in my lungs." On assessment the nurse observes peripheral edema and neck vein distention and auscultates crackles bilaterally. Vital signs are taken and laboratory work is drawn.

1–106. The patient asks the nurse her blood pressure and laboratory values. The nurse's best response is to

A. Tell her they are "a little abnormal" so as not to worry her.
B. Refer her to the physician for the information.
C. Tell her what the values are.
D. Tell her she cannot give out that information.

1–107. In reviewing this patient's laboratory work, the nurse is aware that normal differences resulting from acute tubular necrosis include elevation of all of the following *except*

A. BUN.
B. Calcium.
C. Potassium.
D. Magnesium.

1–108. Interventions for this patient's pulmonary edema include

A. Diuretics.
B. Foley catheter.
C. Phlebotomy.
D. Morphine sulfate.

1–109. Pulmonary artery systolic (PAS) pressure is equal to which of the following pressures?

A. Left ventricular end diastolic pressure (LVEDP).
B. Right ventricular diastolic pressure (RVDP).
C. Right ventricular systolic pressure (RVSP).
D. Right ventricular mean pressure (RVMP).

A patient with left ventricular failure has the following hemodynamic findings:

BP	100/70 mm Hg
MAP	80 mm Hg
Central venous pressure (CVP)	8 mm Hg
Pulmonary artery pressure	20/18 mm Hg
Pulmonary capillary wedge pressure	16 mm Hg
Cardiac output	3.0 l/min
Heart rate	110/min

1–110. He is currently on dopamine at 15 μg/kg/minute and nitroprusside at 2.0 μg/kg/minute. Which of the following nursing interventions will increase the cardiac output?

A. Infuse 250 ml of normal saline.
B. Increase the dopamine infusion to 20 μg/kg/min.
C. Increase the nitroprusside slowly, maintaining a systolic pressure of 100 mm Hg.
D. Give digoxin, 0.25 mg IV push, to increase contractility and slow heart rate.

1–111. Endotracheal/tracheostomy tube cuffs should be kept at what pressure?

A. 10 to 20 cm H_2O.
B. 15 to 25 cm H_2O.
C. 20 to 30 cm H_2O.
D. 25 to 35 cm H_2O.

1–112. A 40-year-old stockbroker of Hispanic descent with a history of surgeries for bleeding ulcers and biliary tract obstruction is a patient on your unit. He has a large, fistulating abdominal wound, multiple tubes, and several IVs. After 7 weeks in the hospital, he refuses any further treatments, blood work, or procedures. The new goal of the critical care nurse will be to

A. Help the patient learn the patient role.
B. Mediate culturally avoided aspects of his illness.
C. Anticipate ongoing emotional breakdown and physical deterioration.
D. Maximize the patient's control of his own recovery.

1–113. While working the night shift, a critical care nurse detects a serious change in a patient's condition. The nurse telephones the attending physician, who fails to come to evaluate the patient. In order to provide legal protection as well as appropriate care for the patient, the nurse must

I. Document the time and response of the physician to the report of the patient's condition.
II. Inform the nursing supervisor of the situation.
III. Continue to monitor the patient's condition and document all changes.
IV. Follow the hospital's policy to contact another physician to evaluate the patient and provide appropriate medical care.

A. I and III.
B. II and IV.
C. I, II, and III.
D. I, II, III, and IV.

1–114. Malignant hyperthermia is

A. Caused by a severe fulminating postoperative infection.
B. A cancerous condition resulting in paroxysmal increased temperatures.
C. A central nervous system disorder manifested by increased core body temperature and muscle flaccidity.
D. A pharmacogenetic disorder caused by the use of potent anesthetics.

Questions 1–115 and 1–116 refer to the following situation.

A 45-year-old male is admitted from the emergency room in respiratory distress. He has a history of ineffective breathing pattern related to polio and has been confined to a wheelchair. He sleeps on a rocking bed and uses glossopharyngeal (frog) breathing when off the bed. His vital signs are: BP 132/76 mm Hg, pulse 120 beats per minute, respirations 36 per minute, and temperature 38.5° C.

1–115. His arterial blood gases in the emergency room on room air are: pH 7.26, Pa_{CO_2} 58 mm Hg; HCO_3 16 mEq/l; Pa_{O_2} 52 mm Hg; Sa_{O_2} 85%; and Ca_{O_2} 16.7 ml/dl. These results show

A. Tissue hypoxia.
B. Acute respiratory failure.
C. Chronic respiratory failure.
D. Respiratory and metabolic alkalosis.

1–116. The most likely physiologic cause of this patient's respiratory distress is

A. Ventilation-perfusion ($\dot{V}/\dot{Q}$) mismatch.
B. Hypoventilation.
C. Shunt.
D. Diffusion limitation.

A 42-year-old male who is undergoing radiation therapy for Hodgkin's disease has been admitted to the intensive care unit for seizures and an acute change in level of consciousness. His temperature is 39.4° C. You have just checked his IV site, which is without redness, swelling, or drainage. His laboratory results include:

WBC	3,200/µl
Differential	
Neutrophils	32% (normal 39–79%)
Eosinophils	0% (normal 0–2%)
Basophils	2% (normal 0–5%)
Monocytes	11% (normal 3–8%)
Leukocytes	55% (normal 10–40%)

1–117. Your care of the IV site should include which of the following:

A. Continue to monitor for signs of inflammation.
B. Change the tubing every 24 hours.
C. Change the IV site and infusion system now.
D. Apply an antibiotic ointment to the site.

1–118. A clinical manifestation that differentiates hyperosmotic hyperglycemic nonketotic coma (HHNK) from diabetic ketoacidosis (DKA) is

A. Hyperglycemia.
B. Serum hyperosmolality.
C. Osmotic diuresis.
D. A normal anion gap.

1–119. A patient with a large anterior wall myocardial infarction 1 month ago is readmitted to the coronary care unit with complaints of chest pain. The pain increases on inspiration and has not been relieved by three doses of nitroglycerin 1/150 sublingually. Initial vital signs are: temperature 38.3°C, BP 140/70 mm Hg, heart rate 110 beats per minute, and sinus tachycardia by ECG. Respiratory rate is 28 per minute and shallow. Which of the following orders is *contraindicated* in the care of this patient?

A. Morphine sulfate, 2 mg IV for chest pain: may repeat times three.
B. Acetaminophen with codeine, 2 tablets each 4 to 6 hours PRN.
C. Heparin, 5,000 units every 12 hours subcutaneously.
D. Aspirin, two tablets (10 grains) every 6 hours p.o.

1–120. Pericarditis is most common in which type of myocardial infarction?

A. Septal infarction.
B. Subendocardial infarction.
C. Transmural infarction.
D. Intramural infarction.

1–121. Turner's sign presents as bruising in which of the following areas?

A. Over the flank and lower back.
B. Around the umbilicus.
C. Behind the ears.
D. Over both iliac crests.

Questions 1–122 and 1–123 refer to the following situation.

A 24-year-old male is admitted following an acute spinal cord injury of C7. An appropriate nursing diagnosis for him is "Alteration in self-concept related to change in body image."

1–122. In planning nursing interventions for him, the best intervention specific to this nursing diagnosis includes

    A. Allow patient to verbalize anxieties and fears.
    B. Permit choices, as appropriate.
    C. Communicate for short periods to avoid overtiring the patient.
    D. Accept the patient's perception of self.

1–123. In caring for this patient, the nurse knows that

    A. A nursing care plan for bowel and bladder care is a priority in the immediate post-injury period.
    B. During the period of spinal shock, he will be at risk for autonomic dysreflexia.
    C. Assessment of respiratory function is unnecessary because the innervation of the diaphragm is well above C7.
    D. Prior to stabilization of the cord by traction or surgery, range of motion of the neck must be performed.

1–124. A 70-kg male is 5 feet, 10 inches tall. He was admitted yesterday with an inferior wall myocardial infarction, and his condition is stable. He reports that he drinks a six-pack of beer every night. This man's history suggests that he is predisposed to a deficiency in

    A. Thiamine.
    B. Vitamin B_{12}.
    C. Zinc.
    D. Vitamin C.

1–125. Laboratory data consistent with the diagnosis of syndrome of inappropriate antidiuretic hormone (SIADH) include

Serum osmolality	Urine osmolality
A. Decreased	decreased
B. Increased	increased
C. Decreased	increased
D. Increased	decreased

1–126. Which of the following changes will have the most impact on coagulation?

    I. Decreased albumin.
    II. Elevated magnesium.
    III. Decreased chloride.
    IV. Increased globulin.

    A. I and II only.
    B. I and III only.
    C. II and IV only.
    D. III and IV only.

1–127. After extubation, a patient develops dyspnea, coughing, wheezing, and stridor. Appropriate actions would include

    A. Racemic epinephrine, aerosol mist, steroids.
    B. Steroids, emergency tracheostomy.
    C. Manual ventilation of the patient, racemic epinephrine.
    D. Sedation, bronchial lavage.

1–128. When instituting transcutaneous pacing, where should the electrode pads be placed?

    A. At the right sternal border and the left lower rib margin.
    B. At the left subscapular region and over the V_3 position.
    C. At the center of the back and over the left sternal border.
    D. At the right subscapular region and the left sternal border.

1–129. To prepare an external pacemaker for use prior to insertion, the nurse should

    I. Set the mA (output) at 5–7 mA.
    II. Turn the rate control to 10 beats above the patient's heart rate.
    III. Turn the sensitivity to the asynchronous mode.
    IV. Turn the sensitivity to the fully demand mode.

    A. II and III only.
    B. I and II only.
    C. I, II, and III only.
    D. I, II, and IV only.

Questions 1–130 and 1–131 refer to the following situation.

A 55-year-old woman presented to the emergency department with nausea, vomiting, crampy abdominal pain, and distention. Her last bowel movement was 7 days ago. Rectal examination reveals mucus only, guaiac negative.

1–130. The nurse suspects the patient has

    A. Acute pancreatitis.
    B. Fulminating hepatitis.
    C. Complete small bowel obstruction.
    D. Duodenal ulcer.

1–131. Other findings to expect in this patient include

    A. Jaundice.
    B. High-pitched tinkling bowel sounds.
    C. Right upper quadrant tenderness.
    D. Hematemesis.

1–132. Pathophysiologic changes associated with a serum phosphorus level of 0.4 mg/dl include decreased ATP production and resultant

    A. Hemolysis.
    B. Increased bacteriocidal activity of WBCs.
    C. Metabolic alkalosis.
    D. Increased myocardial contractility.

1–133. A 19-year-old male underwent an emergency craniotomy for evacuation of a large epidural hematoma following an automobile accident. You notice clear fluid escaping from this patient's nose (rhinorrhea) postoperatively. You are not sure if this fluid is mucus or CSF. Which of the following tests will most likely give the critical care nurse conclusive evidence of the origin of the rhinorrhea?

    A. pH level.
    B. Specific gravity.
    C. Culture and sensitivity.
    D. Dextrostix (Keto-Diastix).

1–134. Which of the following would be an appropriate intervention for the patient with CSF rhinorrhea?

    A. Culture and sensitivity.
    B. Suctioning the nose gently.
    C. Placing a sterile gauze under the nares to collect drainage.
    D. Inserting sterile packing in the nose.

1–135. A 62-year-old female patient with a history of diabetes mellitus is admitted to the intensive care unit following a bowel resection for a large, benign tumor. Admitting vital signs and laboratory data reveal the following:

HR	110 beats/min
RR	24/min
T	102° F
BP	90/60 mm Hg
Cardiac output	7.5 l/min
SVR	750 dynes/sec/cm^{-5}
RBC	4.0 million/μl
Hct	35%
Hgb	11.6 mg/dl
WBC	13,200/μl
Platelets	180,000/μl
Fibrin split products	0

After you administer meperidine (Demerol) to the patient, she complains of "feeling cold" and is shivering. She is breathing normally and her vital signs are unchanged. Blood cultures are done and a Gram stain reveals gram-negative organisms in her blood. This patient is developing

A. Septic shock.
B. Hemorrhagic shock.
C. Diabetic ketoacidosis.
D. Disseminated intravascular coagulation (DIC).

1–136. A laboratory abnormality that may occur during a hypothyroid state is

A. Leukocytosis.
B. Polycythemia.
C. Hyponatremia.
D. Respiratory alkalosis.

Questions 1–137 and 1–138 refer to the following situation.

A patient 6 hours after surgery is on a ventilator and has thick tenacious white sputum.

1–137. What action should be taken?

A. Start antibiotics.
B. Ensure adequate humidification.
C. Send sputum cultures.
D. Perform bronchoalveolar lavage.

1–138. The most appropriate nursing diagnosis for this patient would be

A. Ineffective breathing pattern.
B. Potential for infection.
C. Ineffective airway clearance.
D. Potential for aspiration.

1–139. A patient with a triple-lumen central line has been on continuous CVP monitoring. Currently his waveform appears slightly dampened and the readout says that his CVP is 2 mm Hg. The system appears to zero and calibrate correctly. The next appropriate nursing action would be to

A. Aspirate blood from the stopcock closest to the patient.
B. Ask the patient to take a deep breath and watch the waveform for respiratory variation.
C. Flush the catheter with a syringe filled with 10 ml of normal saline.
D. Raise the transducer to the level of the right atrium.

1–140. Tapping with your finger over the supramandibular portion of the seventh cranial nerve results in twitching in a patient's upper lip. This sign is indicative of

A. Hyperkalemia.
B. Hyponatremia.
C. Hyperphosphatemia.
D. Hypocalcemia.

Questions 1–141 and 1–142 refer to the following situation.

A 52-year-old male was admitted to the intensive care unit complaining of weight loss, fatigue, weakness, muscle cramps, postural dizziness, and diarrhea. He had a history of adrenal insufficiency and was on maintenance hydrocortisone 30 mg per day. His wife died unexpectedly 2 weeks ago, and he has been severely depressed. Physical examination revealed hyperpigmented palms and buccal mucosa.

Vital signs and serum laboratory data:

BP	110/64 mm Hg flat,
	90/60 mm Hg sitting
HR	100/min flat,
	120/min sitting
RR	16/min
K	5.7 mEq/l
Na	128 mEq/l
BUN	22 mg/dl
Glucose	88 mg/dl

1–141. This patient's hyperpigmented buccal mucosa is associated with elevated levels of

   A. Cortisol.
   B. Aldosterone.
   C. Corticotropin releasing hormone (CRH).
   D. Adrenocorticotropic hormone (ACTH).

1–142. A priority intervention for this patient is

   A. Twice-a-day ambulation.
   B. Sodium and water restriction.
   C. Continuous cardiac monitoring.
   D. Foley catheter insertion.

1–143. Which of the following would confirm the diagnosis of ruptured ventricular septum in a patient with acute myocardial infarction?

   A. Large v waves in the pulmonary capillary wedge tracing.
   B. Elevated right ventricular systolic pressures during pulmonary artery catheter insertion.
   C. Pulmonary artery P_{O_2} significantly higher than right atrial P_{O_2}.
   D. Right ventricular diastolic pressure higher than right atrial pressure during pulmonary artery catheter insertion.

1–144. The most effective initial treatment for ventricular septal rupture in the acute myocardial infarction patient is

   A. Immediate surgical intervention.
   B. Immediate insertion of a percutaneous intra-aortic balloon pump.
   C. Blood pressure support with dopamine at 15 µg/kg/minute.
   D. Intubation and mechanical ventilation with PEEP to improve oxygenation and decrease venous return.

1–145. A 58-year-old male has residual encephalopathy from acute hepatic failure. The patient (or his family) should be instructed to

   A. Avoid enemas.
   B. Ensure adequate sodium intake.
   C. Resume over-the-counter medications as needed.
   D. Restrict protein intake.

1-146. An elderly man is admitted to the critical care unit following surgery to remove a malignant tumor. The patient develops adult respiratory distress syndrome (ARDS) and is placed on a mechanical ventilator. When he regains consciousness, the patient indicates to his wife and the nurse that he does not wish to be connected to the ventilator, even if this action would result in his death. The patient's wife verifies that he has made the same statement numerous times in the past. The nurse explains to the patient and his wife that the physician's plan is to wean him from the ventilator and that there is a reasonable chance for recovery. The patient and his wife indicate that they understand, but the patient insists that the ventilator be removed. The attending physician is unwilling to remove the ventilator because he feels he has an obligation to prevent harm to the patient. What ethical principles are in conflict in this situation?

A. Beneficence and justice.
B. Beneficence and autonomy.
C. Autonomy and justice.
D. Autonomy and informed consent.

1-147. In assessing the patient with acute subdural hematoma, the nurse knows that one of the following is a direct effect of the hematoma. It is

A. Transtentorial (uncal) herniation.
B. Bilateral pupillary dilatation.
C. Tachycardia.
D. Decreased arterial blood pressure.

1-148. Subdural hematomas

A. Occur only as a result of head trauma.
B. Are often associated with arterial bleeding.
C. Occur as a result of ruptured intracranial aneurysm.
D. May occur spontaneously.

1-149. Hypercalcemia can be caused by

I. Vitamin D intoxication.
II. Hypomagnesemia.
III. Hyperparathyroidism.

A. I and II.
B. II only.
C. I and III.
D. I only.

Questions 1-150 and 1-151 refer to the following situation.

A patient is admitted with a history of bloody emesis for 2 days. His arterial blood gas results are: pH 7.39, Pa_{CO_2} 36 mm Hg, HCO_3 19 mEq/l, Pa_{O_2} 80 mm Hg, Sa_{O_2} 92%, Ca_{O_2} 13.04 ml/dl on room air. His vital signs are: BP 105/63 mm Hg, pulse 108 beats per minute, respirations 22 per minute, temperature 37.8° C orally. His hemoglobin is 10 gm/dl and his cardiac output is 4.8 per minute.

1-150. The most likely cause of his decreased arterial oxygen content is

A. Decreased Pa_{O_2}.
B. Increased oxygen consumption.
C. Decreased hemoglobin level.
D. Low cardiac output.

1-151. The most efficient way to increase oxygen delivery to the tissues would be to

A. Increase the $F_{I_{O_2}}$.
B. Administer packed red blood cells.
C. Increase the blood pressure.
D. Sedate the patient.

1-152. Stimulation of beta$_1$ receptors will cause

A. Decreased cardiac contractility.
B. Vasoconstriction of all arteries and veins.
C. Increased cardiac automaticity and conductivity.
D. Bronchodilation.

1–153. A patient in the coronary care unit makes sexual advances toward the female nursing staff. It would be most appropriate to respond to the patient by

    A. Telling the patient that you are flattered that he finds you attractive, but that his comments make you uncomfortable.
    B. Simply ignoring the comments.
    C. Telling the patient that you will arrange sexual counseling for him before discharge.
    D. Telling the patient that you are going to tell his wife about his behavior.

1–154. Four days ago, a 44-year-old woman had an emergency ileostomy performed for toxic megacolon. Her ileostomy is draining 1800 ml per day of liquid stool. She is at risk for developing

    A. Metabolic acidosis.
    B. Hyperkalemia.
    C. Metabolic alkalosis.
    D. Hypernatremia.

1–155. It is most likely that a patient admitted following temporal bone fractures will develop which one of the following?

    A. Intracranial hemorrhage.
    B. Subarachnoid hemorrhage.
    C. Subdural hematoma.
    D. Epidural hematoma.

1–156. High serum potassium levels may be further increased by

    A. Acidosis.
    B. Hyponatremia.
    C. Hypercalcemia.
    D. Alkalosis.

1–157. The most important etiologic factor in chronic obstructive pulmonary disease (COPD) is

    A. Family history.
    B. Smoking history.
    C. History of exposure to toxins and pollutants.
    D. Environmental pollution.

1–158. The most appropriate oxygen delivery device to use for a COPD patient is a

    A. Simple face mask.
    B. Nasal cannula.
    C. Venturi mask.
    D. Heated nebulizer.

1–159. A patient is experiencing an anaphylactoid reaction. The signs and symptoms are the result of

    A. Cross-bridging of IgE on the surface of the mast cell.
    B. Deposits of antigen-antibody complexes in mast cells.
    C. The production of autoantibodies.
    D. Direct complement activation of mast cells.

1–160. A patient is transferred to the intensive care unit in atrial fibrillation with a ventricular rate of 118 to 130 beats per minute and has Q waves and ST elevation in the precordial leads of his 12-lead ECG. Respiratory rate is 30 per minute and the ABG shows a pH of 7.25, P_{O_2} of 58 mm Hg, and P_{CO_2} of 50 mm Hg. The blood pressure is 90 mm Hg by palpation. Pulses are 1+ in the upper extremities and trace in the lower extremities. The patient has rales bilaterally half the way up from the lung bases, an S3 gallop, and his skin is cool and moist. This patient is in the clinical state of

    A. Congestive heart failure.
    B. Pulmonary edema.
    C. Cardiogenic shock.
    D. Cor pulmonale.

1–161. Which of the following increases ventricular end-diastolic volume (preload)?

    A. Mitral valve insufficiency.
    B. Hypertension.
    C. Mitral stenosis.
    D. Atrial fibrillation.

1–162. The cerebral cortex is

   A. The outer layer of each hemisphere.
   B. A bundle of nerve fibers.
   C. Deep inside the cerebral hemispheres.
   D. The part of the brain containing the thalamus.

1–163. Early ECG changes associated with hypokalemia include

   A. Peaked, elevated T wave.
   B. Widened QRS complex.
   C. Prolonged PR interval.
   D. Presence of a U wave.

1–164. A male patient is admitted with diffuse chest pain that is referred to the contralateral shoulder and does not change with respirations. This pain is most likely due to

   A. A pleural effusion.
   B. Diaphragmatic inflammation.
   C. Angina.
   D. A fractured rib.

1–165. Which of the following is true of type I second-degree AV block associated with inferior myocardial infarction?

   A. It requires immediate temporary pacemaker insertion.
   B. It is usually temporary, lasting approximately 1 week.
   C. It indicates interventricular septal necrosis.
   D. It occurs from increased vagal tone.

1–166. Which of the following cerebral neurotransmitters is found in decreased amounts in Parkinson's disease?

   A. Acetylcholine.
   B. Norepinephrine.
   C. Serotonin.
   D. Dopamine.

1–167. After admission to the intensive care unit for acute upper GI bleeding, a 67-year-old male has been newly diagnosed with gastric carcinoma. His family members are dazed when they hear about the poor prognosis. The top priority for most families in this situation is to

   A. Be encouraged to express their feelings.
   B. Know the names of staff giving care.
   C. Have their questions answered honestly.
   D. Have a comfortable place nearby to wait between visits.

1–168. Pain and itching in anaphylaxis occur as a result of

   A. The effects of histamine on the mast cells.
   B. Local vascular irritation caused by endotoxins.
   C. Kinin irritation of afferent neurons.
   D. Prostaglandin effects on smooth muscle.

1–169. Ventilator-dependent patients should have ventilation adjusted to maintain a normal

   A. Pa_{O_2}.
   B. pH.
   C. Pa_{CO_2}.
   D. Sa_{O_2}.

1–170. During which phase of reversible acute tubular necrosis does hypernatremia occur?

   A. Early diuresis.
   B. Oliguric.
   C. Late diuresis.
   D. Convalescent.

1–171. A 17-year-old female with myasthenia gravis was admitted to ICU in myasthenic crisis. Her vital signs are stable: BP 136/76 mm Hg, apical pulse 116 beats per minute, and temperature 37° C. She is intubated. A priority assessment of this patient includes

A. Response to routine anticholinergic medications.
B. Response to edrophonium chloride (Tensilon) tests every 4 hours.
C. Determination of CBC and electrolytes every 4 hours.
D. Measurement of vital capacity every 2 to 4 hours.

A 17-year-old female was admitted to ICU 2 days ago, following an automobile accident. Injuries included multiple bruises and lacerations, a left femur fracture, a skull fracture, and multiple rib fractures. She has been unconscious since admission. Vital signs and laboratory data reveal:

BP	90/60 mm Hg
HR	110/min
RR	28/min
24-hour urine output	4,200 ml
24-hour fluid intake	1,800 ml

Serum Values

Na	149 mEq/l
K	4 mEq/l
Osmolality	305 mOsm/l

Urine Values

Osmolality	280 mOsm/l
Specific gravity	1.001

1–172. These findings are most consistent with the development of

A. Brain stem herniation.
B. Diabetes insipidus.
C. Internal hemorrhage.
D. Pneumothorax.

1–173. The following hemodynamic parameters are obtained on a patient in the CCU:

Pulmonary artery diastolic	18 mm Hg
Pulmonary capillary wedge pressure	9 mm Hg
Central venous pressure	5 mm Hg

These findings are consistent with

A. Pericarditis.
B. Mitral regurgitation.
C. Pump failure.
D. Pulmonary embolism.

1–174. Which of the following is *not* a "hallmark" of ARDS?

A. Hypercapnia.
B. Refractory hypoxemia.
C. Increased right-to-left shunt.
D. Decreased functional residual capacity.

1–175. A male patient is unable to assist with the administration of DDAVP (desmopressin acetate) for his diabetes insipidus and therefore vasopressin tannate is ordered. When administering pitressin tannate in oil (vasopressin tannate), the critical care nurse knows to

A. Administer it intravenously.
B. Keep the solution refrigerated until immediately prior to administration.
C. Observe the patient for increased heart rate and cardiac output.
D. Observe the patient for decreased serum osmolality and sodium, indicators of water intoxication.

1–176. Recovery from narcotic-based anesthetic agents is dependent on the

A. Dose given, postoperative renal function, and urinary output.
B. Alveolar ventilation.
C. Solubility coefficient of the agent.
D. Duration of anesthesia.

1–177. Which of the following is true of dilated cardiomyopathy?

   A. The ejection fraction is normal.
   B. It is genetically transmitted.
   C. Dilation of the ventricles is disproportionate to ventricular hypertrophy.
   D. The ventricle is hypercontractile with an increased ejection fraction.

1–178. Yesterday, a 64-year-old male underwent evacuation of subdural hematoma incurred in a motor vehicle accident. Today, the nurse notes that he has developed ecchymosis in the flank area. The nurse suspects that this patient has a

   A. Renal injury.
   B. Ruptured spleen.
   C. Pancreatic injury.
   D. Pelvic fracture.

1–179. Arteriovenous malformation is the result of

   A. Dilation of an intracranial arterial wall.
   B. Vasospasm of cerebral arteries.
   C. Intracranial cerebrospinal fluid leak.
   D. Arterial blood shunted directly into the veins.

1–180. A male patient is admitted from the emergency room producing moderate amounts of frothy, bloody fluid that has an alkaline pH. Based on this assessment, the nurse would expect his initial treatment to be to

   A. Pass a nasogastric tube.
   B. Administer a bronchodilator.
   C. Draw a blood sample for measuring arterial blood gases.
   D. Administer packed RBCs.

1–181. Which of the following are found in *both* acute bacterial endocarditis (ABE) and subacute bacterial endocarditis (SBE)?

   I. Congestive heart failure.
   II. Roth's spots.
   III. Petechiae.
   IV. Temperature elevations of 102° F or greater.

   A. I, II, and III.
   B. I, III, and IV.
   C. II, III, and IV.
   D. I, II, III, and IV.

1–182. If bowel sounds are heard in the chest cavity after abdominochest trauma, the nurse should suspect

   A. The patient is hungry.
   B. A hiatal hernia.
   C. A ruptured hemidiaphragm.
   D. Sound is being referred from the abdomen.

1–183. The critical care nurse knows that the respiratory insufficiency associated with Guillain-Barré syndrome (GBS)

   A. Is caused by involvement of trunk muscles.
   B. Is caused by increased bronchial constriction.
   C. Rarely requires tracheostomy.
   D. Is caused by pulmonary infections.

1–184. A 19-year-old Hispanic male is admitted to the intensive care unit following a motorcycle accident. He has been hypotensive since admission, has had urinary outputs of 30 to 40 ml per hour, and is tachycardic. As you begin your nursing assessment, you notice that the IV site is oozing blood. You also note that the patient is speaking to you in broken Spanish and seems frightened when you attempt to auscultate breath sounds. You make a nursing diagnosis of alteration in individual coping based on which of the following?

    I. The age of the patient.
    II. Possible language barrier.
    III. The stress of the motorcycle accident.
    IV. Decreased cerebral perfusion.

    A. I and II only.
    B. II only.
    C. II and III only.
    D. II and IV only.

1–185. A 59-year-old patient has had a mitral valve replacement for mitral valve stenosis. At 30 years of age, she had a commissurotomy. The patient is on AV sequential pacing at 80 beats per minute in complete capture and has both right atrial and left atrial catheters to transducers. Right atrial pressure had been 18 mm Hg and is now 15 mm Hg. Left atrial pressure had been 20 mm Hg and is now 16 mm Hg. Mean arterial pressure has been constant at 80 to 82 mm Hg. Urine output has decreased over 3 hours from 80 ml, 60 ml, and 20 ml for each hour. Treatment should include which of the following?

    A. Furosemide, 20 mg IV.
    B. Dopamine at 5 µg/kg/minute.
    C. Lactated Ringer's, 250-ml bolus.
    D. No treatment is necessary at present, but the patient's urinary output should continue to be monitored.

1–186. The nurse should anticipate that treatment for a serum phosphorus of 0.4 mg/dl would include

    A. Aluminum hydroxide gel (Amphojel) and calcium supplements.
    B. Aluminum hydroxide gel (Amphojel) and potassium phosphate.
    C. Phospho Soda and calcium supplements.
    D. Potassium phosphate and Phospho Soda.

1–187. The critical care nurse receives report on a craniotomy patient with alteration in fluid volume related to the syndrome of inappropriate antidiuretic hormone (SIADH). The nurse knows to assess for

    A. Urinary output less than 30 ml per hour for 2 consecutive hours.
    B. Specific gravity less than 1.010.
    C. Increased serum osmolality.
    D. Evidence of hypernatremia.

1–188. Last night, a 49-year-old male had an emergency ileostomy performed for toxic megacolon. In the intensive care unit today, his vital signs are stable and he states that his pain medication keeps him free of pain. He is unable to rest. He will not cooperate with routine care, yet uses his call light to summon the nurse whenever s(he) leaves the room. He angrily dismisses his anxious family from his room. The most appropriate initial intervention for this patient's behavior is to

    A. Instruct the family to avoid patient contact for 24 hours.
    B. Insist that the patient cooperate with prescribed care.
    C. Thoroughly clarify the purposes and functions of the intensive care unit.
    D. Set strict limits on use of the call light.

1-189. A patient is admitted to the intensive care unit from the operating room after repair of a fusiform abdominal aortic aneurysm with a tube graft. The patient complains of severe low back pain. The nurse caring for the patient should

A. Administer morphine sulfate, 4 mg IV.
B. Check the dressing for drainage.
C. Check the abdominal girth.
D. Encourage the patient to turn from side to side.

1-190. An 18-year-old male is admitted following a motorcycle accident in which he hit a car broadside. He was wearing a helmet. He is complaining of dyspnea and backache and intense pain in his chest that radiates to his back and is unaffected by respirations. His BP is 90/50 mm Hg, pulse is 115 beats per minute, respirations are 24 per minute, and temperature is 37.8° C. Chest x-ray shows widening of the mediastinum. This most likely represents

A. Ruptured aorta.
B. Ruptured trachea.
C. Flail chest.
D. Ruptured diaphragm.

1-191. After completing the day shift in a busy critical care unit, a nurse is requested to work the next shift owing to the illness of a coworker. Which of the following factors should the nurse consider when making the decision whether to remain for the overtime shift?

I. The nurse has a professional obligation to work overtime, since failing to do so could lead to legal charges of patient abandonment.
II. The nurse has the right to leave; he or she has fulfilled the obligation to the employer by working the assigned shift.
III. The nurse has an obligation to refuse to work overtime if he or she is fatigued, since working while tired could endanger patients.
IV. The nurse who works the extra shift is held accountable to a lower standard of care, because it is assumed that he or she is tired.

A. I and III.
B. II and IV.
C. I and IV.
D. II and III.

1-192. A 43-year-old male patient has just returned from a computed tomography (CT) scan that revealed a noncommunicating hydrocephalus as a result of a tumor. His condition is stable at this time. However, as the nurse caring for him, you anticipate and prepare for which of the following?

A. Increased intracranial pressure.
B. Lumbar puncture to rule out meningitis.
C. Decreased CSF production.
D. Pneumoencephalogram.

1-193. Renal excretion of calcium is increased by

A. Edetate disodium (EDTA).
B. Calcitonin.
C. Plicamycin (mithramycin).
D. Indomethacin.

1–194. A 45-year-old female is admitted to the ICU after a motor vehicle accident. She was not wearing a seat belt and her chest hit the steering wheel. Two days later, weaning is instituted by placing her on a t-piece. Off the ventilator, she became very agitated and restless; her Sa_{O_2} dropped, and her heart rate increased. Upon observation, she displays accessory muscle use and intercostal bulging on expiration, and her sternum depresses on inspiration and bulges on expiration. The nurse identifies her nursing diagnosis as "alteration in breathing pattern." What is the most likely cause of her failure to wean?

A. Pneumothorax.
B. Flail chest.
C. Hemothorax.
D. Pain and anxiety.

1–195. In lower extremity arterial reconstruction, the primary reason for the use of Ace wraps below the knee is to

A. Prevent excessive postoperative edema formation.
B. Promote collateral circulation.
C. Prevent compartment syndrome.
D. Prevent venous thromboembolism.

1–196. Five days ago, a 65-year-old female had a subtotal colectomy with colostomy and single-lobe hepatic resection for metastases. Her gastric pH is now 2.5. She has a new hematemesis of 300 ml. The nurse suspects the patient has developed

A. Gastroesophageal reflux.
B. Hepatic failure.
C. Stress ulcers.
D. Acute pancreatitis.

1–197. A 75-year-old female presents to the emergency department with confusion and lethargy. Her husband reports that she has had "the flu" for 3 days with vomiting and diarrhea. Today she had difficulty walking to the bathroom. Assessment findings include a BP of 80/60 mm Hg and a regular heart rate of 150 beats per minute. Laboratory data include

Serum Na	126 mEq/l
Serum K	4.2 mEq/l
Serum Cl	100 mEq/l
Serum CO_2	14 mEq/l

In planning care for this patient, the IV solution most likely to be ordered would be

A. 0.9% sodium chloride.
B. Dextrose 5% in water.
C. 3% sodium chloride.
D. Dextrose 5% in 0.45% sodium chloride.

1–198. Based on your knowledge of dexamethasone (Decadron), you would question the physician if a craniotomy patient was *not* receiving which one of the following additional medications?

A. Ranitidine hydrochloride.
B. Sodium bicarbonate.
C. Morphine sulfate.
D. Levophed.

1–199. The major cause of morbidity after surgery is

A. Heart disease.
B. Pulmonary problems.
C. Sepsis.
D. Malnutrition.

1–200. Wolff-Parkinson-White syndrome is characterized by which of the following ECG findings?

A. Narrow QRS complex, short PR interval.
B. Inverted P wave with a PR interval less than .12 second.
C. Shortened PR interval with a prolonged initial portion of the QRS.
D. Shortened PR interval with prolongation of the terminal portion of the QRS.

Answers to Core Review Test 1

1–1. (**A**) The MAP depends upon the mean volume of blood ejected from the left ventricle (cardiac output) and the elastic properties of the arterial walls (systemic vascular resistance). Stroke work is a function of stroke volume, mean arterial pressure, and pulmonary capillary wedge pressure. Contractility is a function of left ventricular end-diastolic volume and stroke volume.

Reference: Kinney, M., Packa, D., and Dunbar, S.: AACN's Clinical Reference for Critical Care Nursing, 2nd ed. McGraw-Hill, New York, 1988.

1–2. (**B**) Sodium is the most abundant extracellular cation. Ninety-nine percent of calcium and 99% of magnesium are stored in the bones and teeth; the other 1% is extracellular.

References: Bigelow, L.A.: Fluids, electrolytes, and hemodynamics. In Fincke, M., and Lanros, N.: Emergency Nursing: A Comprehensive Review. Aspen, Rockville, MD, 1986.
Calloway, C.: When the problem involves magnesium, calcium, or phosphate. RN, 50:30–36, 1987.
Chambers, J.K.: Metabolic bone disorders: imbalances of calcium and phosphorus. Nurs Clin North Am, 22:861–872, 1987.

1–3. (**A**) In general, the metabolic action of glucocorticoids provides energy substrate to enable physical exertion. Glucocorticoids are essential for epinephrine- or glucagon-stimulated lipolysis, gluconeogenesis, and glycogenolysis. All of these processes result in increased glucose supply to the tissues. Glucocorticoids also increase cardiac contractility and the work capacity of the skeletal muscles. At pharmacologic levels, glucocorticoids stabilize lysosomal membranes and inhibit the inflammatory process.

Reference: Kohler, P.O., and Jordan, R.M. (eds.): Clinical Endocrinology. John Wiley and Sons, New York, 1986.

1–4. (**D**) The pia mater is the delicate outer covering that adheres to the surface of the brain, carrying branches of the cerebral arteries. Blood vessels in the pia mater form the choroid plexus.

Reference: Alspach, J.G. (ed.): AACN Core Curriculum for Critical Care Nursing, 4th ed. W.B. Saunders, Philadelphia, 1991.

1–5. (**A**) Gas exchange occurs across the alveolar-capillary membrane by passive diffusion. The movement of gas is down a pressure gradient—from a high to a low pressure—to equalize the pressures.

Reference: Shapiro, B.A., Harrison, R.A., Cane, R.D., et al.: Clinical Application of Blood Gases, 4th ed. Year Book Medical Publishers, Chicago, 1989.

1–6. (**C**) Internal respiration occurs at the cellular level. Actual utilization of oxygen occurs within the mitochondria in the cell. Here the oxygen is used with glucose to produce energy, "the fire of life," or adenosine triphosphate (ATP).

Reference: Shapiro, B.A., Harrison, R.A., Cane, R.D., et al.: Clinical Application of Blood Gases, 4th ed. Year Book Medical Publishers, Chicago, 1989.

1–7. (**D**) Having achieved CCRN status obligates a nurse to utilize his or her advanced knowledge to provide a higher standard of care. In a court of law, the CCRN would be held accountable to the standards of a "reasonable and prudent CCRN," rather than a "reasonable and prudent nurse."

Reference: Creighton, H.: Law Every Nurse Should Know, 4th ed. W.B. Saunders, Philadelphia, 1981.

1–8. (**A**) Gastric emptying accelerates in the presence of insulin, aggression, and a large volume of liquids. All of the other factors listed slow gastric emptying.

Reference: Ganong, W.F.: Review of Medical Physiology, 13th ed. Appleton and Lange, Norwalk, CT, 1987.

1–9. (**D**) When a patient receives an infusion of incompatible blood, red cells hemolyze and a hemolytic transfusion reaction occurs. When a hemolytic transfusion reaction occurs, antigen-antibody complexes are formed in the circulation. They cause activation of the complement cascade with release of histamine, serotonin, and bradykinin. These substances cause hypotension and shock. The antigen-antibody complexes and collections of fibrin in the kidney result in renal injury with back pain and hematuria. A patient who is having an allergic transfusion reaction develops pain at the IV site, hives, and palpitations.

Reference: Griffin, J.P.: Hematology and Immunology. Appleton-Century-Crofts, Norwalk, CT, 1986.

1–10. (**C**) Sleep apnea is a condition occurring in many obese, hypertensive patients. Snoring is a symptom of sleep apnea resulting from obstruction, which is common to both overweight and hypertensive persons. The frequency of PVCs generally decreases during sleep, but occurs in sleep apnea from hypoxemia during apneic periods. Sedatives are contraindicated in sleep apnea and may increase apneic periods and hypoxemia. Sedation may further prevent patients from having light sleep periods during which they change position to improve airway clearance. Reinforcing a patient's need to maintain blood pressure control and the positive effects of weight loss will encourage compliance, whereas highlighting possible side effects may discourage patients from maintaining blood pressure control.

Reference: Underhill, S., Woods, S., Froelicher, E., et al.: Cardiac Nursing, 2nd ed. J.B. Lippincott, Philadelphia, 1989.

1–11. (**B**) Cerebral vasospasm is the leading cause of death and disability in patients with aneurysmal subarachnoid hemorrhage (SAH). Vasospasm is caused by the abnormal narrowing of the focal, segmental, or diffuse cerebral arteries locally or distal to the area of aneurysmal rupture. Clinical vasospasm peaks in incidence at about the fourth to seventh day following an SAH. The syndrome causes ischemic consequences characterized by confusion, decreased level of consciousness, worsening headache, increased cerebral vascular resistance, and increasing blood pressure immediately prior to the clinical vasospasm.

Reference: Hickey, J.V.: The Clinical Practice of Neurological and Neurosurgical Nursing, 2nd ed. J.B. Lippincott, Philadelphia, 1986.

1–12. (**A**) Hypervolemic therapy is used to increase CPP, thereby improving cerebral microcirculation in the area of ischemia. Fluid restriction and aggressive diuretic therapy are controversial and may, in fact, aggravate cerebral ischemia. Controlled hypertension may be induced to improve neurologic status.

Reference: Kinney, M.R., Packa, D.R., and Dunbar, S.B.: AACN's Clinical Reference for Critical Care Nursing, 2nd ed. McGraw-Hill, New York, 1988.

1–13. (**D**) Excessive alcohol intake and poor carbohydrate intake can result in a depletion of glycogen stores. In addition, inadequate gluconeogenesis and glucose release are associated with ethanol-induced changes in glucose metabolism. Excessive administration of exogenous insulin is the most common cause of hypoglycemia. Chlorpropamide is an oral sulfonylurea, which stimulates the release of insulin from the pancreas, resulting in a lower blood sugar. Glucocorticoids (hydrocortisone) stimulate lipolysis, gluconeogenesis, and glycogenolysis, resulting in an elevation of serum glucose.

Reference: Hamburger, S., Rush, D.R., and Bosker, G.: Endocrine and Metabolic Emergencies. Robert J. Brady, Bowie, MD, 1984.

1–14. (**B**) Because the only parameter that has changed is the pulmonary artery diastolic pressure, one can assume that the catheter is disrupting pulmonary flow and has possibly caused ischemia in the vessel. Although just pullback of the catheter would relieve the disruption, a catheter in place for 6 days should be removed or replaced.

Reference: Bustin, D.: Hemodynamic Monitoring for Critical Care. Appleton-Century-Crofts, Norwalk, CT, 1986.

1–15. (**A**) The balloon is partially inflated when the tip of the catheter reaches the superior vena cava. It is fully inflated in the right atrium and advanced through the tricuspid valve into the right ventricle. When the catheter is in the pulmonary artery, the balloon is deflated to obtain pulmonary artery systolic and diastolic pressure readings, and then reinflated only long enough to obtain a pulmonary capillary wedge reading.

Reference: Fahey, V.: Vascular Nursing. W.B. Saunders, Philadelphia, 1988.

1–16. (**B**) Diuretic therapy in the treatment of CHF is a common cause of hypokalemia. Almost all diuretics used clinically, except for potassium-sparing diuretics such as spironolactone and amiloride, can produce hypokalemia because of increased renal potassium losses.

References: Schwartz, M.W.: Potassium imbalances. Am J Nurs, *87*:1292–1299, 1987.
Valle, G.A., and Lemberg, L.: Electrolyte imbalances in cardiovascular disease: The forgotten factor. Heart Lung, *17*:324–329, 1988.

1–17. (**C**) ECG changes do not occur rapidly with correction of potassium. U waves disappear, T wave amplitude increases, and QT intervals shorten over time, but these changes are not the best indication of treatment effectiveness. Sudden correction of acidosis can result in a further decrease in potassium. Unless contraindicated, potassium should be diluted in saline, since the infusion of glucose-containing fluids may cause the serum potassium to fall further. If the patient fails to respond to large doses of potassium, hypomagnesemia may be occurring concurrently and needs to be corrected for successful treatment of hypokalemia.

References: Janson, C.L.: Fluid and electrolyte balance. In Rosen, P.: Emergency Medicine: Concepts and Practice. C.V. Mosby, St. Louis, 1988.
Sweetwood, H.: Clinical Electrocardiography for Nurses, 2nd ed. Aspen, Rockville, MD, 1989.

1–18. (**C**) Electrolyte absorption occurs most rapidly in the proximal portion of the small bowel. Although electrolytes are absorbed in all areas of the small and large bowel, disease processes that affect the proximal portion of the small bowel are likely to cause significant disruption in electrolyte absorption.

Reference: Guyton, A.C.: Textbook of Medical Physiology, 7th ed. W.B. Saunders, Philadelphia, 1986.

1–19. (**C**) Pursed-lip breathing adds a form of expiratory retard when a patient is breathing spontaneously. It is thought to improve gas distribution, and most patients find that it eases their dyspnea and allows them to decrease their respiratory rate.

Reference: Kinney, M.R., Packa, D.R., and Dunbar, S.B.: Clinical Reference for Critical-Care Nursing, 2nd ed. McGraw-Hill, New York, 1988.

1–20. (**D**) In obstructive disease, the lungs are distended so that lung volumes and capacities (including compliance) are increased. The FEV is decreased because of the obstruction to flow on expiration.

Reference: West, J.B.: Pulmonary Pathophysiology: The Essentials, 3rd ed. Williams & Wilkins, Baltimore, 1987.

1–21. (**B**) Gram-negative bacteria are the usual cause of septic shock. *Escherichia coli* is the most frequent cause, followed by Klebsiella, Serratia, *Pseudomonas aeruginosa,* Proteus, and Bacteroides. *Staphylococcus epidermidis* and *Streptococcus pneumoniae* are gram-positive bacteria. Gram-positive bacteria can cause septic shock, but not with the same frequency as the gram-negative organisms.

Reference: Wall, S.C.: Septic shock. Nursing '89, *19*:52–60, 1989.

1–22. (**D**) Warm shock is the early phase of septic shock. Vasodilation and decreased peripheral resistance are the result of the release of histamine, bradykinins, and serotonin. Increased cardiac output is the result of activation of the sympathetic nervous system and the release of catecholamines.

Reference: Wall, S.C.: Septic Shock. Nursing '89, *19*:52–60, 1989.

1–23. (**B**) In a comatose patient who has intact connections between cranial nerves VIII and III and VI, the oculocephalic reflex evaluates the integrity of the brain stem by determining reflex movement of the eyeball. The presence of the reflex indicates that the pontine-midbrain level of the brain stem is intact. When the head is rotated, the eyes move in the direction opposite the head movement. When the doll's eye reflex or doll's eye phenomenon is absent, the eyes do not move and therefore remain in the same direction of the passive head movement.

Reference: Hickey, J.V.: The Clinical Practice of Neurological and Neurosurgical Nursing, 2nd ed. J.B. Lippincott, Philadelphia, 1986.

1–24. (**C**) The doll's eye or oculocephalic reflex is tested by briskly rotating, flexing, and extending the unconscious patient's head from side to side; therefore, presence of or suspicion of cervical spine fracture or dislocation is a contraindication. Accommodation without reaction to light is known as Argyll Robertson pupils. The oculovestibular reflex is assessed when the oculocephalic reflex test is inconclusive.

Reference: Hickey, J.V.: The Clinical Practice of Neurological and Neurosurgical Nursing, 2nd ed. J.B. Lippincott, Philadelphia, 1986.

1–25. (**B**) Stress-mediated elevations in circulating glucocorticoids and catecholamines are antagonistic to insulin and can precipitate DKA. Glucocorticoids interfere with glucose uptake and utilization by some tissues. Epinephrine causes inhibition of beta cell insulin secretion. Infection is a common cause of DKA but is not evident in this patient. Considering the patient's history and severity of symptoms, omission of insulin is the most likely cause of DKA.

Reference: Kohler, P.O., and Jordan, R.M. (eds.): Clinical Endocrinology. John Wiley and Sons, New York, 1986.

1–26. (**D**) In the absence of insulin, there is a decreased availability of glucose in fat cells necessary for lipogenesis. As a result, lipolysis occurs, releasing free fatty acids (FFAs). FFAs are oxidized into acetyl-CoA, which is substrate available to enter the Krebs cycle. Excess acetyl-CoA can eventually convert into acetoacetic acid and beta-hydroxybutyric acid. These ketones can be used as cellular energy substrates. However, when their formation exceeds tissue oxidation, ketosis and subsequent acidosis result. Excess ketones are excreted renally (ketonuria) and via the lungs, producing the "fruity" breath odor.

Reference: Hadley, M.E.: Endocrinology, 2nd ed. Prentice-Hall, Englewood Cliffs, NJ, 1988.

1-27. (**A**) The anion gap is calculated in milliequivalents per liter by the following formula: $Na^+ - (Cl^- + HCO_3^-)$. There is a normal range of 12.4 ± 2.0 mEq/l as unmeasured anions such as those on albumin, which are not accounted for by the formula. Addition of strong acid converts HCO_3^- into H_2CO_3, which dehydrates into H_2O and CO_2. CO_2 is eliminated by the lungs. The end result is a lowered HCO_3^-. Bicarbonate as a measured anion is replaced by an unmeasured anion, resulting in a widened anion gap. This patient's anion gap is $132 - (95 + 15) = 22$ mEq/l.

Reference: Kohler, P.O., and Jordan, R.M. (eds.): Clinical Endocrinology. John Wiley and Sons, New York, 1986.

1-28. (**D**) Acetoacetate and 3-hydroxybutyrate (ketones) are unmeasured anions that accumulate in excess as a result of lipolysis induced by an absence of insulin. Accumulation of lactate is usually a consequence of poor tissue perfusion and is not common in diabetic ketoacidosis.

Reference: Kohler, P.O., and Jordan, R.M. (eds.): Clinical Endocrinology. John Wiley and Sons, New York, 1986.

1-29. (**B**) Early (24 to 48 hours) after pacemaker insertion, many people require an increase in the mA of the pacemaker owing to fibrosis at the tip of the pacemaker catheter. The nurse should first turn the mA up to achieve complete capture. The sensitivity does not affect capture, and adjustment of the sensitivity is not indicated.

Reference: Kenner, C., Guzzetta, C., and Dossey, B.: Critical Care Nursing: Body-Mind-Spirit. Little, Brown, Boston, 1985.

1-30. (**C**) Vitamin C deficiency is associated with excessive bruising, petechiae, and spongy, bleeding gums. Iodine deficiency leads to goiter. Iron deficiency is manifested as pallor and listlessness. Vitamin A deficiency presents as dryness of the conjunctiva and mucous membranes, and epidermal hypertrophy.

Reference: Swearingen, P.L., Sommers, M.S., and Miller, K.: Manual of Critical Care: Applying Nursing Diagnoses to Critical Illness. C.V. Mosby, St. Louis, 1988.

1-31. (**C**) The ANA Code for Nurses states, "The nurse provides services with respect for human dignity and the uniqueness of the client unrestricted by considerations of social or economic status, personal attributes or the nature of health problems." Furthermore, the code states, "The nurse exercises informed judgment and uses individual competence and qualifications as criteria in seeking consultation, accepting responsibilities, and delegating nursing activities."

Reference: American Nurses Association: Code for Nurses With Interpretive Statements. American Nurses Association, Kansas City, MO, 1976.

1-32. (**B**) The definition for acute respiratory failure includes both ventilatory failure ($Pa_{CO_2} > 50$ mm Hg) and tissue hypoxia ($Pa_{O_2} < 60$ mm Hg).

Reference: West, J.B.: Pulmonary Pathophysiology, the Essentials, 3rd ed. Williams & Wilkins, Baltimore, 1987.

1-33. (**A**) The upright position allows the diaphragm to descend fully and the chest expands to its fullest capacity, thereby increasing the vital capacity.

Reference: West, J.B.: Pulmonary Pathophysiology, the Essentials, 3rd ed. Williams & Wilkins, Baltimore, 1987.

1–34. (**C**) The patient's passive behavior—
decreased verbalization, depressed
affect, and increased sleeping—reflects hopelessness. Apathy, passive-
ness, and a reluctance to express
feelings are characteristic of powerlessness. The patient does not
have any impairment in verbal communication, nor does the patient express any uncertainties about his
condition or delay decisions. His behavior seems also to be affecting his
wife.

Reference: Cox, H.C.: Clinical Applications of Nursing
Diagnosis. Williams & Wilkins, Baltimore, 1989.

1–35. (**B**) A serum phosphorus of 0.4 mg/
dl indicates hypophosphatemia. Hyperalimentation without phosphate
replacement results in a decreased
intake of this ion. Diabetic ketoacidosis causes hypophosphatemia by
an increased loss due to increased
glucose and osmotic diuresis and
also from the movement of glucose
and phosphorus into the cell by the
administration of insulin. The hypoparathyroid state causes hyperphosphatemia. The causes of phosphate depletion in alcoholics are
complex and may include poor dietary intake, vomiting, diarrhea, use
of antacids that bind phosphate and
reduce its absorption, and calcium
deficiency with secondary hyperparathyroidism.

Reference: Smith, L.H.: Phosphorus deficiency and
hypophosphatemia. In Wyngaarden, J.B., and Smith,
L.H.: Textbook of Medicine, 18th ed. W.B. Saunders,
Philadelphia, 1988.

1–36. (**C**) The rhythm strip shows pacemaker spikes at regular intervals
with beats 1 and 4 having noncap-
ture followed by ventricular escape
beats of low voltage. Beats 2, 3, 5,
6, and 7 demonstrate pacemaker
capture. The ventricular pacemaker
spike is immediately followed by a
ventricular complex.

Reference: Kenner, C., Guzzetta, C., and Dossey, B.:
Critical Care Nursing: Body—Mind—Spirit. Little,
Brown, Boston, 1985.

1–37. (**C**) Calcium plays an important role
in the depolarization of myocardial
cells. The flow of calcium across the
sarcolemma is necessary for contraction and relaxation to occur. Hyperkalemia and hyponatremia decrease cardiac contractility. Mild
hypoxemia may actually increase
contractility through sympathetic
stimulation.

Reference: Bustin, D.: Hemodynamic Monitoring for
Critical Care. Appleton-Century-Crofts, Norwalk,
CT, 1986.

1–38. (**D**) Regardless of the dose of acetaminophen estimated to have been
ingested, acetylcysteine should be
administered immediately if 24
hours or less have elapsed since the
reported ingestion. Acetylcysteine
(Mucomyst) is a mucolytic agent
used as adjunctive treatment for patients with abnormal pulmonary secretions. Although the exact mechanism is unknown, acetylcysteine
prevents or minimizes acetamino-
phen-induced hepatotoxicity by con-
jugating toxic metabolites. Acidosis
is not usually seen in acetaminophen overdoses so bicarbonate is not
indicated. Ipecac syrup is ineffective
after gastric aspiration. Saline cathartics should be avoided because
they may decrease absorption of acetylcysteine.

Reference: McEvoy, G.K., Litvak, K., Mendham, N.A.,
et al. (eds.): American Hospital Formulary Service
Drug Information, 89. American Society of Hospital
Pharmacists, Bethesda, MD, 1989.

1–39. (**A**) Acute ingestion of acetaminophen in doses of 150 mg/kg or more
usually results in hepatotoxicity because toxic metabolites conjugated
in the liver deplete available enzymes and cause liver necrosis.
Acid-base imbalances and agranu-
locytosis are extremely rare complications in acetaminophen overdosage. Although oxyhemoglobinemia
is normal, methemoglobinemia is a
frequent toxic effect of acetaminophen overdosage.

References: McEvoy, G.K., Litvak, K., Mendham,
N.A., et al. (eds.): American Hospital Formulary
Service Drug Information, 89. American Society of
Hospital Pharmacists, Bethesda, MD, 1989.

1–40. (**B**) A neurologic examination typically includes level of consciousness, motor function, cranial nerves, and sensory function. Vital signs, the least reliable indicators of cerebral function, are not usually considered a part of a neurologic examination.

Reference: Alspach, J.G., (ed.): AACN Core Curriculum for Critical Care Nursing, 4th ed. W.B. Saunders, Philadelphia, 1991.

1–41. (**B**) A "blown" pupil is generally seen with cranial nerve III (oculomotor) damage when uncal herniation compresses the cranial nerve against or under the tentorial ridge. This compression causes loss of parasympathetic stimulation, resulting in pupillary dilatation. Central or transtentorial herniation is compression and downward displacement of the cerebral hemispheres, usually causing small pupils (1 to 3 mm). Uncal and central herniation produce very different symptoms in the early period. Central herniation is found more commonly in subacute or chronic disorders, whereas uncal herniation is more commonly found in neurologic emergencies such as epidural hematoma formation.

Reference: Holloway, N.M.: Nursing the Critically Ill Adult. Addison-Wesley, Menlo Park, CA, 1988.

1–42. (**D**) The leads facing the anterior wall of the myocardium are leads V_1 through V_6. The leads facing the inferior wall are leads II, III, and aV_F. Posterior wall infarction is indicated on the ECG by ST depression in leads V_1 and V_2, since none of the leads directly faces the posterior wall. Lateral wall changes occur in leads I and aV_L.

Reference: Andreoli, K., Fowkes, V., Zipes, D., et al.: Comprehensive Cardiac Care, 6th ed. C.V. Mosby, St. Louis, 1987.

1–43. (**A**) The right coronary artery supplies the inferior heart and part of the wall of the right ventricle. It also supplies the sinoatrial (SA) and atrioventricular (AV) nodes in most people. Inferior infarctions generally cause bradydysrhythmias from SA or AV node ischemia. The left anterior descending coronary artery supplies the left ventricle and septum. Anterior wall infarctions are associated with left ventricular failure, bundle branch blocks, and intraventricular conduction disturbances.

Reference: Kenner, C., Guzzetta, C., and Dossey, B.: Critical Care Nursing: Body—Mind—Spirit. Little, Brown, Boston, 1985.

1–44. (**B**) A realistic outcome upon admission would be to impress upon the patient the importance of reporting chest pain immediately. Denial of chest pain is a double-edged sword. Although we do wish the patient to be free of pain, we do not want the patient to deny pain if he has any. A better outcome would be to have the patient rate his chest pain numerically from 0 to 10, with 0 being no pain. Patient teaching regarding signs and symptoms should take place after the stressful admission process. It is unrealistic to expect ST-segment elevation to resolve during admission.

Reference: Underhill, S., Woods, S., Froelicher, E., et al.: Cardiac Nursing, 2nd ed. J.B. Lippincott, Philadelphia, 1989.

1–45. (**A**) The patient is exhibiting defensive behaviors related to his feelings of helplessness and loss of control. Attempting to reason with him or tell him his behavior is unacceptable may increase his hostility and anger. To acknowledge the patient's anger gives the nurse a working point to discuss his feelings and work on their resolution. Sedation will not assist the patient to work through his anger and is a last resort for patient protection from actions that will cause him harm.

Reference: Underhill, S., Woods, S., Froelicher, E., et al.: Cardiac Nursing, 2nd ed. J.B. Lippincott, Philadelphia, 1989.

1–46. (**B**) Hemodialysis is a rapid and efficient method of fluid and solute removal, but it can cause drastic volume changes and fluid shifts with its rapid fluid removal. Peritoneal dialysis is a slow, gradual dialysis treatment requiring little technical support and no anticoagulation. With CAVH, anticoagulation is necessary for the patency of the filter; in this mode of treatment only minimal amounts of protein can be removed. One of the advantages of CAVH is the controlled regulation of fluid balance through a high rate of fluid removal and ease in providing hourly replacement by measuring filter output.

References: Kiely, M.: Continuous arteriovenous hemofiltration. Crit Care Nurs, 4:39–49, 1984.
Palmer, C., Koorejian, K., London, J., et al.: Nursing management of continuous arteriovenous hemofiltration for acute renal failure. Focus Crit Care, 13:21–30, 1986.

1–47. (**A**) TSH secreted by the anterior pituitary gland stimulates the active transport of inorganic iodine into the thyroid gland and ultimately the secretion of T_3 and T_4. Patients with hyperthyroidism have an increase in T_3 and T_4 production rate. These elevated levels of T_3 and T_4 provide negative feedback to the anterior pituitary gland to suppress TSH secretion.

Reference: Kohler, P.O., and Jordan, R.M. (eds.): Clinical Endocrinology. John Wiley and Sons, New York, 1986.

1–48. (**A**) Propranolol is a nonselective beta-adrenergic antagonist indicated for short-term rapid control of tachycardia, arrhythmias, and increased myocardial oxygen consumption. Adverse side effects may include decreased myocardial contractility, congestive heart failure, bronchospasm, and asthma. Propranolol also weakly inhibits the peripheral conversion of T_4 to the more biologically active T_3.

Reference: Kohler, P.O., and Jordan R.M. (eds.): Clinical Endocrinology. John Wiley and Sons, New York, 1986.

1–49. (**B**) During a sustained hyperdynamic state, myocardial oxygen demand may eventually outweigh the supply. Ischemia, infarction, an elevation in afterload, and dysrhythmias may precipitate a fall in the cardiac index. The presence of bibasilar crackles may be a sign of impending heart failure. This patient is prone to fluid volume deficit since she is hyperthermic, diaphoretic, and vomiting. There also may be a hyperglycemia-induced osmotic diuresis. There is no mention of goiter in the data presented, and it is unlikely that one could excessively cool this person.

Reference: Holloway, N.M.: Nursing the Critically Ill Adult, 3rd ed. Addison-Wesley, Menlo Park, CA, 1988.

1–50. (**B**) The blood gases show a trend towards respiratory acidosis even though the pH and Pa_{CO_2} are still within normal limits. This is an ominous sign since asthmatics are usually slightly alkalotic due to reactive airways disease, which stimulates them to increase their respiratory rate and depth. The additional signs of fixed chest and absent breath sounds indicate hyperinflated lungs and little air movement. She should be intubated immediately.

Reference: Kersten, L.D.: Comprehensive Respiratory Nursing: A Decision Making Approach. W.B. Saunders, Philadelphia, 1989.

1–51. (**B**) The therapeutic range is 10 to 20 μg/ml. Levels above this range may result in toxicity ranging from mild caffeine-like side effects to ventricular tachycardia and grand mal seizures.

Reference: Kersten, L.D.: Comprehensive Respiratory Nursing: A Decision Making Approach. W.B. Saunders, Philadelphia, 1989.

1–52. (A) B lymphocytes are responsible for mediating humoral immune responses. Cellular immunity is controlled by T lymphocytes. Type I hypersensitivity reactions are also known as anaphylactic reactions. Cell-mediated hypersensitivity reactions are also known as Type IV hypersensitivity reactions and are responsible for rejection of transplanted tissue.

Reference: Alspach, J.G. (ed.): AACN Core Curriculum for Critical Care Nursing, 4th ed. W.B. Saunders, Philadelphia, 1991.

1–53. (C) T lymphocytes are processed in the thymus gland to recognize the individual's own tissue. Lymphokines are chemical mediators of the immune system that are produced by lymphocytes. The chemical mediators of anaphylaxis are produced primarily by mast cells. Type II hypersensitivity reactions are also known as antibody-dependent mediated immune responses. In this type of reaction, antibodies attach to antigens on the surfaces of cells or in tissues, bringing about tissue injury.

Reference: Gee, G., and Moran, T.A.: AIDS—Concepts in Nursing Practice. Williams & Wilkins, Baltimore, 1988.

1–54. (A) Histopathologic changes that occur in acute spinal cord injury cause progressive edema resulting in small vessel edema and decreased tissue oxygenation. Assessment of reflexes provides an indirect measure of motor ability and, more specifically, determination of spinal shock and differentiation between complete and incomplete spinal cord lesions.

Reference: Alspach, J.G. (ed.): AACN Core Curriculum for Critical Care Nursing, 4th ed. W.B. Saunders, Philadelphia, 1991.

1–55. (D) Poikilothermism, resulting from interruption of sympathetic pathways from the temperature regulating centers in the hypothalamus to the peripheral blood vessels, occurs in some acute spinal cord injured patients. Core temperature may drift to either hypothermia or hyperthermia based on the ambient environmental temperature, requiring vigilant monitoring by the critical care nurse.

Reference: Alspach, J.G. (ed.): AACN Core Curriculum for Critical Care Nursing, 4th ed. W.B. Saunders, Philadelphia, 1991.

1–56. (A) Brown-Séquard syndrome refers to a hemitranssection of the cord resulting in ipsilateral loss of motor, position, and vibratory sensation and contralateral loss of pain and temperature sensation.

Reference: Alspach, J.G. (ed.): AACN Core Curriculum for Critical Care Nursing, 4th ed. W.B. Saunders, Philadelphia, 1991.

1–57. (D) Abdominal tenderness after laparotomy is common not only on the second postoperative day but also into the second post-operative week. Diminished bowel sounds, blood in the stool, and dark purple coloration in the stoma are signs of serious complications and require immediate follow-up.

Reference: Swearingen, P.L., Sommers, M.S., and Miller, K.: Manual of Critical Care: Applying Nursing Diagnoses to Adult Critical Illness. C.V. Mosby, St. Louis, 1988.

1–58. (**A**) Erythropoietin is decreased in chronic renal failure. This hormone stimulates bone marrow to produce red cells. Toxins present in the serum inhibit erythropoiesis and cause an accelerated rate of RBC destruction. Blood loss results from excessive laboratory testing, bleeding from the gastrointestinal (GI) mucosa, and as a result of leaks, rupture, or residual blood remaining in the dialyzer if the patient is being hemodialyzed. Chronic renal failure patients also have folic acid and iron deficiencies that contribute to anemia.

References: Crandall, B.L.: Chronic renal failure. In Ulrich, T.: Nephrology Nursing. Appleton and Lange, Norwalk, CT, 1989.
Lancaster, L.: ESRD: Pathophysiology, assessment and intervention. In Lancaster, L.: The Patient with End Stage Renal Disease, 2nd ed. John Wiley and Sons, New York, 1984.

1–59. (**B**) Decreased glomerular filtration rate (GFR) causes increased phosphates and a subsequent decrease in calcium. The kidney's inability to convert vitamin D to the active metabolite 1,25-dihydroxycholecalciferol (DHCC) results in a decreased absorption of calcium from the intestines, worsening hypocalcemia. Hypocalcemia is the result of increased plasma phosphates and acidosis. Parathormone production is the parathyroid response to an already decreased calcium level.

References: Chambers, J.K.: Metabolic bone disorders: Imbalances of calcium and phosphorus. Nurs Clin North Am, 22:861–872, 1987.
Lancaster, L.: ESRD: Pathophysiology, assessment and intervention. In Lancaster, L.: The Patient with End Stage Renal Disease, 2nd ed. John Wiley and Sons, New York, 1984.

1–60. (**A**) All of the above are complications of endotracheal or tracheostomy tubes, particularly the cuff. The one life-threatening complication is rupture through a major systemic artery such as the innominate artery.

Reference: Kersten, L.D.: Comprehensive Respiratory Nursing: A Decision Making Approach. W.B. Saunders, Philadelphia, 1989.

1–61. (**B**) Balloon dependence is indicated when symptoms of left ventricular failure occur during attempts to wean the patient. The pulmonary artery diastolic pressure of 22 mm Hg is extremely high and reflects increased left ventricular end-diastolic volumes and failure.

Reference: Weeks, L.: Advanced Cardiovascular Nursing. Blackwell, Boston, 1986.

1–62. (**D**) Be honest with the patient and encourage him to talk about his fears. Help the patient identify differences between his condition and the condition of the patient who died. Help him identify with the living. Do not withhold medication, but allow the patient to resolve the issue.

Reference: Kenner, C., Guzzetta, C., and Dossey, B.: Critical Care Nursing: Body—Mind—Spirit. Little, Brown, Boston, 1985.

1–63. (**C**) The normal hemoglobin is 13.3 to 17.7 gm/dl for men and 11.7 to 15.7 gm/dl for women.

Reference: Alspach, J.G. (ed.): AACN Core Curriculum for Critical Care Nursing, 4th ed. W.B. Saunders, Philadelphia, 1991.

1–64. (**C**) When a primary space-occupying lesion exists, brain edema, disruption of CSF reabsorption, and intracranial blood flow compression may occur. Intracranial hemorrhage may also advance the intracranial hypertension. Subarachnoid hemorrhage is more likely a result of a congenital disorder than traumatic injuries.

Reference: Kinney, M.R., Packa, D.R., and Dunbar, S.B.: Clinical Reference for Critical Care Nursing, 2nd ed. McGraw-Hill, New York, 1988.

1-65. (**D**) A decrease in a patient's level of consciousness is considered to be indicative of neurologic deterioration. It is generally the earliest sign of sensitivity to a decreased oxygen supply by the cerebral cortex. Another reason for decreased level of consciousness is compromised terminal arteries, which decrease the oxygen supply to the cerebral cortex.

Reference: Hickey, J.V.: The Clinical Practice of Neurological and Neurosurgical Nursing, 2nd ed. J.B. Lippincott, Philadelphia, 1986.

1-66. (**D**) Evaluating respiratory status is always a priority nursing intervention, regardless of the patient care situation. Although it is important to determine the nature, scope, and extent of a patient's injury, as well as to perform a secondary neurologic examination, respiratory assessment always has a higher priority. Calculation of CPP can be accomplished only after insertion of an intracranial pressure monitoring device. This is usually not a high priority in the first 15 minutes of intervention.

Reference: Caine, R.M., and Bufalino, P.M.: Critically Ill Adults: Nursing Care Planning Guides. Williams & Wilkins, Baltimore, 1988.

1-67. (**C**) The Glasgow Coma Score is used to objectively assess a patient's level of consciousness with responses graded in three categories based on the best response in each of three categories. The first assessment category is eye opening, the second is motor response, and the third is verbal response. A Glasgow Coma Score of 3—3—4 indicates that the patient opens his eyes when spoken to, is not able to follow commands but localizes pain and attempts to remove the noxious stimulus when motor function is tested, and is able to vocalize but is confused, as evidenced by his inability to state who he is, where he is, or the date.

Reference: Alspach, J.G. (ed.): AACN Core Curriculum for Critical Care Nursing, 4th ed. W.B. Saunders, Philadelphia, 1991.

1-68. (**B**) Unconscious patients with motor tract interruption can exhibit abnormal muscle tone or inappropriate motor responses that present as characteristic involuntary (reflex) motor activity or *postures* upon application of a noxious stimulus. Decerebrate posturing results from lesions in the diencephalon, midbrain, or pons. When assessing this, the nurse observes the jaw tightly clenched, the neck extended, arms adducted, elbows extended, forearms pronated, wrists and fingers flexed, legs stiffly extended at the knees, and the feet plantar flexed. The response can occur spontaneously, to environmental stimuli, or to a noxious stimulus.

Reference: Hickey, J.V.: The Clinical Practice of Neurological and Neurosurgical Nursing, 2nd ed. J.B. Lippincott, Philadelphia, 1986.

1-69. (**C**) Unconscious patients with motor tract interruption can exhibit abnormal muscle tone or inappropriate motor responses that present as characteristic movements or *postures* upon application of a noxious stimulus. Decorticate posturing results from lesions of the corticospinal tracts within or near the cerebral hemispheres. When assessing this, the nurse observes adduction of the upper arms with the elbows, wrists, and fingers flexed. The legs are extended and internally rotated. Plantar flexion of the feet is noted.

Reference: Hickey, J.V.: The Clinical Practice of Neurological and Neurosurgical Nursing, 2nd ed. J.B. Lippincott, Philadelphia, 1986.

1–70. (**B**) Decreased excretion and/or increased intake of magnesium can cause an excess in magnesium. However, the most common cause of hypermagnesemia is severe renal failure. When the GFR falls below 30 ml per hour, magnesium is not cleared from the blood and serum levels rise. Addison's disease causes hypermagnesemia by decreasing excretion, and the hypermagnesemia of myxedema is a result of increased intake. Hyperthyroidism causes hypomagnesemia.

Reference: Calloway, C.: When the problem involves magnesium, calcium, or phosphate. RN, *50:*30–36, 1987.

1–71. (**D**) Pulmonary embolus is frequently undiagnosed or misdiagnosed because of the variability in presenting symptoms and extent of pathophysiology. The most definitive test is the angiogram, which detects filling defects in the pulmonary vasculature.

Reference: Kersten, L.D.: Comprehensive Respiratory Nursing: A Decision Making Approach. W.B. Saunders, Philadelphia, 1989.

1–72. (**B**) Ventilation/perfusion mismatch is the cause of hypoxia when pulmonary emboli occur. There is a high ventilation-to-perfusion ratio as ventilation continues to occur in areas with little or no perfusion.

Reference: West, J.B.: Respiratory Physiology: The Essentials, 4th ed. Williams & Wilkins, Baltimore, 1990.

1–73. (**D**) The only use for steroids in treatment of pulmonary emboli has been found to be with fat emboli, and that therapy has not been proven effective.

Reference: Braunwald, E., Isselbacher, K.J., Petersdorf, R.G., et al.: Harrison's Principles of Internal Medicine, 11th ed. McGraw-Hill, New York, 1987.

1–74. (**A**) Cushing's ulcers occur in patients with head injury or intracranial disease. This is probably due to excessive gastric acid secretion. Burns, chronic drug ingestion (e.g., of aspirin or alcohol), and sepsis frequently give rise to stress ulcers. The mechanism causing stress ulcerations is unknown, but a variety of etiologies is postulated.

References: Konopad, E., and Noseworthy, T.: Stress ulceration: A serious complication in critically ill patients. Heart Lung, *17*(4):339–348, 1988.
Luckmann, J., and Sorensen, K.C.: Medical-Surgical Nursing: A Psychophysiologic Approach, 3rd ed. W.B. Saunders, Philadelphia, 1987.

1–75. (**B**) Ascorbic acid (vitamin C) causes a false negative result in the Hemoccult-type slide guaiac test for occult fecal blood. This test is effective in screening for colorectal cancer and for fecal blood with other etiologies (such as colitis, etc.). It is very important to get a medication history including over-the-counter drugs prior to administering the test because in addition to the above, iron supplements, iodine, and aspirin cause a false positive result on the Hemoccult-type slide guaiac test.

Reference: Sleisenger, M.H., and Fordtran, J.S.: Gastrointestinal Disease: Pathophysiology, Diagnosis, Management, 4th ed. W.B. Saunders, Philadelphia, 1989.

1–76. (**A**) Medications that cause delayed myocardial repolarization (prolonged QT interval), such as procainamide and quinidine, may cause torsades de pointes. Digoxin may shorten the QT interval. Propranolol and verapamil act on the AV node, and their effect on the QT interval is solely rate related.

Reference: Underhill, S., Woods, S., Froelicher, E., et al.: Cardiac Nursing, 2nd ed. J.B. Lippincott, Philadelphia, 1989.

1-77. (**C**) Medications that cause delayed myocardial repolarization (prolonged QT interval), such as procainamide and quinidine, may cause torsades de pointes. Isoproterenol increases the rate of sinus node discharge and shortens the refractory period.

Reference: Underhill, S., Woods, S., Froelicher, E., et al.: Cardiac Nursing, 2nd ed. J.B. Lippincott, Philadelphia, 1989.

1-78. (**D**) Dialysis disequilibrium syndrome is related to the osmotic gradient produced across the blood-brain barrier by the efficient removal of urea from the blood. Because urea is not removed from the brain tissue, it draws in water from the extracellular fluid and causes cerebral edema.

References: Lancaster, L.: The patient receiving hemodialysis. In Lancaster, L.: The Patient With End Stage Renal Disease, 2nd ed. John Wiley and Sons, New York, 1984.
Sauer, S.N., and Nolander, M.E.: The pediatric renal patient. In Ulrich, B.T.: Nephrology Nursing: Concepts and Strategies. Appleton and Lange, Norwalk, CT, 1989.
Thompson, J., McFarland, G.K., Hirsch, J.E., et al.: Mosby's Manual of Clinical Nursing, 2nd ed. C.V. Mosby, St. Louis, 1989.

1-79. (**A**) Use of a larger dialyzer causes a greater risk because it provides a more rapid clearance. Treatment includes shortening the treatment and slowing the blood flow rate through the dialyzer until BUN and electrolytes are lower to decrease risk of dialysis disequilibrium syndrome. Saline IV has no effect on dialysis disequilibrium syndrome.

References: Lancaster, L.: The patient receiving hemodialysis. In Lancaster, L.: The Patient With End Stage Renal Disease, 2nd ed. John Wiley and Sons, New York, 1984.
Thompson, J., McFarland, G.K., Hirsch, J.E., et al.: Mosby's Manual of Clinical Nursing, 2nd ed. C.V. Mosby, St. Louis, 1989.

1-80. (**B**) Brain tumors are classified according to their histologic features and grade of malignancy from I to IV. Grade IV tumors are considered the most malignant. Location and accessibility of the tumor are of clinical and surgical significance.

Reference: Alspach, J.G. (ed.): AACN Core Curriculum for Critical Care Nursing, 4th ed. W.B. Saunders, Philadelphia, 1991.

1-81. (**B**) CHF is unlikely in a 24-year-old basically healthy adult. Fat emboli could produce the symptoms and ABGs, but not the chest x-ray findings. The most likely cause is ARDS.

Reference: West, J.B.: Pulmonary Pathophysiology: The Essentials, 3rd ed. Williams & Wilkins, Baltimore, 1987.

1-82. (**D**) The Pa_{CO_2} is at the upper limit of normal, but the pH is still within normal limits. The main problem is continuing hypoxemia on high levels of oxygen, hence the name "refractory" hypoxemia.

Reference: Kinney, M.R., Packa, D.R., and Dunbar, S.B.: Clinical Reference for Critical-Care Nursing, 2nd ed. McGraw-Hill, New York, 1988.

1-83. (**B**) Since the hypoxemia is due to collapsed alveoli, shunting of blood through nonventilated areas, and fluid and debris in the interstitial space, the only therapy shown to have an effect is PEEP. PEEP holds the alveoli open at end-expiration and prevents their collapse, thereby decreasing the pressure required to initiate inspiration. In addition, the increased pressure in the alveoli pushes fluid from the alveoli into the lung interstitial space, and the fluid is then carried away by the lymphatic system and capillaries.

Reference: West, J.B.: Pulmonary Pathophysiology: The Essentials, 3rd ed. Williams & Wilkins, Baltimore, 1987.

1–84. (**D**) In order to determine that negligence has occurred, all of the above criteria must be proven. The duty to provide care is implied when the provider-client relationship is established. An omission does not constitute negligence unless it can be shown to have been the probable cause of harm.

References: American Heart Association: Textbook of Advanced Cardiac Life Support. American Heart Association, Dallas, 1987.
Creighton, H.: Law Every Nurse Should Know, 4th ed. W.B. Saunders, Philadelphia, 1981.

1–85. (**D**) Propranolol is a rapid-acting beta-blocking agent that should effect a decrease in rate to maintain cardiac output. Carotid massage generally does not break atrial fibrillation-flutter in mitral valve disease. Cardioversion is contraindicated following digitalization.

Reference: Kenner, C., Guzzetta, C., and Dossey, B.: Critical Care Nursing: Body—Mind—Spirit. Little, Brown, Boston, 1985.

1–86. (**A**) Class I antiarrhythmics interact with sodium channels (blockade). Class II antiarrhythmics (e.g., propranolol) are beta$_1$-adrenergic blockers. Class III drugs (e.g., bretylium) cause potassium channel blockade. Class IV antiarrhythmics (e.g., verapamil) are calcium channel blockers.

Reference: Anderson, J.: Critical Care Cardiology. Karger, New York, 1988.

1–87. (**B**) Cold agglutinins are antibodies that cause a patient's blood to coagulate if blood colder than body temperature is infused. Therefore, the patient will not tolerate the administration of blood that is significantly colder than the body temperature. The patient with cold agglutinins must have blood warmed for safe administration. Keeping the patient warm will have no effect. Blood should not be administered without a filter.

Reference: Alspach, J.G. (ed.): AACN Core Curriculum for Critical Care Nursing, 4th ed. W.B. Saunders, Philadelphia, 1991.

1–88. (**B**) Epidural hematomas classically display a brief period of unconsciousness, followed by a lucid interval of varying duration, finally followed by rapid deterioration of level of consciousness with complaints of a severe headache.

Reference: Alspach, J.G. (ed.): AACN Core Curriculum for Critical Care Nursing, 4th ed. W.B. Saunders, Philadelphia, 1991.

1–89. (**B**) Lactated Ringer's or normal saline is rapidly administered to counteract potential hypovolemic shock associated with hemorrhage into the pancreas. Meperidine is the drug of choice for pain relief, because drugs such as morphine cause spasms at the ampulla of Vater and sphincter of Oddi, which may cause biliary obstruction and exacerbate acute pancreatitis. Dextrose solutions stimulate inflamed pancreatic cells to secrete more pancreatic juice; the goal for these patients is to inhibit secretion of pancreatic juice. Vasopressors are contraindicated until hypovolemia has been ruled out.

Reference: Fain, J.A., and Amato-Vealey, E.: Acute pancreatitis: A gastrointestinal emergency. Crit Care Nurse, 8(5):47–64, 1989.

1–90. (**B**) Crush syndrome results in destruction of large muscles, which releases myoglobin molecules into the circulating blood volume. These molecules filter into the tubules but are too large to pass through the system, where they cause intracellular obstruction.

Reference: Norris, M.: Acute tubular necrosis: Preventing complications. Dimen Crit Care Nurs, 8:16–26, 1989.

1–91. (**B**) ARDS and pulmonary edema cause alveolar filling by transudate—fluid coming into the alveoli from the capillaries. In chronic bronchitis, the alveoli are not involved, but the bronchi and airways are filled with mucus.

Reference: West, J.B.: Pulmonary Pathophysiology: The Essentials, 3rd ed. Williams & Wilkins, Baltimore, 1987.

1–92. (**D**) The primary reason for turning and repositioning ventilator-dependent patients is to mobilize and drain secretions. Secretions in the base of the lung are difficult to drain unless the patient is frequently repositioned.

Reference: Kinney, M.R., Packa, D.R., and Dunbar, S.B.: Clinical Reference for Critical-Care Nursing, 2nd ed. McGraw-Hill, New York, 1988.

1–93. (**A**) The bundle of His travels through the septum from the AV node to the right and left bundle branches. The Purkinje system extends from the right and left bundles into the subendocardial layers of the ventricles. Bachmann's bundle transmits impulses from the SA node to the left atrium. The internodal pathways travel between the SA and AV nodes.

Reference: Kinney, M., Dear, C., Packa, D., et al.: AACN's Clinical Reference for Critical Care Nursing, 2nd ed. McGraw-Hill, New York, 1988.

1–94. (**B**) Junctional escape rhythms generally have a rate of 40 to 60 beats per minute. Accelerated junctional rhythms have a rate of 60 to 100 beats per minute. Junctional tachycardia has a rate of 100 to 160 beats per minute. Accelerated junctional tachycardia has a rate of 160 to 220 beats per minute.

Reference: Underhill, S., Woods, S., Froelicher, E., et al.: Cardiac Nursing, 2nd ed. J.B. Lippincott, Philadelphia, 1989.

1–95. (**A**) In acute bacterial meningitis, the CSF analysis will reveal increased WBCs (1000–2000 mm^3 or more), increased protein (100–500 mg/dl), and decreased glucose (<40 mg/dl). CSF will appear cloudy and bacteria will be present on Gram stain and culture. RBCs are not found in normal CSF. Normally CSF is clear, WBCs will be between 0 to 5 cells per mm^3, protein is between 15 to 45 mg/dl, and glucose between 60 to 80 mg/dl. Normally the specific gravity of CSF is 1.007.

References: Alspach, J.G. (ed.): AACN Core Curriculum for Critical Care Nursing, 4th ed. W.B. Saunders, Philadelphia, 1991.
Hickey, J.V.: The Clinical Practice of Neurological and Neurosurgical Nursing, 2nd ed. J.B. Lippincott, Philadelphia, 1986.

1–96. (**B**) Renin is a proteolytic enzyme secreted into the blood by the kidney, specifically by a specialized area of the nephron known as the juxtaglomerular apparatus.

References: Lancaster, L.: ESRD: Pathophysiology, assessment and intervention. In Lancaster, L.: The Patient with End Stage Renal Disease, 2nd ed. John Wiley and Sons, New York, 1984.
Ulrich, B.: Renal anatomy and physiology. In Ulrich, B.: Nephrology Nursing: Concepts and Strategies. Appleton and Lange, Norwalk, CT, 1989.

1–97. (**A**) Cimetidine and ranitidine do *not* affect the metabolism of gentamicin. It should be noted that the drugs are *not* compatible for parenteral infusion, however. Cimetidine and ranitidine significantly inhibit metabolism of theophylline, lidocaine HCl, and procainamide, so that a 50% reduction in their dosage is indicated.

Reference: Chernow, B.: The Pharmacologic Approach to the Critically Ill Patient, 2nd ed. Williams & Wilkins, Baltimore, 1988.

1–98. (**C**) The normal SV_{O_2} is 60% to 80%. Patients are maintained on higher flows of oxygen and have higher than normal SV_{O_2} levels to promote wound healing. An SV_{O_2} of 87% is acceptable.

Reference: Jaquith, S.: The oximetric opticath: What is it and how can it facilitate nursing management of the critically ill patient? Crit Care Nurs, *4:*55–68, 1984.

1–99. (**B**) When blood flow decreases, as in low cardiac output states, the tissues extract more oxygen. Venous oxygen therefore decreases, causing a wide a-vD$_{O_2}$ (a-vD$_{O_2}$ = arterial oxygen content − venous oxygen content).

Reference: Daily, E., and Schroeder, J.: Techniques in Bedside Hemodynamic Monitoring, 3rd ed. C.V. Mosby, St. Louis, 1985.

1–100. (**C**) At this point, ignoring or forcing the issue would not help the situation and may worsen it. After verbalization, the patient may be willing to look at the stoma and care for the tracheostomy by discharge.

Reference: Kersten, L.D.: Comprehensive Respiratory Nursing: A Decision Making Approach. W.B. Saunders, Philadelphia, 1989.

1–101. (**B**) The patient's hematocrit, hemoglobin, WBC, and BUN are all normal, thus ruling out anemia, infection, and uremia. However, the patient has a decreased fibrinogen (normal 200–400 mg/dl) and an elevated fibrin split products (normal <10 μg/ml) and is developing a coagulopathy.

Reference: Von Rueden, K.T., and Walleck, C.A.: Advanced Critical Care Nursing. Aspen, Rockville, MD, 1989.

1–102. (**D**) A simple answer addressing the expressed concerns will help allay anxiety. Gaining a more precise understanding of the patient's questions will help you plan your care to meet her specific needs.

Reference: Doenges, M., and Moorhouse, M.: Nursing Diagnosis with Interventions. F.A. Davis, Philadelphia, 1988.

1–103. (**A**) Status epilepticus is characterized by recurrent generalized seizure activity during which consciousness is not regained. These recurrent tonic-clonic (grand mal) seizures are generalized, symmetric seizures that affect the whole body. Absence seizures (petit mal) are so named because the patient experiences a brief loss of contact with the environment. Akinetic seizures are manifested by a brief loss of muscle tone. Myoclonic seizures are sudden, brief muscular contractions that usually involve the arms.

Reference: Alspach, J.G. (ed.): AACN Core Curriculum for Critical Care Nursing, 4th ed. W.B. Saunders, Philadelphia, 1991.

1–104. (**D**) Patients who are experiencing seizures are most at risk for airway obstruction and injury. Once jaws have clenched, it is not appropriate to pry them open, since teeth may be broken in the process, causing airway obstruction. The patient who is experiencing a seizure should be protected against injury. The airway should be suctioned gently if necessary, a tongue depressor inserted between the teeth of a patient whose jaws are not clenched, constricting clothing loosened, use of restraints avoided, and the patient's movements guided.

Reference: Hickey, J.V.: The Clinical Practice of Neurological and Neurosurgical Nursing, 2nd ed. J.B. Lippincott, Philadelphia, 1986.

1–105. (**B**) Desmopressin is a synthetic analogue of arginine vasopressin (ADH). It is conveniently and effectively administered intranasally. The dosage required to promote antidiuresis is 5 to 20 μg. Mannitol may be indicated to promote diuresis when increased intracranial pressure is present. Phenytoin may exacerbate the diuresis. Oxytocin is the other neurohypophyseal hormone, and it has mild antidiuretic effects.

Reference: Kohler, P.O., and Jordan, R.M. (eds.): Clinical Endocrinology. John Wiley and Sons, New York, 1986.

1–106. (C) Patients with end-stage renal disease are usually well aware of their vital signs and laboratory values and need to know this information to decrease their anxiety.

Reference: Crandall, B.L.: Chronic renal failure. In Ulrich, T.: Nephrology Nursing. Appleton and Lange, Norwalk, CT, 1989.

1–107. (B) As renal failure progresses, the ability of the kidney to filter phosphorus decreases and serum concentrations of phosphorus rise. Because serum phosphorus and ionized calcium are in equilibrium, this results in a fall in the level of calcium. Magnesium is elevated because of the inability to excrete this electrolyte.

Hyperkalemia is a life-threatening complication of renal failure. Once the glomerular filtration rate falls sufficiently to reduce daily urine output to 500 ml, serum potassium levels rise rapidly.

Urea is the major end product of protein metabolism and is filtered at the glomerulus. Urea is reabsorbed throughout the renal tubule, especially when the kidney is attempting to conserve salt and water.

Reference: Crandall, B.L.: Acute renal failure. In Ulrich, T.: Nephrology Nursing. Appleton and Lange, Norwalk, CT, 1989.

1–108. (D) Diuretics are not effective when there is inadequate renal function to respond to the effects of a diuretic. A Foley catheter is not indicated because urinary output will not increase in response to therapy. A phlebotomy is contraindicated, since most chronic renal failure patients are anemic. Because morphine sulfate decreases venous return and left ventricular filling volume (preload), it is helpful in relieving pulmonary congestion.

Reference: Chambers, J.K.: Metabolic bone disorders: Imbalances of calcium and phosphorus. Nurs Clin North Am, 22:861–872, 1987.

1–109. (C) Up to the point of closure of the pulmonic valve, right ventricular and pulmonary artery systolic pressures are usually equal.

Reference: Bustin, D.: Hemodynamic Monitoring in Critical Care. Appleton-Century-Crofts, Norwalk, CT, 1986.

1–110. (C) This patient has elevated pulmonary artery and capillary wedge pressures. If the systemic vascular resistance were calculated from the MAP, CVP, and cardiac output, it would equal 1887. The left ventricle must work hard to eject against this afterload. Reduction of afterload (decreased SVR) with increased nitroprusside would increase the cardiac output. Increased fluid and a higher dose of dopamine would further stress the left ventricle. Since the patient is already on maximum inotropic support with dopamine, administration of digoxin would not affect cardiac output.

Reference: Daily, E., and Schroeder, J.: Techniques in Bedside Hemodynamic Monitoring, 3rd ed. C.V. Mosby, St. Louis, 1985.

1–111. (B) The capillary filling pressure of the tracheal wall is 27 to 29 cm H_2O pressure. The cuff pressure should be less than this but greater than 15 cm H_2O, since aspiration has been observed to occur in animals at that pressure.

Reference: Millar, S.: Procedure Manual for Critical Care, 2nd ed. W.B. Saunders, Philadelphia, 1985.

1–112. (D) It is critically important that patients be able to participate in their own recovery. The patient who is demoralized by prolonged illness is unable to recognize his or her own power to influence recovery. The expert nurse will maximize the patient's control and participation in recovery.

Reference: Holloway, N.M.: Nursing the Critically Ill Adult, 3rd ed. Addison-Wesley, New York, 1988.

1–113. (**D**) If a physician fails to respond appropriately to notification of a change in a patient's condition, the nurse is legally obligated to ensure that designated supervisors are informed and that action is taken to provide medical evaluation and care for the patient. The nurse's documentation that the physician was notified and failed to respond provides no care for the patient and therefore no legal protection for the nurse. Notification and documentation are important, but they are incomplete steps unless the physician responds appropriately to the nurse's call.

Reference: Yob, M.O.: Communication issues: A potential source of liability for nurses. Focus Crit Care, 2:78–79, 1988.

1–114. (**D**) Malignant hyperthermia (MH) is a pharmacogenetic disorder usually caused by potent inhalation anesthetic agents and depolarizing muscle relaxants. Stress is also a contributing factor and may precipitate a crisis in the absence of surgery. The disorder causes symptoms of tachycardia, muscular rigidity, and acute hyperthermia, with reported temperatures as high as 112°F. The primary defect in MH is the result of increased calcium ion levels, which may not be pumped back into the sarcoplasmic reticulum—the calcium-storing sacs. Immediate interventions include discontinuation of anesthetic agents, administration of 100% oxygen, obtaining ABGs, administration of dantrolene sodium and procainamide, and cooling measures. Ongoing interventions include monitoring and treating cardiovascular complications, acid-base imbalances, urinary output, and central nervous system deficits. Patient and family counseling is encouraged.

Reference: Caine, R., Molla, K., and Reynolds, R.: Malignant hyperthermia: A critical care challenge. Dimen Crit Care Nurs, 5(3):144–154, 1986.

1–115. (**B**) The pH, in conjunction with the Pa_{CO_2} and HCO_3, is most consistent with acute respiratory failure. There may be tissue hypoxia, but that is a clinical, not laboratory, diagnosis. The pH would be closer to normal (compensated) in chronic respiratory failure. The HCO_3 is low because it is starting to compensate for the acidosis.

Reference: Shapiro, B.A., Harrison, R.A., Cane, R.D., et al.: Clinical Application of Blood Gases, 4th ed. Year Book Medical Publishers, Chicago, 1989.

1–116. (**A**) The combination of hypoxemia and hypercapnia with his history is most indicative of a ventilation-perfusion mismatch. A $\dot{V}/\dot{Q}$ mismatch usually occurs owing to pneumonia or atelectasis, when mucus or debris fills an area of lung resulting in decreased ventilation to a portion of the perfused area. A shunt indicates widespread mismatching; he is not at that point—a shunt is usually associated with ARDS and the Pa_{O_2} would be lower. Hypoventilation occurs owing to depression of the central drive to breathe, and the Pa_{CO_2} would be higher. A diffusion limitation is associated with fibrotic lung disease, and the Pa_{O_2} would be lower.

Reference: Shapiro, B.A., Harrison, R.A., Cane, R.D., et al.: Clinical Application of Blood Gases, 4th ed. Year Book Medical Publishers, Chicago, 1989.

1–117. (**C**) Neutrophils, eosinophils, and basophils are granulocytes. In patients who are granulocytopenic, fever may be the only sign of an infection. Because this IV site may be the source of infection, the site and tubing should be changed.

Reference: Alspach J.G. (ed.): AACN Core Curriculum for Critical Care Nursing, 4th ed. W.B. Saunders, Philadelphia, 1991.

1–118. (**D**) Hyperglycemia and an osmotic diuresis with subsequent hyperosmolality and dehydration are signs associated with both DKA and HHNK. Lipolysis and free fatty acid production is not as accelerated in patients with HHNK as in those who develop DKA. Therefore, patients with HHNK do not develop metabolic acidosis and their anion gap remains normal.

Reference: Hamburger, S., Rush, D.R., and Bosker, G.: Endocrine and Metabolic Emergencies. Robert J. Brady, Bowie, MD, 1984.

1–119. (**C**) Post-myocardial infarction syndrome (late pericarditis or Dressler's syndrome) is considered to be an autoimmune phenomenon that responds well to anti-inflammatory agents such as aspirin or indomethacin. Pain control may be effected with codeine or morphine. Heparin is contraindicated because it predisposes the patient to cardiac tamponade.

Reference: Underhill, S., Woods, S., Froelicher, E., et al.: Cardiac Nursing, 2nd ed. J.B. Lippincott, Philadelphia, 1989.

1–120. (**C**) Transmural and epicardial infarctions are associated with the development of pericarditis. It is felt that transmural infarcts that extend into the epicardium result in local inflammation and exudation. In addition, dyskinesis of the damaged myocardium may further increase pericardial friction, inflammation, and subsequent exudation.

Reference: Underhill, S., Woods, S., Froelicher, E., et al.: Cardiac Nursing, 2nd ed. J.B. Lippincott, Philadelphia, 1989.

1–121. (**A**) Turner's sign is bruising over the flank and lower back in the presence of retroperitoneal hematoma. It is frequently present following fractures of the pelvis and may be noted if the parenchyma of the kidney is ruptured enough to cause a retroperitoneal hematoma. Bruising around the umbilicus is known as Cullen's sign, and bruising behind the ears is known as Battle's sign.

Reference: Cook, L.: Genitourinary injuries and renal management. In Cardona, V.D., Hurn, P.D., and Mason, P.J.: Trauma Nursing: From Resuscitation to Rehabilitation. W.B. Saunders, Philadelphia, 1988.

1–122. (**D**) Patients with disturbed self-concept and altered self-perception require that the nurse accept the patient's beliefs about himself in a nonjudgmental manner. Whereas the other interventions are important for providing emotional support to any patient, they are not specific to this diagnosis and are more appropriate for the patient with anxieties, fears, or feelings of powerlessness.

Reference: Alspach, J.G. (ed.): AACN Core Curriculum for Critical Care Nursing, 4th ed. W.B. Saunders, Philadelphia, 1991.

1–123. (**A**) Patients with C7 injuries may experience spinal shock, a period of areflexia, and flaccid paralysis below the level of the lesion. Urinary retention may lead to urinary reflux and autonomic dysreflexia after the spinal shock phase has subsided. An intermittent urinary catheterization program should be instituted as soon as possible to ensure continuity of urinary drainage and prevention of complications. Loss of respiratory function is associated with complete cord transsection at C1 to C4 and possibly C5. C7 lesions cause quadriplegia, but biceps muscles are intact and patients have diaphragmatic breathing. Assessment of respiratory function is always necessary, regardless of the level of the injury.

Reference: Alspach, J.G. (ed.): AACN Core Curriculum for Critical Care Nursing, 4th ed. W.B. Saunders, Philadelphia, 1991.

1–124. (**A**) Although his weight does not indicate reduced dietary intake, as an alcoholic, the patient is predisposed to deficiencies of thiamine and folate. Patients with chronic high alcohol intake demonstrate impaired active transport of thiamine. Folate deficiency through increased urinary losses further reduces thiamine absorption. If liver disease is present, there is also a defect in thiamine storage and metabolism. Severe thiamine deficiency is often overlooked as a cause of lactic acidosis in the alcoholic patient. The strict vegetarian patient or one with ileal resection is predisposed to vitamin B_{12} deficiency. Zinc deficiency is seen in patients with severe malabsorption or chronic diarrhea. Vitamin C deficiency is seen in burn patients and patients who avoid all fruits, juices, and vegetables.

References: Sleisinger, M.H., and Fordtran, J.S.: Gastrointestinal Disease: Pathophysiology, Diagnosis, Management, 4th ed. W.B. Saunders, Philadelphia, 1989.
Swearingen, P.L., Sommers, M.S., and Miller, K.: Manual of Critical Care: Applying Nursing Diagnosis to Adult Critical Illness. C.V. Mosby, St. Louis, 1988.

1–125. (**C**) Free water retention elevates the water-to-electrolyte ratio and results in a lower serum osmolality. Water-to-electrolyte ratio in the renal filtrate decreases as water is reabsorbed from the collecting duct. The result is an elevation in the urine osmolality.

Reference: Holloway, N.M.: Nursing the Critically Ill Adult, 3rd ed. Addison-Wesley, Menlo Park, CA, 1988.

1–126. (**A**) Adequate amounts of calcium are necessary for normal coagulation to occur. Calcium levels are decreased with decreased albumin levels and elevated magnesium levels.

Reference: Alspach, J.G. (ed.): AACN Core Curriculum for Critical Care Nursing, 4th ed. W.B. Saunders, Philadelphia, 1991.

1–127. (**A**) The signs and symptoms are indicative of stridor and tracheal swelling with stenosis. Racemic epinephrine and steroids decrease the swelling, and the aerosol mist helps to soothe the inflamed trachea.

Reference: Kinney, M.R., Packa, D.R., and Dunbar, S.B.: Clinical Reference for Critical-Care Nursing, 2nd ed. McGraw-Hill, New York, 1988.

1–128. (**B**) Pads should not be placed at *cardiopulmonary resuscitation (CPR)* or *defibrillator* paddle sites. Placing the electrode pads at V_3 and at the left subscapular sites decreases trapezius and pectoral muscle stimulation, permits access to the sternum for CPR, and clears defibrillator paddle placement sites.

Reference: Parsons, C.: Transcutaneous pacing—meeting the challenge. Focus Crit Care, *14:*13–19, 1987.

1–129. (**D**) The standard setting to initiate pacing is 5 to 7 mA, which is then adjusted to provide the minimal mA necessary to pace the patient. Setting the rate 10 beats above the patient rate suppresses the patient's pacemaking site. The demand mode prevents competition, because extrasystoles may occur during insertion.

Reference: Millar, S., Sampson, L., and Soukup, M.: AACN Procedure Manual for Critical Care, 2nd ed. W.B. Saunders, Philadelphia, 1985.

1–130. (**C**) The four cardinal signs for complete small bowel obstruction are pain, vomiting, absolute constipation, and abdominal distention.

Reference: Luckmann, J., and Sorensen, K.C.: Medical-Surgical Nursing: A Psychophysiologic Approach, 3rd ed. W.B. Saunders, Philadelphia, 1987.

1–131. (**B**) Crampy abdominal pain, vomiting, distention, and absolute constipation are the cardinal signs of small bowel obstruction. They are usually accompanied by high-pitched, metallic peristaltic bowel sounds as the bowel attempts to force material through the obstructed area. Jaundice is an expected finding in hepatitis or pancreatitis. Right upper quadrant tenderness, especially on deep inspiration, is a classic sign for acute cholecystitis or acute liver pathology. Although vomiting is extremely common in patients with small bowel obstruction, the emesis rarely contains red blood cells.

Reference: Luckmann, J., and Sorensen, K.C.: Medical-Surgical Nursing: A Psychophysiologic Approach, 3rd ed. W.B. Saunders, Philadelphia, 1987.

1–132. (**A**) Hemolysis results from the change in the shape of the RBC as a result of decreased ATP and 2,3–DPG. When ATP levels in the erythrocyte fall below 15% of normal, the cells become spherocytic and rigid and are trapped and destroyed in the spleen. With decreased ATP production, bacteriocidal activity decreases, metabolic acidosis develops, and myocardial contractility decreases.

References: Chambers, J.K.: Metabolic bone disorders: imbalances of calcium and phosphorus. Nurs Clin North Am, 22:861–872, 1987.
Janson, C.L.: Fluid and electrolyte balance. In Rosen, P.: Emergency Medicine: Concepts and Practice. C.V. Mosby, St. Louis, 1988.
Smith, L.H.: Phosphorus deficiency and hypophosphatemia. In Wyngaarden, J.B., and Smith, L.H.: Textbook of Medicine, 18th ed. W.B. Saunders, Philadelphia, 1988.

1–133. (**D**) Because the rhinorrhea may be cerebrospinal fluid, the nurse should test for the presence of glucose using a Keto-Diastix or other device for assessing the glucose content of the drainage.

Reference: Hickey, J.V.: The Clinical Practice of Neurological and Neurosurgical Nursing, 2nd ed. J.B. Lippincott, Philadelphia, 1986.

1–134. (**C**) The patient with CSF rhinorrhea has an open communication between the external environment and the meninges. Packing anything into the nose may increase the risk of infection. Suctioning is usually contraindicated without a specific order.

Reference: Caine, R.M., and Bufalino, P.M.: Nursing Care Planning Guides for Adults. Williams & Wilkins, Baltimore, 1987.

1–135. (**A**) The presence of gram-negative organisms in the blood stream places this patient at risk for developing septic shock. The increased cardiac output and decreased systemic vascular resistance (SVR) further indicate that the patient is in the hyperdynamic or warm phase of septic shock.

References: Doenges, M., and Moorhouse, M.: Nursing Diagnosis with Interventions. F.A. Davis, Philadelphia, 1988.
Wall, S.C.: Septic shock. Nursing '89, 19:52–60, 1989.

1–136. (**C**) Hyponatremia is of dilutional origin secondary to impairment of renal water excretion. There may be inappropriate ADH secretion or a cortisol deficiency. Pseudohyponatremia may occur when plasma triglyceride levels are elevated. In this case, plasma osmolality would be normal.

Reference: Hamburger, S., Rush, D.R., and Bosker, G.: Endocrine and Metabolic Emergencies. Robert J. Brady, Bowie, MD, 1984.

1–137. (**B**) Inadequate humidification causes secretions to thicken. The lavage only temporarily relieves the problem, and it is not likely at this point that an infection has started.

Reference: Kinney, M.R., Packa, D.R., and Dunbar, S.B.: Clinical Reference for Critical-Care Nursing, 2nd ed. McGraw-Hill, New York, 1988.

1–138. **(C)** Thick secretions are difficult to remove from an endotracheal tube by suctioning, leading to the nursing interventions aimed at clearing the airway. The breathing pattern would not be the problem at this point, and even though these patients are always at risk for aspiration and infection, these diagnoses are not the most appropriate at this time.

Reference: Gettrust, K.V., Ryan, S.C., and Engleman, D.S.: Applied Nursing Diagnosis: Guides for Comprehensive Care Planning. John Wiley and Sons, New York, 1985.

1–139. **(B)** The most noninvasive measure to check for CVP accuracy is to note the respiratory variation. The waveform should dip during deep inspiration. Flushing the catheter with saline may dislodge a thrombus formed at the tip of the catheter. A transducer at a level lower than the right atrium would give a falsely elevated reading.

Reference: Underhill, S., Woods, S., Froelicher, E., et al.: Cardiac Nursing, 2nd ed. J.B. Lippincott, Philadelphia, 1989.

1–140. **(D)** The sign described is known as Chvostek's sign and is a manifestation of hypocalcemia. Calcium acts as a conveyor of nerve stimulation to muscles. Hypocalcemia is manifested by dysfunction of both nerve conduction and muscle contraction.

References: Calloway, C.: When the problem involves magnesium, calcium, or phosphate. RN, 50:30–36, 1987.
Chambers, J.K.: Metabolic bone disorders: Imbalances of calcium and phosphorus. Nurs Clin North Am, 22:861–872, 1987.

1–141. **(D)** Adrenocorticotropic hormone (ACTH) secretion is regulated by steroids via a negative feedback mechanism. Consequently, when steroid levels fall secondary to primary adrenal insufficiency (Addison's disease), ACTH secretion increases, resulting in elevated plasma levels. ACTH stimulates melanocytes, causing hyperpigmentation primarily of the buccal mucosa, palmar creases, and scar tissue.

Reference: Hadley, M.E.: Endocrinology, 2nd ed. Prentice-Hall, Englewood Cliffs, NJ, 1988.

1–142. **(C)** Hyperkalemia is a common sign of adrenal insufficiency, since there is hemoconcentration and decreased renal potassium secretion. Hyperkalemia may correct with fluid and steroid therapy and may become subnormal. Hyperkalemia and hypokalemia are associated with dysrhythmias, warranting continuous cardiac monitoring.

Reference: Hamburger, S., Rush, D.R., and Bosker, G.: Endocrine and Metabolic Emergencies. Robert J. Brady, Bowie, MD, 1984.

1–143. **(C)** Shunting of oxygenated blood into the right ventricle through the septal defect increases the oxygen content of pulmonary artery blood. V waves signify mitral valve conditions. Elevated right ventricular pressures can be found in many conditions, including pulmonary hypertension, right ventricular failure, and pulmonary valve stenosis.

Reference: Daily, E., and Schroeder, J.: Techniques in Bedside Hemodynamic Monitoring, 3rd ed. C.V. Mosby, St. Louis, 1985.

1–144. **(B)** Intra-aortic balloon counterpulsation is generally used to decrease the left-to-right shunting in ventricular septal rupture. Surgery is associated with high mortality rates when performed early in myocardial infarction complicated by septal rupture. Increased afterload from dopamine infusion would increase left-to-right shunting through the VSD. Oxygenation is better controlled by decreasing the left-to-right shunt.

Reference: Daily, E., and Schroeder, J.: Techniques in Bedside Hemodynamic Monitoring, 3rd ed. C.V. Mosby, St Louis, 1985.

1–145. (**D**) Protein loads cause accumulation of ammonia in patients with hepatic dysfunction. This occurs because in hepatic disease the liver no longer converts the ammonia formed from protein metabolism to urea, and the unbound ammonia circulates. Excess ammonia is toxic to nerve cells and leads to impaired mentation and sensory-perceptual alterations. Enemas are beneficial to remove intestinal contents and ammonia-producing bacteria. Sodium is restricted because it exacerbates ascites formation and peripheral edema. Because many over-the-counter medications are hepatotoxic, all medications should be cleared with the patient's physician prior to administering.

References: Sleisinger, M.H., and Fordtran, J.S.: Gastrointestinal Disease: Pathophysiology, Diagnosis, Management, 4th ed. W.B. Saunders, Philadelphia, 1989.
Swearingen, P.L., Sommers, M.S., and Miller, K.: Manual of Critical Care: Applying Nursing Diagnoses to Adult Critical Illness. C.V. Mosby, St. Louis, 1988.

1–146. (**B**) An ethical dilemma exists between the duty of the physician to do good and prevent harm (beneficence) and the right of the patient to refuse treatment (autonomy). There is no indication that the conditions of informed consent (mental competence, voluntariness, and the provision of adequate information relevant to the patient's ability to understand) were not met. The principle of justice refers to the fair treatment of all people and has no bearing on this situation.

References: Douglas, S., and Larson, E.: There's more to informed consent than information. Focus Crit Care, 2:43–47, 1986.
Johnson, P.T.: Critical care visitation: An ethical dilemma. Crit Care Nurs, 6:72–78, 1988.

1–147. (**A**) Transtentorial herniation is most often associated with epidural and acute subdural hematoma formation because diffuse brain swelling shifts the intracranial structures. In transtentorial herniation, the medial aspect of the temporal lobe (also called the uncus) shifts toward the midline until it finally shifts over the edge of the tentorium cerebelli, causing ipsilateral, not bilateral, pupillary involvement. Herniation syndromes are rostral to caudal (head to tail) events manifesting symptoms associated with increasing intracranial pressure (i.e., increased arterial blood pressure, bradycardia, and altered respiratory patterns).

Reference: Cardona, V.D., Hurn, P.D., Mason, P.J.B., et al.: Trauma Nursing: From Resuscitation Through Rehabilitation. W.B. Saunders, Philadelphia, 1988.

1–148. (**D**) Subdural hematomas may be either acute, subacute, or chronic. The venous bleeding associated with subdural hematomas accumulates below the dura mater, and the patient presents with changes in sensorium from as early as immediately to several months following injury. However, head injury is not the only cause of subdural hematomas; they may also occur spontaneously as a result of coagulation disorders or administration of anticoagulation medications.

Reference: Alspach, J.G. (ed.): AACN Core Curriculum for Critical Care Nursing, 4th ed. W.B. Saunders, Philadelphia, 1991.

1–149. (**C**) Vitamin D intoxication causes increased absorption of calcium. Hyperparathyroidism stimulates renal tubular reabsorption of calcium. Celiac disease and hypomagnesemia cause hypocalcemia.

Reference: Chambers, J.K.: Metabolic bone disorders: Imbalances of calcium and phosphorus. Nurs Clin North Am, 22:861–872, 1987.

1–150. (**C**) The primary determinant of oxygen content is the hemoglobin level. The other factors will affect oxygen transport to the tissues to varying degrees, but the hemoglobin has the greatest effect.

Reference: West, J.B.: Respiratory Physiology, the Essentials, 3rd ed. Williams & Wilkins, Baltimore, 1985.

1–151. (**B**) The major determinants of oxygen delivery are hemoglobin and cardiac output. This patient's blood pressure is low but within normal limits, whereas his hemoglobin is low and his oxygen content is in the venous range.

Reference: Snyder, J.V., and Pinsky, M.R.: Oxygen Transport in the Critically Ill. Year Book Medical Publishers, Chicago, 1987.

1–152. (**C**) There are four types of sympathetic receptors: alpha (vasoconstriction of all arteries and veins), beta$_1$ (increased automaticity and conductivity), beta$_2$ (bronchodilation), and dopa (coronary artery vasodilation).

Reference: Hurst, C.: Dysrhythmia Interpretation Based on Cardiac Suppression and Irritability. J.B. Lippincott, Philadelphia, 1986.

1–153. (**A**) The best approach is to be honest with the patient. The anxiety produced by fear of inadequacy often manifests itself as aggressive sexual behavior. Ignoring the comments or telling the patient that you will tell his wife or arrange sexual counseling will increase the patient's anxiety.

Reference: Underhill, S., Woods, S., Froelicher, E., et al.: Cardiac Nursing, 2nd ed. J.B. Lippincott, Philadelphia, 1989.

1–154. (**A**) The likely imbalances to develop from excess drainage from a new ileostomy are metabolic acidosis, sodium deficit, potassium deficit, and fluid volume deficit. The metabolic acidosis occurs owing to a reduction in plasma bicarbonate (HCO_3) when alkali is lost in large amounts of stool output. Loss of extracellular fluid through the ileostomy causes a sodium deficit. Lower gastrointestinal output is also potassium-rich, and high output results in potassium deficit. Excessive output will also lead to a volume deficit if untreated.

References: Luckmann, J., and Sorensen, K.C.: Medical-Surgical Nursing: A Psychophysiologic Approach, 3rd ed. W.B. Saunders, Philadelphia, 1987.
Swearingen, P.L., Sommers, M.S., and Miller, K.: Manual of Critical Care: Applying Nursing Diagnoses to Adult Critical Illness. C.V. Mosby, St. Louis, 1988.

1–155. (**D**) Epidural hematomas are more likely following temporal bone fractures. If fractured, the temporal bone, one of the thinnest bones in the body, may cause a significant inward displacement of bone, resulting in a major intravascular disruption of the middle meningeal artery.

Reference: Alspach, J.G. (ed.): AACN Core Curriculum for Critical Care Nursing, 4th ed. W.B. Saunders, Philadelphia, 1991.

1–156. (**A**) Acidosis causes potassium to shift from the cells to the extracellular fluid. Acidosis may increase serum potassium levels profoundly and increase myocardial irritability. Alkalosis, hyponatremia, and hypercalcemia decrease serum potassium.

References: Crandall, B.L.: Chronic renal failure. In Ulrich, T.: Nephrology Nursing, Appleton and Lange, Norwalk, CT, 1989.
Schwartz, M.W.: Potassium imbalances. Am J Nurs, *87*:1292–1299, 1987.

1–157. (**B**) Smoking is the most important causative factor in COPD.

Reference: Kersten, L.D.: Comprehensive Respiratory Nursing: A Decision Making Approach. W.B. Saunders, Philadelphia, 1989.

1–158. (**C**) The most appropriate and safest device would be the Venturi mask. The other devices allow the oxygen level to be increased, whereas the percentage of oxygen is fixed on the Venturi. This prevents accidentally increasing the FI_{O_2} and eliminating the hypoxic drive, which is the stimulus to breathe in COPD. Increasing the flow rate will only increase delivery; the ratio of air to oxygen remains the same.

Reference: West, J.B.: Pulmonary Pathophysiology: The Essentials, 3rd ed. Williams & Wilkins, Baltimore, 1987.

1–159. (**D**) A few antigenic substances such as contrast media cause the activation of the complement cascade. Protein fragments C3a and C5a, formed as a result of complement activation, act directly on the mast cell to trigger the release of the chemical mediators of anaphylaxis. This is known as an "anaphylactoid reaction." Most antigenic substances cause IgE to be produced. The IgE then attaches to the surface of mast cells. Further contact with the antigen results in IgE cross-bridging on the surface of the mast cell and the release of chemical mediators. This is known as an "anaphylactic reaction." Antigen-antibody complexes are formed and deposited in various tissues during type III hypersensitivity reactions, also known as immune-complex–mediated hypersensitivity. Glomerulonephritis is an example of this type of reaction. The production of autoantibodies results in injury to one's own tissues and results in autoimmune diseases.

Reference: Dickerson, M.A.: Anaphylaxis and anaphylactic shock. Crit Care Nurs Q, 11:68–74, 1988.

1–160. (**C**) Cardiogenic shock may be precipitated by myocardial infarction, as demonstrated by Q waves and ST elevation, and severe congestive failure, as demonstrated by rales, hypoxia, and atrial fibrillation. In cardiogenic shock the heart is unable to maintain adequate cardiac output, and compensatory mechanisms such as vasoconstriction, evidenced by cool, clammy skin, are inadequate to maintain blood pressure and tissue perfusion. Lactic acidosis and diminished pulses are further evidence of diminished perfusion. In cardiogenic shock a cycle develops whereby compensatory mechanisms further decrease tissue perfusion and suppress myocardial contractility.

Reference: Weeks, L.: Advanced Cardiovascular Nursing. Blackwell, Boston, 1986.

1–161. (**A**) Mitral valve insufficiency increases end-diastolic volume by permitting backflow of blood into the ventricle. Hypertension increases afterload. Mitral valve stenosis decreases preload by inhibiting ventricular diastolic filling. Atrial fibrillation prevents efficient ventricular filling and causes a loss of atrial kick, which assists late diastolic filling.

Reference: Daily, E., and Schroeder, J.: Techniques in Bedside Hemodynamic Monitoring, 3rd ed. C.V. Mosby, St. Louis, 1985.

1–162. (**A**) The cerebrum consists of two hemispheres that are connected by the corpus callosum. The cerebral cortex is the outer layer of each of the hemispheres, which are each divided into four lobes. Bundles of nerve fibers called cerebral tracts are found within the interior of the cerebrum. Deep inside the cerebral hemispheres are the basal ganglia. The diencephalon is located between the cerebrum and the midbrain and has several structures around the third ventricle. The most important of these structures are the thalamus and the hypothalamus.

Reference: Holloway, N.M.: Nursing the Critically Ill Adult. Addison-Wesley, Menlo Park, CA, 1988.

1–163. (**D**) U waves are small, low-voltage waves sometimes seen following the T wave. U waves are made more prominent with potassium deficiency, but digitalis, quinidine, hypercalcemia, and exercise can increase their amplitude. A peaked and elevated T wave, widened QRS complex, and prolonged PR interval are ECG manifestations of hyperkalemia. Widened QRS complexes can occur with hypokalemia but are usually a later manifestation.

References: Marriott, H.: Practical Electrocardiography, 8th ed. Williams & Wilkins, Baltimore, 1988.
Sweetwood, H.: Clinical Electrocardiography for Nurses, 2nd ed. Aspen, Rockville, MD, 1989.

1–164. (**B**) The lung is free of sensory nerve fibers so the pain would not be well localized there. Pain from the chest wall due to a fractured rib or pleural effusion is well localized and exacerbated by a deep breath. Pain that is inflammatory and originating in the mediastinum is substernal and dull. Diaphragmatic pain is referred to the contralateral shoulder.

Reference: Kinney, M.R., Packa, D.R., and Dunbar, S.B.: Clinical Reference for Critical-Care Nursing, 2nd ed. McGraw-Hill, New York, 1988.

1–165. (**B**) Type I second-degree AV block associated with inferior infarction is usually caused by ischemia of the AV node and lasts approximately 7 days. Increased vagal tone is usually associated with first-degree AV block. Interventricular septal necrosis is more common with anterior infarction.

Reference: Weeks, L.: Advanced Cardiovascular Nursing. Blackwell, Boston, 1986.

1–166. (**D**) Dopamine is found in the substantia nigra and corpus striatum. It acts primarily as an inhibitory transmitter and is decreased in Parkinson's disease. Acetylcholine may be associated with drinking behavior, and norepinephrine may also be found in drinking behavior as well as feeding behavior, temperature control, and rapid eye movement (REM) sleep. Serotonin is involved in sleep behavior.

Reference: Alspach, J.G. (ed.): AACN Core Curriculum for Critical Care Nursing, 4th ed. W.B. Saunders, Philadelphia, 1991.

1–167. (**C**) Several researchers have validated and ranked the needs of family members of critically ill patients. One of the top needs is to have questions answered honestly. The other responses are of low importance to family members of critically ill patients with poor prognosis.

References: Holloway, N.M.: Nursing the Critically Ill Adult, 3rd ed. Addison-Wesley, New York, 1988.
Simpson, T.: Research review: Needs and concerns of families of critically ill adults. Focus Crit Care, 16(5):388–397, 1989.

1–168. (**C**) Kinins have a direct effect on afferent neurons, which may account for the pain and itching associated with an anaphylactic reaction. Histamine is a vasoactive substance that causes dilation of vessels and increased capillary permeability. It is also a bronchoconstrictor. Endotoxins are the toxic substances generally released by gram-negative bacteria. They are believed to trigger the body's defense mechanisms, which may result in the development of septic shock. Prostaglandins are vasoactive mediators produced when arachidonic acid is released from cell membranes. They contribute to the decreased systemic vascular resistance seen in septic shock.

References: Dickerson, M.A.: Anaphylaxis and anaphylactic shock. Crit Care Nurs Q, 11:68–74, 1988.
Littleton, M.T.: Pathophysiology and assessment of sepsis and septic shock. Crit Care Nurs Q, 11:40–47, 1988.

1–169. (**B**) Alveolar ventilation is adjusted to keep the pH within normal range, no matter what the Pa_{CO_2} may be. Oxygenation is not manipulated by changing the rate or tidal volume.

Reference: West, J.B.: Pulmonary Pathophysiology: The Essentials, 3rd ed. Williams & Wilkins, Baltimore, 1987.

1–170. (**B**) Hypernatremia occurs when the glomerular filtration rate is reduced and the kidney is unable to excrete sodium. In the diuretic phase, hyponatremia may occur because of the loss of sodium, which is associated with increased urinary output.

References: Chambers, J.K.: Fluid and electrolyte problems in renal and urologic disorders. Nurs Clin North Am, 22:815–825, 1987.
Jett, M., Lancaster, L., and Small, S.: Renal disorders. In Renal and Urologic Disorders. Springhouse, Springhouse, PA, 1984.

1–171. (**D**) The two major concerns associated with myasthenia gravis are myasthenic crisis and cholinergic crisis. Myasthenic crisis is characterized by changes in vital signs, severe generalized weakness, and impending respiratory failure. Myasthenic crisis in a known patient is often precipitated by underdosage of medication or stress. Cholinergic crisis, usually associated with overdosage of the anticholinesterase medications used to treat myasthenia gravis, is characterized by increased salivation, sweating, lacrimation, abdominal cramping, diarrhea, and muscle fasciculations.

References: Alspach, J.G. (ed.): AACN Core Curriculum for Critical Care Nursing, 4th ed. W.B. Saunders Company, Philadelphia, 1991.
Caine, R.M., and Bufalino, P.M.: Nursing Care Planning Guides for Adults. Williams & Wilkins, Baltimore, 1987.

1–172. (**B**) Signs that are characteristic of diabetes insipidus include a diuresis despite an elevated serum osmolality and urine osmolality lower than serum osmolality. When fluid intake lags behind urine output, dehydration and hypovolemic symptoms appear, such as an elevated serum sodium, decreased BP, and elevated heart and respiratory rates. A history of head trauma is commonly associated with the development of diabetes insipidus.

Reference: Kohler, P.O., and Jordan, R.M. (eds.): Clinical Endocrinology. John Wiley and Sons, New York, 1986.

1–173. (**D**) Normally pulmonary artery diastolic (PAD) and pulmonary capillary wedge pressures (PCWP) are equal. When the PAD is greater than the PCWP, a right-to-left pressure gradient exists. When the difference is greater than 6 mm Hg, it is significant for pulmonary disease such as COPD or pulmonary embolism. Mitral valve dysfunction elevates both PAD and PCWP but does not cause a pressure gradient. Pump failure increases PAD, PCWP, and CVP. Pericarditis increases the CVP. Pulmonary embolism does not affect the CVP unless it progresses to cause right heart failure.

Reference: Bustin, D.: Hemodynamic Monitoring. Appleton-Century-Crofts, Norwalk, CT, 1986.

1–174. (**A**) Hypercapnia may occur, especially in the later stages of the disease. However, it does not always occur, and so is not considered one of the "hallmarks" that identify the syndrome.

Reference: Kinney, M.R., Packa, D.R., and Dunbar, S.B.: Clinical Reference for Critical-Care Nursing, 2nd ed. McGraw-Hill, New York, 1988.

1–175. (**D**) Vasopressin tannate is administered only intramuscularly. To administer the drug, the nurse must first warm the solution and shake it thoroughly for 2 to 3 minutes prior to withdrawing it from the ampule. The major side effects of this drug result from water intoxication, characterized by decreased serum sodium and osmolality. Cardiovascular side effects include decreased heart rate and cardiac output with an increase in blood pressure and dysrhythmias.

Reference: Hartshorn, J., and Hartshorn, E.: Pharmacology update: Vasopressin in the treatment of diabetes insipidus. J Neurosci Nurs, *20*(1):58–59, 1988.

1–176. (**A**) Recovery from narcotic-based anesthetic agents is dependent on the dose given, postoperative renal function, and urinary output. Recovery from inhaled anesthetics is dependent on alveolar ventilation, solubility coefficient of the anesthetic agent, and duration of anesthesia.

Reference: Alspach, J.G. (ed.): AACN Core Curriculum for Critical Care Nursing, 4th ed. W.B. Saunders, Philadelphia, 1991.

1–177. (**C**) Dilated cardiomyopathy is associated with alcohol abuse, hypertension, viral infections, and myocardial toxins, unlike hypertrophic cardiomyopathy, which may be genetically transmitted. In dilated cardiomyopathy the ventricular chamber size is greatly increased, but because the muscle mass of the ventricle does not increase, impaired contraction, reduced ejection fraction, and increased end-diastolic volumes result. In restrictive cardiomyopathy, the ejection fraction is often normal.

Reference: Underhill, S., Woods, S., Froelicher, E., et al.: Cardiac Nursing, 2nd ed. J.B. Lippincott, Philadelphia, 1989.

1–178. (**C**) Ecchymosis in the flank area is a sign of retroperitoneal bleeding related to a pancreatic injury. A renal injury is characterized by a hematoma in the flank area. A ruptured spleen is characterized by an irritable diaphragm and pain referred to the left shoulder. Pelvic fractures are characterized by ecchymosis of the scrotum (or labia). Potentially fatal injuries from blunt abdominal trauma are frequently masked by more obvious wounds.

References: Luckmann, J., and Sorensen, K.C.: Medical-Surgical Nursing: A Psychophysiologic Approach, 3rd ed. W.B. Saunders, Philadelphia, 1987.
Semonin-Holleran, R.: Critical nursing care for abdominal trauma. Crit Care Nurs, *8*(3):48–59, 1988.

1–179. (**D**) An arteriovenous malformation results from arterial blood bypassing the capillary network and shunting directly into the veins. Shunting of the blood may cause ischemia, cerebral atrophy, and local infarction. Dilation of an intracranial arterial wall causes a cerebral aneurysm that may ultimately weaken the arterial wall and rupture.

Reference: Alspach, J.G. (ed.): AACN Core Curriculum for Critical Care Nursing, 4th ed. W.B. Saunders, Philadelphia, 1991.

1–180. (**C**) Blood from the lungs is alkaline, whereas blood from the stomach is acidic from contamination by digestive enzymes. Food particles should be obtained only from the stomach. Since the fluid from this patient is hemoptysis and coming from the lungs, the initial treatment would be to obtain an arterial blood gas determination to assess the extent of the lung damage.

Reference: Kersten, L.D.: Comprehensive Respiratory Nursing: A Decision Making Approach. W.B. Saunders, Philadelphia, 1989.

1–181. (**A**) Temperature elevations greater than 102° F are associated with an acute infectious process. Temperature elevations in subacute bacterial endocarditis are low-grade. Petechiae and Roth's spots occur from microemboli, common to both forms of endocarditis. Congestive heart failure occurs in endocarditis from damage to valves and associated structures. It is the most common cause of death in both forms of endocarditis.

Reference: Weeks, L.: Advanced Cardiovascular Nursing. Blackwell, Boston, 1986.

1–182. (**C**) Bowel sounds should not be heard in the chest but can be present when the diaphragm has been ruptured as a consequence of blunt trauma.

Reference: Alspach, J.G. (ed.): AACN Core Curriculum for Critical Care Nursing, 4th ed. W.B. Saunders, Philadelphia, 1991.

1–183. (**A**) Respiratory paralysis is the result of trunk muscle involvement and possible vagal dysfunction that prevents bronchial constriction or dilation. If hypoxia occurs as a result of respiratory insufficiency, or if the patient's vital capacity falls below 800 ml, the patient will require a tracheostomy. Respiratory insufficiency is found in approximately 50% of patients with GBS and causes a mortality rate between 10% and 20%.

Reference: Hickey, J.V.: The Clinical Practice of Neurological and Neurosurgical Nursing, 2nd ed. J.B. Lippincott, Philadelphia, 1986.

1–184. (**C**) The patient's possible difficulty understanding the nurse and the stress of the motorcycle accident contribute to the alteration in coping.

Reference: Von Rueden, K.T., and Walleck, C.A.: Advanced Critical Care Nursing. Aspen, Rockville, MD, 1989.

1–185. (**C**) In mitral valve disease, right atrial and left atrial pressures are maintained at higher levels because normal filling pressures for these patients are elevated. Increased right atrial pressures are also induced to provide greater contractility, utilizing the Frank Starling principle.

Reference: Kenner, C., Guzzetta, C., and Dossey, B.: Critical Care Nursing: Body—Mind—Spirit. Little, Brown, Boston, 1985.

1–186. (**D**) A serum phosphorus of 0.4 mg/dl indicates hypophosphatemia. Aluminum hydroxide gel (Amphojel) and calcium supplements are used in the treatment of hyperphosphatemia. Phospho Soda is an oral phosphate preparation. Monobasic potassium phosphate is an intravenous phosphate and is the treatment for this abnormally low phosphorus.

References: Rice, V.: Magnesium, calcium and phosphate imbalances: Their clinical significance. Crit Care Nurse, *3*:90–111, 1983.
Smith, L.H.: Phosphorus deficiency and hypophosphatemia. In Wyngaarden, J.B., and Smith, L.H.: Textbook of Medicine, 18th ed. W.B. Saunders, Philadelphia, 1988.

1–187. (**A**) A high urine specific gravity (greater than 1.020) with a urinary output of less than 30 ml per hour for 2 consecutive hours is indicative of SIADH. The nurse should also assess laboratory findings, particularly BUN, creatinine, electrolytes, and osmolality. Patients with SIADH will be hyponatremic (serum sodium less than 135 mEq/l) with a serum osmolality less than 275 mOsm/l. SIADH is treated with water restriction and hypertonic saline administration based on the serum sodium level.

References: Caine, R.M., and Bufalino, P.M.: Critically Ill Adults: Nursing Care Planning Guides. Williams & Wilkins, Baltimore, 1988.
Holloway, N.M.: Nursing the Critically Ill Adult. Addison-Wesley, Menlo Park, CA, 1988.

1–188. (**C**) Thorough explanation of the purposes and functions of the intensive care unit will begin the process of reducing the stress of unexpected critical illness. Reduced stress is evidenced by ability to rest, participation in care, appropriate use of the call bell, and involvement with family. Other interventions include involving family members in care, providing familiar personal items nearby, and responding promptly to patient needs and requests.

References: Swearingen, P.L., Sommers, M.S., and Miller, K.: Manual of Critical Care: Applying Nursing Diagnosis to Adult Critical Illness. C.V. Mosby, St. Louis, 1988.

1–189. (**C**) Severe back pain may be the first symptom of retroperitoneal bleeding in the patient with an abdominal aortic aneurysm repair. Increase in the abdominal girth is a sign of retroperitoneal bleeding. The surgical site is anterior and probably would not demonstrate significant drainage associated with back pain. The nurse should evaluate the pain prior to giving pain medication, particularly when the pain is not incisional.

Reference: Fahey, V.: Vascular Nursing. W.B. Saunders, Philadelphia, 1988.

1–190. (**A**) A ruptured aorta is a complication of blunt trauma to the chest. The leak of blood into the mediastinum increases the intrathoracic pressure, stimulates the respiratory rate, and causes pain in his chest and back. An aortogram will need to be done immediately and emergency surgery performed.

Reference: Alspach, J.G. (ed.): AACN Core Curriculum for Critical Care Nursing, 4th ed. W.B. Saunders, Philadelphia, 1991.

1–191. (**A**) The legal and ethical issue faced by the nurse in this situation is one of two conflicting obligations—the duty to remain and the duty to refuse to remain if impaired by fatigue. If the nurse chooses to work the extra shift, he or she will be held accountable to the same standards of patient care that would apply under normal circumstances. Whether all obligations to the employer have been fulfilled by working the assigned shift depends upon the contractual agreement between the nurse and the institution.

Reference: Gaines, C., and Carter, D.: Overtime: A professional responsibility? Focus Crit Care, 4:270–273, 1989.

1–192. (**A**) There are two types of hydrocephalus—communicating and noncommunicating. Communicating or nonobstructive hydrocephalus is often caused by bacterial meningitis. With this type of hydrocephalus, lumbar puncture or pneumoencephalogram is generally not contraindicated. A mass or tumor that causes a noncommunicating or obstructive hydrocephalus gives rise to a decreased CSF reabsorption, resulting in increased intracranial pressure.

Reference: Alspach, J.G. (ed.): AACN Core Curriculum for Critical Care Nursing, 4th ed. W.B. Saunders, Philadelphia, 1991.

1–193. (**A**) Edetate disodium (EDTA), because of its affinity for calcium, produces a lowering of the serum calcium level during intravenous infusion. The chelates formed are excreted in the urine. Plicamycin (mithramycin) and calcitonin decrease bone absorption of calcium. Indomethacin lowers serum calcium but only when hypercalcemia is associated with tumors that produce prostaglandin.

References: Chambers, J.K.: Metabolic bone disorders: Imbalances of calcium and phosphorus. Nurs Clin North Am, 22:861–872, 1987.
Kastrup, E.K.: Drug Facts & Comparisons. J.B. Lippincott, Philadelphia, 1988.

1–194. (**B**) The force of the chest hitting the steering wheel fractured the cartilage between the ribs and sternum, disrupting the integrity of the chest wall. During spontaneous inspiration, the negative intrathoracic pressure causes the sternum to collapse inward and prevents an adequate inspiration.

Reference: West, J.B.: Pulmonary Pathophysiology, the Essentials, 3rd ed. Williams & Wilkins, Baltimore, 1987.

1–195. (**A**) Edema slows wound healing. Severe edema may impede blood flow through the graft. A benefit of antiembolism stockings and Ace wraps is the promotion of venous return, thus decreasing venous stasis.

Reference: Fahey, V.: Vascular Nursing. W.B. Saunders, Philadelphia, 1988.

1–196. (**C**) A major surgical procedure and gastric pH below 3.5 are highly suggestive of acute GI bleeding from stress ulceration. Although the pathophysiology of stress ulceration is not totally understood, critically ill patients remain at high risk for development of stress ulcers. Gastroesophageal reflux is evidenced by heartburn and reflux of normal gastric secretions. Hepatic failure and pancreatitis are possible etiologies of stress ulcer, but there is no evidence of these disease processes in this patient.

References: Konopad, E., and Noseworthy, T.: Stress ulceration: A serious complication in critically ill patients. Heart Lung, *17*(4):339–348, 1988.
Sleisinger, H.H., and Fordtran, J.S.: Gastrointestinal Disease: Pathophysiology, Diagnosis, Management, 4th ed. W.B. Saunders, Philadelphia, 1989.

1–197. (**A**) 0.9% Sodium chloride solution replaces sodium and water. Whereas hypertonic (3%) sodium chloride can be administered in cases of severe hyponatremia, it must be used with extreme caution, especially in elderly patients. If the body does not have time to distribute the incoming volume to its cells and extracellular spaces, hypovolemia or hypernatremia may develop.

Reference: Barta, M.: Correcting electrolyte imbalances. RN, *50*(2):30–34, 1987.

1–198. (**A**) Dexamethasone (Decadron), an anti-inflammatory corticosteroid, is used in the treatment and prevention of cerebral edema. Dexamethasone, a very potent drug, is often prescribed preoperatively and continued postoperatively. The nurse must be watchful for signs of toxic effects and side effects associated with steroid administration. In particular, the drug must never be abruptly withdrawn and a gradual tapering of the dose must be observed. Additionally, because the drug is irritating to the GI tract, it should be administered with antacids such as aluminum hydroxide (Mylanta) or with drugs used to reduce gastric secretions, such as cimetidine (Tagamet) or ranitidine hydrochloride (Zantac).

Reference: Hickey, J.V.: The Clinical Practice of Neurological and Neurosurgical Nursing, 2nd ed. J.B. Lippincott, Philadelphia, 1986.

1–199. (**B**) Surgery, especially of the thoracoabdominal region, is a significant physical insult to the body. Any predisposition to pulmonary disease is exacerbated and exaggerated after surgery.

Reference: Alspach, J.G. (ed.): AACN Core Curriculum for Critical Care Nursing, 4th ed. W.B. Saunders, Philadelphia, 1991.

1–200. (**C**) In Wolff-Parkinson-White syndrome, the PR interval is shortened (less than .12 second) and a delta wave is present. The delta wave is the prolonged initial segment of the QRS, which is caused by early depolarization of the septum via the anomalous pathway.

Reference: Andreoli, K., Fowkes, V., Zipes, D., et al.: Comprehensive Cardiac Care, 6th ed. C.V. Mosby, St. Louis, 1987.

CORE
REVIEW
TEST
2

2-1. During exercise stress testing, which of the following is considered an ischemic response?

  A. T wave inversion immediately following exercise.
  B. ST depression of 1 to 2 mm.
  C. Tachycardia greater than 120 beats per minute.
  D. Increased T wave amplitude.

2-2. Ventilation occurs

  A. In the alveolus.
  B. Across the alveolar-capillary membrane.
  C. At the mitochondria.
  D. By diaphragmatic contraction.

2-3. In which of the following structures does reabsorption of cerebrospinal fluid take place?

  A. Meninges.
  B. Arachnoid villi.
  C. Dura mater.
  D. Subarachnoid space.

2-4. Intrarenal failure involving tubular damage may be caused by

  A. Transfusion reactions.
  B. Papillary necrosis.
  C. Decreased cardiac output.
  D. Prostatic obstruction.

2-5. Before his coronary artery bypass graft surgery, a 57-year-old male weighed 160 pounds. Twenty-four hours after surgery, his weight is 168 pounds. This patient has a fluid excess of approximately

  A. 1 liter.
  B. 2 liters.
  C. 4 liters.
  D. 8 liters.

2–6. The hemodynamic parameter that clinically measures afterload is

    A. Central venous pressure (CVP).
    B. Mean arterial pressure (MAP).
    C. Systemic vascular resistance (SVR).
    D. Left ventricular end-diastolic pressure (LVEDP).

2–7. The main therapeutic objective for a near-drowning victim includes

    A. Decreasing neurologic stimuli.
    B. Preventing infection.
    C. Increasing the functional residual capacity.
    D. Replacing fluid volume.

2–8. Primary glomerular injury as a cause for acute renal failure can be the result of

    A. Systemic lupus erythematosus.
    B. Gentamicin.
    C. Abdominal aortic aneurysm repair.
    D. Hemoglobinuria due to intravascular hemolysis.

2–9. A 27-year-old male developed a subdural hematoma following an automobile accident. It is likely that he sustained a contrecoup effect. A contrecoup effect occurs when

    A. The cerebellum and brain stem are damaged.
    B. Brain herniation occurs following injury.
    C. Injury occurs on one side of the brain and the opposite side is also affected.
    D. The optic nerve is compressed against the uncus, causing herniation.

2–10. Which of the following are requisites of informed consent?

    I. The patient must have the capacity to reason and make judgements.
    II. The decision must be made voluntarily and without coercion.
    III. The patient must have a clear understanding of the risks and benefits of proposed treatment.
    IV. The patient's family must agree with the decision.

    A. I, II, and III.
    B. I and IV.
    C. II and III.
    D. II, III, and IV.

2–11. A 32-year-old man is admitted to the intensive care unit after being found unconscious in his apartment. His vital signs are: BP 122/68 mm Hg, pulse 130 beats per minute, respirations 36 per minute, temperature 37.3° C orally. His skin is warm and dry with bounding pulses and cherry red in color. Pulse oximeter shows 96% saturation on 100% nonrebreather mask. His arterial blood gases (ABGs) return as pH 7.30, Pa_{CO_2} 30 mm Hg, HCO_3 18 mEq/l, Pa_{O_2} 150 mm Hg, Sa_{O_2} 65%. What accounts for the difference between the arterial blood gas saturation and the pulse oximeter results?

    A. Pulse oximeter is broken.
    B. Arterial blood gas results are incorrect.
    C. Pulse oximeter measures only what is bound to hemoglobin.
    D. The oxygen dissociation curve has shifted.

2–12. Hypocalcemia produces which of the following changes in the ECG?

    A. ST elevation.
    B. Prolonged QT interval.
    C. Prolonged PR interval.
    D. Shortened QT interval.

2–13. Antacids act by

A. Suppressing volume and concentration of gastric acid secretion.
B. Binding and neutralizing intraluminal hydrogen ions.
C. Forming a protective barrier over gastric mucosa.
D. Stimulating phospholipid formation in the gastric mucosal barrier.

2–14. A 41-year-old female develops status epilepticus. She is receiving phenytoin (Dilantin), 100 mg IV every 8 hours. In assessing the response to the drug, the critical care nurse knows

A. This dosage is excessive, causing severe sedation.
B. This dosage is too low.
C. To stop the drug if the patient's QT segment widens.
D. To observe for hypertension related to drug administration.

2–15. When hyponatremia is associated with fluid overload, treatment includes

I. Diuretics.
II. Fluid restriction.
III. Isotonic saline IV.

A. I only.
B. I and II.
C. III only.
D. II only.

2–16. A patient admitted to the intensive care unit after treatment for cardiac arrest and electromechanical dissociation has the following laboratory and hemodynamic findings 3 hours after successful resuscitation:

Mean arterial pressure (MAP)	80 mm Hg
PCWP	16 mm Hg
CVP	12 mm Hg
Hct	29%

Therapy at this time should include which of the following?

A. Infusion of one unit of packed RBCs.
B. Administration of furosemide, 20 mg IV push.
C. Continuous infusion of dobutamine at 10 μg/kg/min.
D. Continuous infusion of dopamine at 10 μg/kg/min.

2–17. The process that involves the attraction of neutrophils, monocytes, and leukocytes to the site of injury is

A. Chemotaxis.
B. Emigration.
C. Opsonization.
D. Agglutination.

2–18. Which of the following statements accurately describes autoregulation?

A. It is dependent on the patient's arterial blood pressure, pulse rate, and Pa_{O_2}.
B. It is a response to injury and stress as the result of hypothalamic stimulation of the antidiuretic hormone (ADH).
C. It is the perfusion of cerebral blood flow over and above the brain's metabolic needs.
D. It refers to the brain's ability to maintain a constant rate of blood flow over a wide range of perfusion pressures despite changes in arterial and intracranial pressures.

2–19. Clubbing of the fingers indicates

   A. A long-term smoking history.
   B. Cardiopulmonary disease.
   C. Peripheral vascular disease.
   D. A nervous disorder.

2–20. What is the effect of tissue plasminogen activator (t-PA) on cardiac enzymes in myocardial infarction?

   I. CPK levels peak in 13 to 14 hours.
   II. CPK levels peak in 24 to 36 hours.
   III. CPK levels are generally lower in patients in whom t-PA is used.
   IV. CPK levels are generally higher in patients in whom t-PA is used.

   A. I, III.
   B. II, III.
   C. II, IV.
   D. I, IV.

2–21. The most frequently used type of ventilator is

   A. Pressure-cycled.
   B. Volume-cycled.
   C. Negative pressure.
   D. Time-cycled.

2–22. One treatment for increased intracranial pressure is barbiturate coma therapy. When evaluating the effectiveness of this treatment, the critical care nurse knows that this treatment

   A. Increases cerebral metabolism.
   B. Must be used in conjunction with assisted ventilation.
   C. Increases cerebral blood flow, thus reducing intracranial pressure.
   D. Will require continued monitoring of the usual neurologic parameters and reflexes.

2–23. A 41-year-old man has Crohn's disease with regional ileitis. He has developed acute hypovolemia due to high-volume fistula drainage. Which of the following operative therapies is indicated?

   A. Transverse colostomy.
   B. Temporary ileostomy.
   C. Mesenteric embolectomy.
   D. Pyloroplasty and vagotomy.

2–24. A patient develops the dysrhythmia illustrated below and becomes hypotensive.
The nurse should immediately

   A. Set up for the insertion of a temporary pacemaker.
   B. Administer atropine, 0.5 mg IV push.
   C. Administer lidocaine, 1 mg/kg IV push.
   D. Initiate a continuous IV infusion of isoproterenol at 2 to 10 μg/minute.

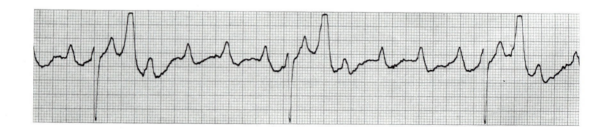

Questions 2–25 and 2–26 refer to the following situation.

A 51-year-old male has been diagnosed as having diabetes insipidus (DI).

2–25. As the critical care nurse assigned to this patient, you know that DI

A. Results in decreased urine production.
B. Is characterized by a urine specific gravity of more than 1.020.
C. Is an impairment of the posterior pituitary.
D. Is an impairment of the anterior pituitary.

2–26. The physician orders vasopressin (Pitressin) for this patient. This medication will be used to

A. Decrease water excretion.
B. Increase blood flow to the coronary beds.
C. Decrease motility of the GI tract.
D. Increase water excretion.

2–27. A common side effect of the beta$_2$-adrenergic sympathomimetic drugs is

A. Tachycardia.
B. Hypotension.
C. Nausea.
D. Dizziness.

2–28. In describing the effect of ventilation on pulmonary capillary wedge pressure measurement, which of the following is true?

A. The waveform is elevated during spontaneous inspiration.
B. The waveform is depressed during delivery of a mechanical breath.
C. Discontinuation of artificial ventilation to perform readings may cause false elevation of the measurement.
D. Discontinuation of artificial ventilation is the only method to obtain an accurate wedge pressure measurement.

2–29. Family members should be instructed to assess the patient with hypothyroidism for the development of

A. Insomnia and a sense of impending doom.
B. Nervousness and a poor attention span.
C. Compulsiveness and rapid speech.
D. Paranoia and delusions.

2–30. In planning nursing care to maintain the airway and gas exchange for the patient undergoing emergency treatment for increasing intracranial pressure, the following is usually most important:

A. Avoid hypercapnia in the patient.
B. Encourage the patient to cough vigorously.
C. Firmly pack gauze in the nares if there is drainage.
D. Suction the patient nasotracheally.

2–31. A change in serum protein concentration of 1 gm/dl results in a 0.8 mg/dl change in

A. Potassium.
B. Calcium.
C. Magnesium.
D. Sodium.

2–32. Adequate fluid therapy and hydration are essential in asthmatics to

A. Assure adequate intravascular volume.
B. Decrease airway responsiveness to stimuli.
C. Thin secretions.
D. Decrease mucosal edema.

2–33. For which of the following intensive care unit patients would you expect human leukocyte antigen (HLA) testing to be done?

   A. A patient undergoing a heart transplant.
   B. A patient who has received a transfusion of whole blood.
   C. A patient who has a septicemia.
   D. A patient who has been exposed to HIV.

2–34. Which of the following is a common manifestation of tumors of the left and descending segments of the colon?

   A. Weight loss.
   B. Anemia.
   C. Dyspepsia.
   D. Obstructive symptoms.

2–35. Cerebral vasospasm associated with cerebral aneurysm is treated with various drug protocols. Which of the following protocols is *not* used to modify and control vasospasm?

   A. Aminophylline-isoproterenol (Isuprel).
   B. Serotonin antagonists.
   C. Calcium channel blockers.
   D. Anticholinesterase drugs.

2–36. Which of the following is true of the action potential during the absolute refractory period (Phases 0, 1, and 2 of the action potential) in myocardial cells?

   A. A stimulus other than one from the sinoatrial (SA) node may elicit another action potential.
   B. Only a stimulus from the SA node will elicit another action potential.
   C. Only a stimulus from the ventricle will elicit another action potential.
   D. No stimulus can elicit an action potential.

2–37. Clinical manifestations of respiratory muscle fatigue include

   A. Decreased Pa_{CO_2}, increased work of breathing.
   B. Decreased respiratory rate and Pa_{CO_2}.
   C. Increased Pa_{CO_2} and accessory muscle use.
   D. Increased respiratory rate, decreased inspiration-expiration ratio (I:E).

2–38. In chronic renal failure patients, therapeutic agent(s) that will temporarily reverse the symptoms of hypermagnesemia is (are)

   A. Diuretics.
   B. Saline.
   C. Phosphate.
   D. Calcium gluconate.

2–39. Cerebellopontine angle tumors arise from

   A. Cranial nerve V.
   B. Cranial nerve VI.
   C. Cranial nerve VII.
   D. Cranial nerve VIII.

2–40. The sinoatrial (SA) node receives its blood supply from the

   A. Right coronary artery in 90% of hearts.
   B. Right coronary artery in 55% of hearts, the circumflex in 45% of hearts.
   C. Circumflex artery in 45% of hearts, the left anterior descending artery in 55% of hearts.
   D. Circumflex artery in 30% of hearts, the right coronary artery in 60% of hearts, and the left anterior descending artery in 10% of hearts.

2–41. A 12-lead ECG that shows Q waves and ST elevations in leads V_2 through V_4 indicates

   A. Occlusion of the left anterior descending artery.
   B. Occlusion of the circumflex artery.
   C. Occlusion of the right coronary artery.
   D. Prinzmetal's angina.

2–42. During the inflammatory response

  A. Antibodies and immunoglobulins cause changes in capillary permeability.
  B. Basophils and eosinophils capture and engulf invading organisms.
  C. Necrotic debris is removed and tissue repair begins.
  D. Macrophages isolate the invading organisms and transport them to the liver for destruction.

Questions 2–43 and 2–44 refer to the following situation.

A 26-year-old male who sustained head injury is on a ventilator at FI_{O_2} 0.3, V_T 750, respiratory rate 14 per minute, PEEP 0, with a compliance of 48 cm H_2O. His pulse oximeter reading is 95%.

2–43. During the shift, the nurse notices his saturation has decreased to 90%, compliance decreased to 35 cm H_2O, and temperature increased to 38.5° C rectally. His lungs have rales and rhonchi bilaterally that do not clear with suctioning; he has increased sputum production and it has changed from thick white to a grey-green color, and he is now triggering the respirator to 28 breaths per minute. The most likely cause of these changes is

  A. Pleural effusion.
  B. Pneumonia.
  C. Pneumothorax.
  D. ARDS.

2–44. The most appropriate action to take first is to

  A. Start broad-spectrum antibiotic therapy.
  B. Send sputum cultures.
  C. Send blood cultures.
  D. Increase the respiratory rate on the ventilator.

2–45. To be effective in discussing sexual and reproductive functioning in patients with renal failure, the nurse must understand that

  A. Institution of hemodialysis will result in a return to normal sexual and reproductive function.
  B. Hormone levels (testosterone in males and ovarian hormone secretion in females) are decreased with chronic renal failure.
  C. There is no psychological basis for the dysfunction.
  D. No treatment modality can result in normalization of these functions.

2–46. Which of the following is a priority in protecting the patient with seizures against injury?

  A. Using a tongue blade during a seizure.
  B. Assuring that restraints are secured to the patient.
  C. Positioning the patient to prevent aspiration of secretions.
  D. Determining if the patient is incontinent.

2–47. An elderly male is being treated with gentamicin and cefoxitin. He is also receiving tube feedings. The nurse suspects the patient will develop

  A. Anemia.
  B. Jaundice.
  C. Diarrhea.
  D. Peripheral neuritis.

2–48. Which of the following are indications for the insertion of a temporary transvenous pacemaker?

  I. Acute inferior infarction with Mobitz type I second degree AV block.
  II. Acute inferior infarction with Mobitz type II second degree AV block.
  III. Acute anterior infarction with Mobitz type I second degree AV block.

  A. II only.
  B. I and II.
  C. I and III.
  D. II and III.

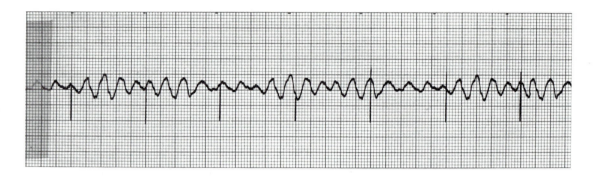

2–49. The above rhythm resulted from R on T phenomena in a patient who has a temporary pacemaker. The nurse should immediately

A. Increase the pacemaker sensitivity.
B. Increase the pacemaker mA (output).
C. Increase the pacemaker rate.
D. Defibrillate the patient.

Questions 2–50 and 2–51 refer to the following situation.

A 58-year-old male with a history of chronic obstructive lung disease (COPD) and a 2-day course of shortness of breath, productive cough, and fever has arterial blood gases of pH 7.36, Pa_{CO_2} 50 mm Hg, HCO_3 28 mEq/l, Pa_{O_2} 58 mm Hg, and Sa_{O_2} 78% on room air. His A-a gradient is 30. He is placed on FI_{O_2} 0.4 by mask and the next set of blood gases indicate pH 7.33, Pa_{CO_2} 58 mm Hg, HCO_3 27 mEq/l, Pa_{O_2} 83 mm Hg, and Sa_{O_2} 90% with an A-a gradient of 130.

2–50. The patient's A-a gradient indicates his oxygenation status is

A. Deteriorating.
B. Improving.
C. Staying the same.
D. Unable to be assessed.

2–51. The patient's worsening acidosis is probably due to

A. Sepsis.
B. Reduced hypoxic drive.
C. Tissue hypoxia.
D. Lactic acidosis.

2–52. The chronic excessive ingestion of licorice can cause

A. Hypercalcemia.
B. Hyponatremia.
C. Hyperphosphatemia.
D. Hypokalemia.

2–53. Which one of the following drugs must be kept at the bedside of the patient with myasthenia gravis?

A. Protamine sulfate.
B. Neostigmine.
C. Atropine.
D. Tensilon.

2–54. When teaching a patient about the drugs used to treat myasthenia gravis, the nurse knows to teach about which one of the following classifications of medications used to treat the disease?

A. Anticholinesterase.
B. Cholinesterase.
C. Anticholinergics.
D. Antibiotics.

2–55. The patient died peacefully after he was removed from the ventilator, according to his wishes. The critical care nurses met to discuss strategies to improve their role as patient advocates in future situations. The nurses agreed that they should promote patient autonomy. Which of the following actions would protect patients and be consistent with the expressed values of the nurses?

A. Request that the ethics committee be consulted before any elderly person is placed on a ventilator.
B. Request that all patients sign Living Wills when they are admitted to the hospital.
C. Ask the medical staff to discuss with their patients the type of care they would wish to receive under extreme circumstances.
D. Ask nursing administration to write a policy restricting the admission of elderly cancer patients to the critical care area.

2–56. Clay-colored stools are associated with

A. Upper GI tract bleeding.
B. Absence of bile pigments.
C. Megadose iron supplementation.
D. An eroding pancreatic tumor.

Questions 2–57 and 2–58 refer to the following situation.

A patient is admitted to the intensive care unit from the operating room after repair of a fusiform abdominal aortic aneurysm with a tube graft. His heart rate is 110 beats per minute with sinus tachycardia. BP by arterial line is 110/76 mm Hg. Blood loss in the operating room was 1,200 ml. The patient received 4,000 ml of lactated Ringer's and 3 units of packed RBCs during the procedure. His hematocrit after the second unit of blood was 28%. Central venous pressure (CVP) is 4 mm Hg, pulmonary artery diastolic (PAD) and wedge (PCWP) pressures are equal at 8 mm Hg. Skin is cool and dry, and core temperature is 34.4° C. Warming blankets are placed on the patient.

2–57. Which of the following fluid orders is most appropriate at this time?

A. 5% dextrose in water (D5W) at 75 ml/hour.
B. 5% dextrose in lactated Ringer's (D5LR) at 200 ml/hour.
C. 0.45% normal saline at 100 ml/hour.
D. One unit of packed RBCs infused over 2 hours.

2–58. After 2 hours the following hemodynamic parameters are obtained on the patient: BP 88/64 mm Hg, heart rate 100 beats per minute, PAD 10 mm Hg, CVP 6 mm Hg, Hct 31%. His urine output has been 20 ml per hour for 2 hours. The patient's values remained as above after a 500-ml fluid challenge. The most appropriate intervention at this point would be to

A. Administer furosemide, 20 mg IV.
B. Infuse dopamine at 5 µg/kg/hour.
C. Place the patient in modified Trendelenburg position.
D. Infuse one unit of packed cells slowly over 2 hours.

Questions 2–59 and 2–60 refer to the following situation.

A 52-year-old male was admitted to the intensive care unit complaining of weight loss, fatigue, weakness, muscle cramps, postural dizziness, and diarrhea. He had a history of adrenal insufficiency and was on maintenance hydrocortisone, 30 mg per day. His wife died unexpectedly 2 weeks ago, and since then he has been severely depressed. Physical examination revealed hyperpigmented palms and buccal mucosa.

Vital signs and serum laboratory data:

BP	110/64 mm Hg flat, 90/60 mm Hg sitting
Heart rate	100/min flat, 120/min sitting
Respiratory rate	16/min
K	5.7 mEq/l
Na	128 mEq/l
BUN	22 mg/dl
Glucose	88 mg/dl

2–59. Signs that are indicative of mineralocorticoid deficiency in this patient are

    A. Hypoglycemia and fatigue.
    B. Hyperkalemia and depression.
    C. Azotemia and hyperpigmentation.
    D. Hyponatremia and postural hypotension.

2–60. Appropriate nursing diagnoses for this patient include all of the following *except*

    A. Fluid volume deficit related to aldosterone deficiency.
    B. Impaired oral mucous membrane integrity related to hyperpigmentation.
    C. Impaired physical mobility related to fatigue, weakness, and postural dizziness.
    D. Potential for dysrhythmia related to hyperkalemia.

2–61. Magnesium plays a role in all of the following intracellular activities *except*

    A. Depolarization of myocardial cells.
    B. Acetylcholine release.
    C. RNA stabilization.
    D. Glycogen breakdown.

2–62. To reduce trauma to the pulmonary artery and its capillaries while performing hemodynamic monitoring, the nurse should

    A. Inflate the catheter balloon with the minimum amount of air necessary to obtain a pulmonary capillary wedge waveform.
    B. Withdraw air from the balloon as soon as the pulmonary capillary waveform occurs.
    C. Perform the wedging procedure only when the patient's clinical picture has changed.
    D. Monitor only the pulmonary artery diastolic reading after the initial pulmonary artery diastolic and wedge readings are obtained.

2–63. A 60-year-old female with chronic obstructive lung disease (COPD) from alpha$_1$-antitrypsin deficiency is admitted from the emergency room in respiratory distress. She has oxygen by simple face mask at 6 l per minute, she is lethargic, and her vital signs are: BP 108/70 mm Hg, pulse 110 beats per minute, respirations 10 per minute. Arterial blood gases are obtained and the results show

    A. Decreased Pa$_{O_2}$.
    B. Decreased pH.
    C. Increased pH.
    D. Decreased HCO$_3$.

2–64. The difference between high- and low-flow oxygen devices is that

    A. High flow devices are easier to use.
    B. The F$_{I_{O_2}}$ is more variable with low flow devices.
    C. High flow systems deliver only high F$_{I_{O_2}}$.
    D. Low flow systems deliver the total inspired gas.

2–65. The parent steroid from which all adrenal steroids are synthesized is

    A. Cortisol.
    B. Cholesterol.
    C. Aldosterone.
    D. Progesterone.

2–66. Ongoing, routine assessment of a patient on Coumadin includes

    A. Partial thromboplastin time (PTT).
    B. Prothrombin time (PT).
    C. Fibrin split products.
    D. Fibrinogen.

Questions 2–67 and 2–68 refer to the following situation.

A 33-year-old male is admitted to the intensive care unit 3 weeks after a mild respiratory infection, with paralysis of the lower extremities and trunk and weakness of the upper extremities. A diagnosis of Guillain-Barré syndrome (GBS) is made.

2–67. The nurse knows to assess the patient for which one of the following major life-threatening complications of GBS?

A. Cerebral edema.
B. Cardiac dysrhythmias.
C. Respiratory arrest.
D. Deep vein thrombosis.

2–68. This patient will go through a process of grieving related to his diagnosis. The nurse determines that he is in the stage of *denial*. This stage is

A. An attempt to postpone dying until specific tasks are completed.
B. An adaptive coping mechanism to delay the pain and shock and to enable the patient to deal better with reality.
C. A realization that many losses are imminent.
D. A sense of unfairness of the diagnosis.

2–69. Which of the following calcium-reducing agents has the side effect of deposition of calcium in soft tissues?

A. Edetate disodium (EDTA).
B. Sodium bicarbonate.
C. Plicamycin (Mithracin).
D. Phosphate.

2–70. The primary goal in caring for a patient with ruptured esophageal varices is to

A. Maintain esophageal tissue perfusion.
B. Restore circulating blood volume.
C. Correct portal hypertension.
D. Prevent ammonia intoxication.

2–71. Bleeding esophageal varices may be treated by intravenous infusion of

A. Oxytocin (Pitocin).
B. Corticotropin (ACTH).
C. Heparin (Liquaemin).
D. Vasopressin (Pitressin).

2–72. Physical assessment findings indicative of right ventricular infarction would include

A. Bibasilar rales.
B. Flat neck veins with the patient's head raised 45°.
C. Jugular venous distention.
D. Auscultation of an S_4 heart sound.

2–73. Which of the following is the earliest clinical sign of right ventricular failure?

A. 2+ pitting edema of the ankles.
B. Palpable hepatomegaly.
C. Rales.
D. Jugular venous distention.

2–74. Acidosis causes the oxyhemoglobin dissociation curve to shift to the right, which results in

A. Oxygen binding loosely to hemoglobin.
B. Less oxygen dissolved in plasma.
C. Oxygen binding tighter to hemoglobin.
D. More oxygen dissolved in plasma.

2–75. A postoperative patient has been receiving steroids for the last 6 months. This will influence the nurse's plan of care, because steroid administration can cause

A. Increased platelet adhesion, resulting in clotting.
B. Enhanced oxygen binding to hemoglobin, resulting in anemia.
C. Decreased monocyte function, resulting in infection.
D. Increased release of heparin, resulting in bleeding.

2–76. The secretion of antidiuretic hormone (ADH) is stimulated by

A. Hypervolemia.
B. Hypertension.
C. Decreased plasma osmolality.
D. Decreased venous return.

2–77. A 41-year-old woman has acute viral hepatitis. Her serum ammonia level is 120 µg/dl. The nurse can expect drug therapy to include which of the following?

   A. Chloramphenicol.
   B. Hydrochlorothiazide.
   C. Neomycin.
   D. Rifampin.

Questions 2–78 and 2–79 refer to the following situation.

A 37-year-old female is admitted with subarachnoid hemorrhage (SAH).

2–78. As the critical care nurse caring for this patient, you know to

   A. Limit fluid to treat vasospasm.
   B. Restrain the patient to avoid injury.
   C. Ensure a quiet, dark environment.
   D. Avoid sedatives such as phenobarbital because they increase intracranial pressure.

2–79. As the nurse caring for this patient, you would question the following order:

   A. Restrict television, radio, and reading.
   B. Apply bilateral thigh-high antiembolic stockings.
   C. Administer a gentle cleansing enema.
   D. Elevate the head of the bed 30°.

2–80. In simultaneous sampling of the ultrafiltrate and the blood of patients on continuous arteriovenous hemofiltration, which of the following substances will have a different composition in the two samples?

   A. Calcium.
   B. Sodium.
   C. Potassium.
   D. Urea.

2–81. A patient has been managed in the intensive care unit for malignant hypertension. For 3 days the patient has been on an IV infusion of nitroprusside at a rate of 75 to 100 µg/minute. Formerly alert and cooperative, the patient is becoming confused and combative. His systolic BP had been maintained at 130 mm Hg, but it is now 150 mm Hg and climbing. The nurse should immediately

   A. Place soft restraints on the patient.
   B. Increase the nitroprusside by 3 µg/minute.
   C. Draw thiocyanate levels.
   D. Draw an arterial blood gas.

2–82. A patient who was originally admitted with a BP of 250/160 mm Hg is in the intensive care unit on a nitroprusside infusion. Her BP is currently 150/80 mm Hg. Although she no longer has a headache, she continues to complain of blurred vision and is unable to read. The nurse should instruct the patient

   A. That her longstanding hypertension has caused irreversible changes in her eyes and that corrective lenses will be necessary.
   B. That it will take some time for her eyesight to clear completely, when the edema or swelling in portions of her eyes resolves.
   C. That visual changes are common with extreme elevations in blood pressure, and until her blood pressure has been normal for a few days it will be hard to tell if any permanent damage has occurred.
   D. That blurred vision is a side effect of nitroprusside, and when she is weaned from the infusion her eyesight will return to normal.

2–83. A possible complication of thyroid-ectomy is

A. Hyperkalemia.
B. Hypocalcemia.
C. Hypernatremia.
D. Hypoglycemia.

2–84. A patient has an elevated erythrocyte sedimentation rate. This test is used to determine

A. The presence of inflammation.
B. Platelet function.
C. A patient's response to a decreased RBC count.
D. The compatibility of a possible tissue graft.

Questions 2–85 and 2–86 refer to the following situation.

A 56-year-old man is admitted with respiratory distress. He admits to a 40-year history of smoking and has worked in a coal mine for 36 years. He has had some progressive dyspnea but has been able to function well at home up to this time. He has a productive cough and has been coughing up blood in the last 2 days. He looks wasted and has had a 20-pound weight loss in the last couple of months.

2–85. What most likely is the patient's problem?

A. Chronic bronchitis.
B. Lung cancer.
C. Pulmonary embolus.
D. Emphysema.

2–86. The patient's therapy most likely will be

A. Antibiotic therapy.
B. Pulmonary rehabilitation program.
C. Heparin.
D. Lobectomy.

2–87. That portion of the neurologic system responsible for hormonal secretion by the pituitary gland is the

A. Neurohypophysis.
B. Adenohypophysis.
C. Hypothalamus.
D. Thalamus.

2–88. Under what circumstances can an employer be held legally responsible for negligent actions of a nurse?

A. Only if the nurse is not qualified for work assigned by the employer.
B. Only if the nurse has failed to act in accordance with hospital policy.
C. Only if the institution continues to employ a nurse accused of negligence.
D. Even if the hospital itself is not at fault.

2–89. Two days after successful coronary artery bypass graft surgery, a 60-year-old male complains of unrelenting epigastric pain and nausea. He reports that he has gallstones. His serum amylase and lipase levels are elevated. The nurse should suspect that the patient has developed

A. Acute pancreatitis.
B. Hepatic failure.
C. Graft occlusion.
D. Peptic ulcer.

2–90. A 58-year-old male with chronic obstructive pulmonary disease (COPD) is admitted in respiratory distress. His chest x-ray shows a dilated right heart and ECG changes show peaked P waves in leads II, III, and aVF; right axis deviation; and T wave inversion in V_1 to V_3. This clinical picture is most likely due to

A. An acute right ventricular infarction.
B. Ischemic heart damage.
C. Cor pulmonale.
D. Fluid overload.

2–91. Which of the following ECG intervals varies with the heart rate?

A. ST segment.
B. PR interval.
C. QRS interval.
D. QT interval.

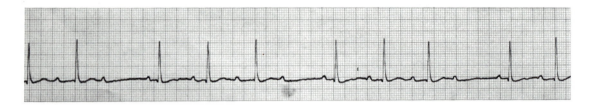

2–92. The above rhythm strip demonstrates which dysrhythmia?

    A. Mobitz type I second degree AV block (Wenckebach).
    B. Mobitz type II second degree AV block.
    C. Sinus exit block.
    D. First degree AV block with sinus exit block.

Questions 2–93 through 2–95 refer to the following situation.

A 63-year-old male patient is maintained on hemodialysis 3 times a week. He presents to the emergency department with complaints of lethargy, nausea, diarrhea, weakness, and numbness of the extremities. Associated findings include a serum potassium of 7.5 mEq/l and tall peaked T waves and widening of the QRS complex on the ECG recording.

2–93. Immediate interventions for this patient include

    I. Administration of IV sodium bicarbonate and calcium.
    II. Administration of IV hypertonic glucose and insulin.
    III. Hemodialysis.

    A. III only.
    B. I and II only.
    C. II and III only.
    D. I, II, III.

2–94. Following emergency interventions, this patient is admitted to the intensive care unit. Cation exchange resin has been administered by means of retention enemas. Several hours later, ECG monitoring demonstrates a lengthened QT interval, broadening of the T wave, and the appearance of a U wave. The nurse should anticipate that the serum potassium will most likely be

    A. 7.0 mEq/l.
    B. 2.5 mEq/l.
    C. 4.0 mEq/l.
    D. 5.5 mEq/l.

2–95. A social worker visits the patient and his wife after his transfer from the intensive care unit to evaluate their potential service needs. The patient's wife becomes angry with the social worker and refuses to discuss possible financial assistance. Her anger may be the result of

    I. Stress of her husband's chronic illness.
    II. Her need to assume responsibilities that were previously her husband's.
    III. The economic impact of long-term illness and disability.

    A. I, II, III.
    B. II and III only.
    C. I only.
    D. III only.

2–96. A low cortisol level would be most reliable as an indicator of adrenal insufficiency when measured at

    A. 12 a.m.
    B. 8 a.m.
    C. 1 p.m.
    D. 4 p.m.

2–97. You are caring for a patient with increased intracranial pressure. On the basis of your knowledge of increased intracranial pressure, you would question a physician order for which of the following tests?

    A. Computed axial tomography.
    B. Magnetic resonance imaging.
    C. Arterial blood gas sampling.
    D. Lumbar puncture.

2–98. When formulating a nursing care plan for the patient with the nursing diagnosis "alteration in tissue perfusion: cerebral, related to an increase in brain tissue, intracranial blood volume, and CSF volume," the critical care nurse knows that an expected outcome would be

    A. Cerebral perfusion pressure (CPP) will be maintained above 50 mm Hg.
    B. Intracranial pressure (ICP) will be maintained above 25 mm Hg.
    C. pH will be maintained above 7.50.
    D. P_{CO_2} will be maintained above 40 mm Hg.

2–99. A patient is admitted to the intensive care unit with *Pneumocystis carinii* pneumonia. The patient has AIDS and this is the patient's first admission with the diagnosis. As you explain the intubation procedure, the patient looks up at you and asks, "Am I going to die here?" Your response is

    A. Silence, because you know that people with this type of pneumonia die very quickly.
    B. "You're not going to die. This tube will help you breathe better."
    C. "You seem frightened. I don't know if you're going to die, but we will do everything we can to help you."
    D. "You should not worry about that. Not every one dies."

2–100. A 62-year-old female patient with a history of diabetes mellitus is admitted to the intensive care unit following a bowel resection for a large, benign tumor. Admitting vital signs and laboratory data reveal the following:

Heart rate	110/min
Respiratory rate	24/min
Temperature	102° F
BP	90/60 mm Hg
Cardiac output	7.5 l/min
SVR	750 dynes/sec/cm^{-5}
RBC	4 million/µl
Hct	35%
Hgb	11.6 mg/dl
WBC	13,200/µl
Platelets	180,000/µl
Fibrin split products	0

After you administer meperidine (Demerol) to the patient, she complains of "feeling cold" and is shivering. She is breathing normally and her vital signs are unchanged. Blood cultures are done and a Gram stain reveals gram-negative organisms in her blood.

Four hours later, the patient's vital signs and laboratory data include the following:

Heart rate	148/min
Respiratory rate	26/min
Temperature	98.2° F
BP	80/60 mm Hg
Cardiac output	3.5 l/min
SVR	1600 dynes/sec/cm^{-5}
S$\bar{v}$O$_2$	89%
RBC	4 million/µl
Hct	34%
Hbg	11.8 gm/dl
WBC	14,000/µl
Platelets	190,000/µl
Fibrin split products	<10 µg/ml

This information indicates

    A. The patient is developing a coagulopathy.
    B. Hypodynamic (cold) septic shock is developing.
    C. The patient is immunosuppressed.
    D. Peripheral circulation is good.

2–101. Respiratory muscle fatigue is caused by

A. Decreased work of breathing.
B. Increased demand for ventilation.
C. Hyperkalemia.
D. Hypothermia.

2–102. A physical finding specific for a true ventricular aneurysm is

A. Muffled heart tones.
B. Palpation of a sustained ventricular impulse separate from the apical impulse.
C. Palpation of pulsus paradoxus.
D. Palpation of a heave along the sternal border.

2–103. Palpation of the apical impulse (PMI) 1 centimeter lateral to the left sternal border is most likely in which of the following?

A. Arterial hypertension.
B. Left ventricular hypertrophy.
C. Pregnancy.
D. Chronic obstructive pulmonary disease (COPD).

2–104. The cellular functions of the liver include all of the following *except*

A. Drug detoxification.
B. RBC formation.
C. Bile production.
D. Protein metabolism.

2–105. Which of the following is a cause of primary hypernatremia?

A. Hyperglycemia.
B. Hyperaldosteronism.
C. Mannitol administration.
D. Watery diarrhea.

2–106. Nursing interventions for a patient with complete spinal cord transsection with the nursing diagnosis "Powerlessness related to total physical dependency" include all of the following *except*

A. Encourage verbal expression of having no control over the situation.
B. Permit expression of frustration and sadness, and allow crying.
C. Teach the patient about health maintenance activities.
D. Tell the patient that, in time, he or she will gain more control.

2–107. Immediately after coronary artery bypass surgery, a patient has a paced heart rate of 70 beats per minute, BP of 110/80 mm Hg by arterial line, and pulmonary artery wedge pressure (PAWP) of 18 mm Hg. Core temperature is 34.4° C. The patient is on a dobutamine drip at 10 μg/kg/minute. Treatment of the elevated pulmonary capillary wedge pressure (PCWP) would consist of

A. Administration of furosemide, 10 mg IV push.
B. Administration of nitropaste, 2 inches topically.
C. Continuous infusion of nitroglycerin at 80 μg/minute.
D. Application of warming blankets to induce vasodilation.

2–108. A patient is pain-free after coronary artery bypass graft surgery, but has pathologic Q waves and ST elevations on his 12-lead ECG during a followup office visit and is referred to a medical center for cardiac catheterization. Cardiac catheterization shows 90% occlusion of the right coronary artery graft. Laboratory studies performed prior to the procedure include coagulation studies that are all within normal range, Hct 35%, and normal renal function studies. Creatine kinase (CK) enzymes are within normal range. Which of the following therapies is appropriate for this patient?

A. Systemic infusion of streptokinase.
B. Systemic tissue plasminogen activator (t-PA) therapy.
C. Percutaneous balloon angioplasty (PCTA).
D. Emergency coronary artery bypass grafting.

2–109. Restrictive lung disease shows which of the following pulmonary function patterns?

A. Decreased TLC, FRC, RV, and FVC.
B. Increased FRC, RV, TLC, decreased FVC.
C. Increased compliance, FVC.
D. Decreased TLC, increased FVC.

2–110. *Comparison* of static and dynamic compliance pressures is useful to determine

A. Baseline values for the patient.
B. Which aspects of the pulmonary system are changing.
C. Progression of the lung disease.
D. Resistance of the ventilator system.

2–111. Hyponatremia caused by the syndrome of inappropriate secretion of antidiuretic hormone (SIADH) is associated with

A. Hypovolemia and elevated urine osmolarity.
B. Hypovolemia and decreased urine osmolarity.
C. Hypervolemia and elevated urine osmolarity.
D. Hypervolemia and decreased urine osmolarity.

2–112. A potential complication associated with balloon tamponade of bleeding esophageal varices is

A. Bradycardia.
B. Bowel obstruction.
C. Asphyxiation.
D. Portal hypertension.

2–113. The ascending reticular activating system is essential for

A. Alert wakefulness, focusing attention, and controlling skeletal musculature.
B. Arousal from sleep and facilitating activity of the motor neurons.
C. Controlling skeletal musculature and facilitating activity of the motor neurons.
D. Arousal from sleep, alert wakefulness, and perceptual association.

2–114. A patient's laboratory results reveal a WBC of 17,000/μl with a "shift to the left." This result indicates

I. A normal response to infection.
II. An increased number of immature neutrophils.
III. The patient is at risk for developing a coagulopathy.
IV. A decreased number of mature basophils.

A. I only.
B. I and II only.
C. II and III only.
D. IV only.

2–115. Anticipated complications of an acute *anterior* wall myocardial infarction would include

   A. Sinus bradycardia.
   B. Mobitz type I heart block (Wenckebach).
   C. Pump failure.
   D. Papillary muscle rupture.

2–116. Which of the following would be found in a patient with a ruptured ventricular septum?

   I. Right ventricular oxygen saturation of 45%.
   II. Right ventricular oxygen saturation of 75%.
   III. A palpable thrill at the left sternal border.
   IV. Right ventricular systolic pressure of 50 mm Hg.

   A. II only.
   B. III and IV only.
   C. I, III, IV.
   D. II, III, IV.

2–117. Which of the following factors is considered in ethical decisions to withhold or withdraw treatment?

   A. The patient's age and medical diagnosis.
   B. The expressed or implied wishes of the individual.
   C. The written hospital policies.
   D. The risk-to-benefit ratio of the treatment and the physician's personal value system.

2–118. A patient's arterial-venous oxygen content difference $C(a - \bar{v})O_2$ has increased from 4 gm/dl to 8 gm/dl. This indicates that

   A. Cardiac output is adequate.
   B. Lung function has improved.
   C. Oxygen delivery has decreased.
   D. Metabolic rate has decreased.

Questions 2–119 and 2–120 refer to the following situation.

A 16-year-old victim of a motor vehicle accident is presently on a ventilator with a rate of 10 per minute, V_T 650, $F_{I_{O_2}}$ 0.40, PEEP 0. Her blood gases are within normal limits for these settings.

2–119. While doing an assessment, the nurse observes that the patient has nasal flaring during inspiration. This is an indication of

   A. Increased alveolar ventilation.
   B. Air hunger.
   C. Anxiety.
   D. Pneumothorax.

2–120. The correct action the nurse should then take to eliminate nasal flaring and accessory muscle use would be to

   A. Increase the $F_{I_{O_2}}$.
   B. Provide sedation.
   C. Increase the flow rate.
   D. Increase the tidal volume.

2–121. Which of the following is *not* a likely complication associated with fulminating meningococcal meningitis?

   A. Pulmonary embolus.
   B. Waterhouse-Friderichsen syndrome.
   C. Disseminated intravascular coagulation (DIC).
   D. Encephalitis.

Questions 2–122 and 2–123 refer to the following situation.

A hemodialysis patient has been treated for ulcer disease.

2–122. The cause of GI problems in end-stage renal disease (ESRD) is most likely

   A. Inflammation of the GI tract.
   B. Decreased perfusion of the GI tract.
   C. Increased gastric acid secretion.
   D. The medication regime.

2–123. The patient has been using excessive amounts of aluminum hydroxide gel (Mylanta) in an attempt to relieve his gastric symptoms. A laboratory value that might be expected with use of aluminum hydroxide gel is

A. Magnesium > 2.5 mEq/l.
B. Calcium < 8.5 mEq/l.
C. Sodium < 136 mEq/l.
D. Potassium > 5.5 mEq/l.

2–124. A patient who has had an anterior wall myocardial infarction 7 weeks ago continues to have ST elevations of 5 mm and frequent premature ventricular contractions. He is currently being weaned from his lidocaine infusion and has been started on procainamide by mouth. Plans for continued treatment of this patient should include

A. Cardiac catheterization.
B. Intra-aortic balloon pump insertion.
C. Transfer to telemetry.
D. Percutaneous balloon angioplasty.

2–125. A patient who has received streptokinase infusion for acute myocardial infarction complains of mild shortness of breath 1 hour after completion of therapy. The nurse auscultates clear breath sounds. Temperature is 37.8° C. The nurse should

A. Draw arterial blood gases.
B. Increase nasal oxygen delivery from 4 liters to 6 liters.
C. Perform a 12-lead ECG.
D. Obtain vials of diphenhydramine and methylprednisolone and remain with the patient for close monitoring.

2–126. The normal daily volume of gastric secretions is approximately

A. 500 to 900 ml.
B. 1000 to 1400 ml.
C. 1500 to 3000 ml.
D. 3500 to 4500 ml.

2–127. The pH of gastric contents aspirated from a patient's nasogastric tube is 2.8. The nurse should expect to administer

A. An antacid.
B. Sucralfate (carafate).
C. An antiemetic.
D. An antihistamine (H_1 antagonist).

2–128. Functions of the lung include all of the following *except*

A. Gas exchange.
B. Reservoir.
C. Humidification.
D. Filtration.

Questions 2–129 and 2–130 refer to the following situation.

A 20-year-old female, 3 days after surviving a motor vehicle accident, develops respiratory failure and is placed on a ventilator. Her nursing diagnosis is impaired gas exchange.

2–129. A pulmonary artery catheter is placed and pressures obtained are: PA systolic/diastolic 34/18 mm Hg, mean 23 mm Hg, PCWP 8 mm Hg. The abnormal pulmonary artery pressures are most likely due to

A. Pulmonary edema.
B. Congestive heart failure.
C. Blood loss.
D. Hypoxic vasoconstriction.

2–130. Arterial blood gases are drawn and the results are: pH 7.32, Pa_{CO_2} 30 mm Hg, HCO_3 14 mEq/l, Pa_{O_2} 60 mm Hg, Sa_{O_2} 89%, Ca_{O_2} 17.5 ml/dl, on FI_{O_2} 0.35, SIMV 12, V_T 750, PEEP 0. The hypoxemia is most likely due to

A. A diffusion defect.
B. Alveolar hypoventilation.
C. Low inspired oxygen tension.
D. A ventilation/perfusion ($\dot{V}/\dot{Q}$) mismatch.

2–131. In continuous arteriovenous hemofiltration, ultrafiltration rates can
be decreased by

A. Lowering the level of the collection device.
B. Increasing systemic blood flow.
C. Lengthening the ultrafiltrate
tubing.
D. Maintaining the hematocrit at
less than 40%.

**Questions 2–132 through 2–134 refer to
the following situation.**

A 56-year-old right-handed male patient
is admitted with an astrocytoma. On computed tomography scan the tumor is revealed to be in the left frontal cerebral
hemisphere.

2–132. The nurse anticipates which of the
following symptoms in this patient?

A. Expressive aphasia.
B. Paresthesia.
C. Visual hallucinations.
D. Loss of left-right discrimination.

2–133. The patient is unable to deal with
his diagnosis and the nurse assesses
him to be in situational crisis. The
most likely cause for this is

A. He feels threatened.
B. He has a distorted perception of
the diagnosis.
C. He perceives a lack of personal
control over the event.
D. A lack of adequate cerebral perfusion sufficient to promote adequate thought processes.

2–134. The patient's prognosis is poor. In
determining his psychological level
of grieving, the nurse determines
that he is in the stage of *bargaining*.
This stage is

A. An attempt to postpone dying
until specific tasks are completed.
B. An adaptive coping mechanism
to delay the pain and shock and
to enable the patient to deal better with reality.
C. A realization that many losses
are imminent.
D. A sense of unfairness of the diagnosis.

2–135. The effects of slow reactive substance of anaphylaxis (SRS-A), kinins, and histamine in an anaphylactic reaction are

I. Bronchoconstriction.
II. Hypotension.
III. Edema.
IV. Supraventricular tachydys-
rhythmias.

A. I and IV only.
B. II and III only.
C. I, II, and III only.
D. II, III, and IV only.

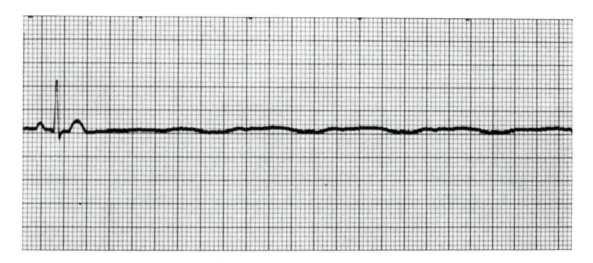

2–136. An alarm sounds in the coronary care unit at 2:00 a.m. Staff response is immediate. The above rhythm is on the monitor.

The nurse calls the patient's name and he does not respond. The nurse should next

A. Defibrillate the patient with 400 joules.
B. Defibrillate the patient with 200 joules.
C. Perform a precordial thump.
D. Shake the patient to see if he responds.

2–137. A patient with atrioventricular (AV) dissociation has a temporary pacemaker inserted as an emergency and he is admitted to the coronary care unit for continuous monitoring until a permanent pacemaker can be inserted. During the admission assessment of the patient, a pericardial friction rub is noted. The nurse should

A. Obtain an order for a chest x-ray *stat*.
B. Immediately position the patient on his left side.
C. Increase the mA of the pacemaker.
D. Turn the sensitivity dial all the way to "asynchronous."

Questions 2–138 through 2–140 refer to the following situation.

A 28-year-old female is admitted to your facility following an automobile accident in which she sustained a head injury.

2–138. On assessment, you note that the patient has decreased ability to concentrate and a flat affect. You know that this is most likely due to injury of the

A. Occipital lobe.
B. Temporal lobe.
C. Parietal lobe.
D. Frontal lobe.

2–139. This patient has been demonstrating respiratory dysrhythmias. She begins to demonstrate the following pattern: sustained, rapid, regular, and deep hyperpnea. As the nurse caring for her, you know that this respiratory pattern is most likely due to a lesion involving the

A. Basal ganglia.
B. Midbrain.
C. Posterior fossa.
D. Rostral medulla.

2–140. Later, you are assessing this patient and discover otorrhea. Which nursing intervention is appropriate at this time?

A. Apply pressure to the area.
B. Check the patient for bowel sounds.
C. Assess the drainage for the presence of glucose.
D. Pack the ear firmly with sterile dressings.

2–141. Patients with adult respiratory distress syndrome (ARDS) frequently cough up pink frothy sputum. This is due to

   A. Left heart failure.
   B. Pulmonary microhemorrhages.
   C. Alteration in Starling forces.
   D. Pulmonary emboli.

Questions 2–142 and 2–143 refer to the following situation.

A critical care nurse is assessing a peritoneal dialysis patient and notes cloudy effluent in the drainage bag and a decreased volume of return fluid. On physical examination, the nurse elicits rebound tenderness, and the patient complains of severe, diffuse abdominal pain.

2–142. The most likely cause of this patient's signs and symptoms is

   A. Cold or acidic dialysate.
   B. Peritoneal infection.
   C. Rapid infusion of dialysate.
   D. Air under the diaphragm.

2–143. The decrease in dialysate return in this patient is most likely the result of

   A. Positioning of the catheter.
   B. Increased absorption of dialysate.
   C. Fibrin occluding the catheter.
   D. Position of the patient.

2–144. A potential immediate postoperative complication of pancreatectomy is

   A. Anastomotic leak.
   B. Pseudocyst.
   C. Mesenteric thrombosis.
   D. Coagulopathy

Questions 2–145 through 2–147 refer to the following situation.

A 22-year-old female is admitted to your unit complaining of nausea and a sudden severe headache rated a 9 on a pain scale of 1 to 10, with 1 being the least and 10 being the worst. As you are bathing her you note that she is becoming increasingly unarousable. You note generalized seizure activity. Clinical signs indicate an intracerebral aneurysm.

2–145. In evaluating this patient's symptoms, the critical care nurse knows that the most likely reason for her abrupt change in level of consciousness is

   A. A subarachnoid hemorrhage.
   B. An alteration in her electrolyte and fluid balance.
   C. The usual postictal behavior following seizure activity.
   D. Vasodilatation of cerebral vessels.

2–146. The patient continues to be unresponsive and has right hemiplegia. She has hypertensive episodes and nuchal rigidity. In evaluating these clinical findings, the nurse knows that the patient's aneurysm is a grade

   A. I.
   B. II.
   C. III.
   D. IV.

2–147. The patient has now spent 10 days in your unit. Initially, she responded to antifibrinolytic treatment for intracerebral aneurysm. In determining the efficacy of this treatment, the nurse knows to assess for

   A. Hydrocephalus resulting from increased intracranial pressure.
   B. Neurologic deficits caused by vasospasm.
   C. Evidence of rebleeding because of lysis of the clot.
   D. Seizure activity as a side effect of the medication.

2–148. Which of the following statements best describes the pathophysiology of disseminated intravascular coagulation (DIC)?

A. Intravascular thrombin promotes fibrin clot formation and platelet aggregation; clots are lysed and clotting factors are consumed excessively.
B. Antithrombin is formed as fibrin clots break down, resulting in thrombin inactivation of clotting factors and anticoagulation.
C. Increased production of fibrin split products results in enhanced clot breakdown, fibrin neutralization, and consumption of clotting factors.
D. Plasminogen activators cause increased coagulation with subsequent consumption of clotting factors, clot shrinkage, and lysis with bleeding.

2–149. Which of the following transfusions would you anticipate for the patient with DIC?

A. Packed RBCs, platelets.
B. Plasmanate, cryoprecipitate.
C. Whole blood, albumin.
D. Platelets, fresh frozen plasma.

2–150. The physiologic factors that predispose patients to thrombosis include all of the following *except*

A. Bedrest.
B. Chemotherapy.
C. Polycythemia.
D. Trauma.

2–151. The nursing diagnosis "Decreased cardiac output related to an acute pulmonary embolus" indicates that

A. Pulmonary vascular resistance (PVR) is decreased.
B. An embolectomy is needed immediately.
C. Preload to the left ventricle is decreased.
D. Mini-dose heparin is indicated.

2–152. Integumentary characteristics associated with myxedema include

A. Diaphoresis and thick hair.
B. Pitting edema and thin nails.
C. Brittle nails and velvety smooth skin.
D. Nonpitting edema and cool, dry skin.

Questions 2–153 and 2–154 refer to the following situation.

A 60-year-old female was admitted to the ICU with a diagnosis of thyroid storm and complaining of dyspnea, nausea, and vomiting. She had a history of angina and hyperthyroidism, and underwent cardiac catheterization 3 weeks ago. The family stated that she had become increasingly agitated and inattentive in the last few weeks. She is restless, tremulous, and diaphoretic with flushed skin, and has bibasilar crackles. Her heart rate is 150 per minute and her ECG shows normal sinus rhythm with an occasional premature ventricular contraction (PVC).

Vital signs and laboratory data are:

BP	170/80 mm Hg
Temperature	104° F
Respiratory rate	32/min
Cardiac index	4.7 l/min/m²
Serum glucose	320 mg/dl
WBC	6,000/mm³
Neutrophils	50%
Band cells	3%

2–153. Signs and symptoms that are indicative of an augmented adrenergic state in this patient include

A. Bibasilar crackles and diaphoresis.
B. Nausea and narrow pulse pressure.
C. Elevated cardiac index and tachycardia.
D. Decreased cardiac index and hyperglycemia.

2–154. A *priority* nursing intervention for this patient would be

A. Continuous reorientation.
B. Applying hand restraints.
C. Monitoring heart rhythm.
D. Assessing for the presence of bowel sounds.

2–155. In the treatment of hypercalcemia, bone reabsorption of calcium can be decreased by

   A. Corticosteroids.
   B. Calcitonin.
   C. Immobilization.
   D. IV sodium chloride.

2–156. A patient is extremely anxious about his impending cardiac surgery. He had been scheduled for surgery 10 days prior, but had not adjusted his medications as his physician had instructed. He is convinced that the reason surgery was postponed is because he is so "sick" he will probably die. His medications at the time that surgery was postponed were: isosorbide dinitrate, 40 mg QID; digoxin, 0.125 mg daily; aspirin, one tablet with each meal; and propranolol, 10 mg QID. In preparing the patient for surgery, which of the following approaches would be most appropriate?

   A. Explain to the patient that aspirin damages platelets and that surgery was postponed so that he would not bleed after surgery.
   B. Focus on postoperative routines and have the patient demonstrate coughing and deep breathing and flexion and extension of his feet, as you reinforce that these are necessary after surgery.
   C. Instruct the patient that if he follows all the instructions and does all of the exercises the doctor tells him to, he will do just fine.
   D. Tell the patient that anxiety is normal before surgery, but that he will do very well after surgery and he should stop worrying.

2–157. In examining a patient with constrictive pericarditis, the nurse would expect to palpate

   A. Pulsus magnus.
   B. Pulsus alternans.
   C. Pulsus parvus.
   D. Pulsus paradoxus.

2–158. Which of the following confirms the clinical diagnosis of myocarditis?

   A. ECG changes suggestive of acute MI without enzyme elevation.
   B. Endomyocardial biopsy.
   C. Cardiac catheterization.
   D. New onset of congestive failure of unknown etiology in young adults 20 to 40 years old.

2–159. A patient has had chest pain for a total of 2 hours. The ECG shows ST segment elevations in leads II, III, and aV_F as well as first degree AV block and one premature ventricular contraction (PVC) each 6 seconds. The heart rate is 64 beats per minute. The patient has had angina in the past and an inconclusive exercise stress test. This patient is probably a candidate for

   A. Emergency coronary artery bypass graft.
   B. Percutaneous transluminal coronary angioplasty.
   C. Tissue plasminogen activator therapy.
   D. Temporary pacemaker insertion.

2–160. In a patient with head injury, hyperventilation associated with alterations in respiratory functioning

   A. Raises mean thoracic pressure, decreases venous return and cardiac output.
   B. Decreases mean thoracic pressure, increases venous return and cardiac output.
   C. Raises mean thoracic pressure, increases venous return, and decreases cardiac output.
   D. Decreases mean thoracic pressure, decreases venous return, and increases cardiac output.

2–161. A patient has a subarachnoid screw in place for intracranial pressure monitoring. Which one of the following is the most clinically significant of all the pressure waveforms seen?

   A. A waves.
   B. B waves.
   C. C waves.
   D. F waves.

2–162. A 36-year-old male had a percutaneous liver biopsy 2 hours ago. His platelet count this morning was 130,000/mm³. Which of the following actions is most appropriate at this time?

A. Monitor for abdominal distention.
B. Position the patient on his left side.
C. Ambulate the patient.
D. Auscultate lung fields for diminished breath sounds on the right side.

2–163. Which of the following sets of laboratory values suggests acute hepatic failure?

	Total Bilirubin (mg/dl)	SGOT (units/l)	Serum Albumin (gm/dl)
A.	2.0	300	2.0
B.	1.2	30	6.0
C.	0.5	280	4.5
D.	0.1	10	1.8

2–164. During intra-aortic balloon pump therapy, premature inflation of the intra-aortic balloon causes

A. Reduced coronary artery filling.
B. Increased left ventricular afterload.
C. Decreased peak systolic pressure.
D. Decreased assisted end-diastolic pressure.

2–165. The dysrhythmia depicted on the rhythm strip below would best be termed

A. Mobitz type I second degree AV block (Wenckebach).
B. High-grade second degree AV block.
C. Third degree AV block.
D. Idiojunctional rhythm.

Questions 2–166 and 2–167 refer to the following situation.

A 56-year-old male is recovering from triple coronary artery bypass surgery when he develops perioral and digital paresthesias, dyspnea, and wheezing. His ECG shows a lengthened ST segment and prolonged QT interval.

2–166. The most likely electrolyte abnormality associated with these ECG findings would be

A. Calcium   7.5 mg/dl.
B. Potassium   3.0 mEq/l.
C. Sodium   126 mEq/l.
D. Magnesium   7 mEq/l.

2–167. Treatment of this patient's electrolyte abnormality will include the intravenous administration of

A. Normal saline.
B. Furosemide.
C. Monobasic potassium phosphate.
D. 10% calcium gluconate.

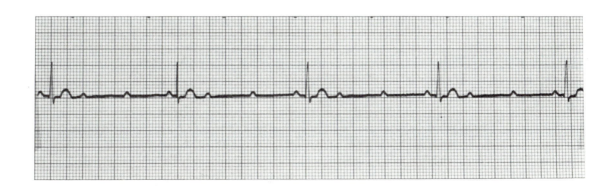

2–168. A 62-year-old male is admitted in respiratory distress. He has a history of working in a paint factory for 35 years, but no smoking history. His arterial blood gases normally are: pH 7.38, Pa_{CO_2} 42 mm Hg, HCO_3 20 mEq/l, Pa_{O_2} 68 mm Hg, Sa_{O_2} 91%. Physical examination shows a thin, cachectic man with signs of recent weight loss, skin warm and pink and dry, increased anteroposterior diameter of the chest, distant breath sounds, and dyspnea at rest. Laboratory values show WBC 12,000/µl, hemoglobin 16 gm/dl, hematocrit 48% with a slight shift to the left. This clinical picture is characteristic of

   A. Congestive heart failure.
   B. Chronic bronchitis.
   C. Emphysema.
   D. Asthma.

2–169. When assessing for the optimal level of PEEP to achieve an acceptable arterial oxygen pressure (Pa_{O_2}), the PEEP is increased until

   A. Hemodynamic compromise occurs.
   B. A pneumothorax occurs.
   C. A pressure of 20 cm H_2O is reached.
   D. Pulmonary vascular resistance is decreased.

Questions 2–170 and 2–171 refer to the following situation.

An 80-year-old male has lived alone since the death of his wife. His only living relative is a grandniece with whom he has had minimal contact. Several years earlier, the patient sustained a stroke, which left him with left hemiparesis, interfering with his ability to care for himself. He was admitted to the hospital for surgical treatment of an intestinal obstruction resulting from a malignant tumor. He understood the palliative nature of the procedure and was anxious to regain physical comfort so he could return home to enjoy his remaining months of life. During the preoperative phase, the patient suffered another stroke, which caused right-sided paralysis and required the use of mechanical ventilation to keep him alive. During the next several weeks, attempts to wean him from the ventilator were unsuccessful and he expressed the desire to be removed from the ventilator and allowed to die. The attending physician was unwilling to discontinue the ventilator, stating, "He is too ill and depressed to make a competent decision. Besides, I took an oath to preserve life."

2–170. Which of the following statements can be inferred from this situation?

   A. The physician values beneficence over autonomy.
   B. The decision whether to continue mechanical ventilation should be made by the patient's grandniece.
   C. The patient's desire to be removed from the ventilator constitutes a suicide wish.
   D. The removal of the ventilator would be an act of murder in the eyes of the law.

2–171. Which of the following actions would be reasonable if the nurse believed that the patient was competent and that his autonomy should be honored?

   I. The nurse should document the patient's expressed wishes in the medical record.
   II. The nurse should maintain open communication with the physician about the patient's care and suggest a second medical opinion.
   III. The nurse should immediately begin action to obtain a court order to remove the patient from the ventilator.
   IV. The nurse should follow established administrative channels to take the patient's case before the institutional ethics committee.

   A. I and III.
   B. I, II, and IV.
   C. III.
   D. I, III, and IV.

2–172. Which of the following is the most reliable diagnostic indicator in determining the consequences of myocardial contusion?

   A. Serial CPK-MB fractions.
   B. Radionuclide imaging.
   C. Serial 12-lead ECG.
   D. Development of a pericardial friction rub that decreases on daily examination.

2–173. When a diabetic patient is admitted comatose directly to the intensive care unit, the intervention of choice is to obtain a blood sample for analysis and

   A. Wait for the results before beginning treatment.
   B. Administer a 44 to 88 mEq/l IV bolus of sodium bicarbonate.
   C. Administer 2 to 12 units of insulin IV.
   D. Administer an IV bolus of glucose, 25 to 50 gm in a 50% solution.

2–174. CNS depression in the patient with diabetic ketoacidosis is best correlated with the

   A. Blood ketone levels.
   B. Degree of acidosis.
   C. Degree of hyperosmolality.
   D. Degree of hyperkalemia.

2–175. Which of the following medications is appropriate in the treatment of obstructive hypertrophic cardiomyopathy?

   A. Digoxin.
   B. Nitroglycerin.
   C. Sodium nitroprusside.
   D. Propranolol.

2–176. A patient is being treated with gentamicin and penicillin after he developed a change in his prosthetic valve murmur, indicating the development of endocarditis. The patient is on continuous ECG monitoring and it has been noted that his PR interval is increasing. BP and heart rate have not changed significantly. Current ECG findings include a heart rate of 84 beats per minute with a PR interval of 0.22 second. BP is 116/70 mm Hg. The patient's white cell count has increased from 18,000/mm³ to 21,000/mm³. The most likely cause of these findings is

   A. Abscess formation.
   B. Meningitis.
   C. Congestive heart failure.
   D. Cerebral infarction.

2–177. The most common early signs of acute subdural hematoma that progressively worsen include

   A. Headache and contralateral pupil dilatation.
   B. Drowsiness and fixed contralateral pupil dilatation.
   C. Headache, confusion, and ipsilateral pupil dilatation.
   D. Drowsiness, confusion, and contralateral pupil dilatation.

2–178. Basilar skull fractures are of particular concern because they may result in

A. Transsection of the spinal cord.
B. Jugular venous compression.
C. Seizures.
D. Meningitis.

Questions 2–179 and 2–180 refer to the following situation.

A patient is admitted to the intensive care unit with night sweats, seizures, and unexplained weight loss.

2–179. The patient's enzyme-linked immunosorbent assay (ELISA) and western blot tests are positive. What will your patient teaching include?

A. Avoid receiving blood transfusions in the future.
B. Information about safe sex practices.
C. Avoid bruising and injury.
D. Taking antibiotics to prevent infection.

2–180. Which of the following types of precautions should be followed when caring for a patient with a positive western blot test?

A. Wear a gown, gloves, a mask, and goggles when giving the patient a bath.
B. Break needles to prevent possible reuse by anyone else.
C. Put the patient in reverse isolation to prevent infection.
D. Handle blood specimens with gloved hands.

2–181. Mixed venous blood gases are obtained from the

A. Pulmonary artery.
B. Right atrium.
C. Right ventricle.
D. Left atrium.

2–182. A 62-year-old male is admitted to the intensive care unit, after surgery, from the recovery room. As he is awakening, he is restless and agitated, triggering the ventilator frequently, and has increased pulse rate and BP with nasal flaring and use of accessory muscles. Lungs are clear bilaterally. The last pain medication he received was 30 minutes ago. The most appropriate action would be

A. Sedation.
B. Increase oxygen flow rate.
C. Set up for a chest tube.
D. Increase the $F_{I_{O_2}}$.

2–183. A patient is admitted in acute oliguric renal failure. A peritoneal dialysis catheter was inserted 2 hours ago and hourly peritoneal dialysis with 2 l of dialysate was begun. The nurse notes that 1,500 ml of cloudy yellow fluid was returned for each cycle. The patient suddenly is incontinent of approximately 700 ml of watery diarrhea. The nurse suspects

A. Dialysis disequilibrium syndrome.
B. Pseudomembranous colitis.
C. Bowel perforation.
D. Dumping syndrome.

Questions 2–184 and 2–185 refer to the following situation.

A 27-year-old male has been in ICU for several days following a severe motor vehicle accident in which he sustained multiple fractures and crush injuries to his lower extremities. His urine output has now decreased and the nurse notes edema of his ankles, feet, back, sacrum, and periorbital areas. On auscultation of lung fields, crackles are heard in both bases. Urinalysis results include

Specific gravity	1.010
Osmolarity	250 mOsm/l
Urea	300 mg/dl
Creatinine	60 mg/dl
Potassium	21 mEq/24 hr

2–184. The patient is placed on hemodialysis using a subclavian access. Complications of hemodialysis include

A. Disequilibrium syndrome.
B. Hyperglycemia.
C. Hypernatremia.
D. Protein loss.

2–185. The patient becomes angry and hostile toward his family and staff members. He becomes noncompliant with medical treatment. The best response from the nurse would be to

A. Avoid discussion of his accident and treatment for now.
B. Encourage verbalization and answer questions simply and honestly.
C. Tell him everything will be fine soon.
D. Provide him self-learning packets and educational material on dialysis.

2–186. The clinical significance of a contusion is that

A. Loss of consciousness may be transient.
B. It is reversible.
C. Retrograde amnesia occurs.
D. Laceration of the brain may occur.

2–187. SIADH may result in the development of cerebral edema owing to

A. Hypokalemia.
B. Hyponatremia.
C. Hypercalcemia.
D. Hyperglycemia.

2–188. Auscultation of a patient's abdomen reveals loud, high-pitched, tinkling bowel sounds. The patient complains of nausea and crampy abdominal pain. The nurse suspects that this patient has

A. Paralytic ileus.
B. Ascites.
C. Mesenteric thrombosis.
D. Intestinal obstruction.

2–189. The primary management goal for the patient with spinal cord injury upon arrival at the acute care hospital is to

A. Transfer the patient from stretcher to bed.
B. Minimize the extent of spinal cord damage.
C. Reduce cervical swelling.
D. Elevate the head to reduce intracranial hypertension.

2–190. A 32-year-old female, 6 days after craniotomy for an acoustic neuroma, is complaining of a headache that is becoming increasingly worse; her temperature is 103° F, and she is complaining of nausea. Upon physical examination, she is found to be tachycardic and has nuchal rigidity. Brudzinski's and Kernig's signs are positive. The critical care nurse anticipates a diagnosis of

A. Increased intracranial pressure.
B. Guillain-Barré syndrome.
C. Cerebral vascular accident.
D. Meningitis.

Questions 2–191 and 2–192 refer to the following situation.

A patient has reddish-brown urine following femoral artery revascularization.

2–191. Which of the following laboratory values is diagnostic for this finding?

A. BUN 20 mg/dl.
B. Moderate urinary ketones.
C. Hct 30.4%.
D. CPK total 3,400 IU.

2–192. Which of the following treatment orders would the nurse anticipate for the patient?

A. D5/.45 normal saline with 50 mEq/l of sodium bicarbonate at 200 ml/hour.
B. Furosemide, 20 mg IV push.
C. Acetazolamide (Diamox), 500 mg via nasogastric tube.
D. No treatment is required.

2–193. A 28-year-old female was in a motor vehicle accident 7 days ago. She had emergency surgery to repair a ruptured spleen and liver laceration. A C6 fracture has resulted in symmetric flaccid motor paralysis. Her bowel sounds are active in all quadrants. She is receiving full-strength enteral nutrition. The nurse will

A. Firmly stimulate the anal sphincter and rectum QID.
B. Restrict intake of bulk-building additives.
C. Provide strenuous passive range of motion.
D. Establish a regular time for bowel elimination.

2–194. The serum glucose value most consistent with the diagnosis of hyperosmolar hyperglycemic nonketotic coma (HHNK) is

A. 100 to 250 mg/dl.
B. 251 to 400 mg/dl.
C. 401 to 550 mg/dl.
D. 551 to 700 mg/dl.

2–195. A patient with a chest wound in the lung from a knife attack is intubated and on a ventilator at FI_{O_2} 0.4, V_T 800 ml, respiratory rate 18 per min, intermittent mandatory ventilation (IMV), PEEP 5 cm H_2O. He has a chest tube in place to 20 cm H_2O suction. He becomes agitated and combative, and pulls the dressing off his knife wound. What would be the most appropriate initial action to take?

A. Sedate the patient.
B. Restrain the patient.
C. Cover the wound with a dressing immediately.
D. Increase the suction on the chest tube.

2–196. The nursing priority for a patient having an anaphylactoid reaction to an IV contrast agent will be to

A. Administer oxygen and diphenhydramine (Benadryl) IM.
B. Discontinue the IV and encourage oral fluids.
C. Stop the infusion of the contrast agent and place a tourniquet above the IV site.
D. Start a dopamine drip and give a *stat* dose of aminophylline.

Questions 2–197 and 2–198 refer to the following situation.

A 17-year-old female was admitted to the intensive care unit 2 days ago, following an automobile accident. Injuries included multiple bruises and lacerations, a left femur fracture, a skull fracture, and multiple rib fractures. She has been unconscious since admission. Vital signs and laboratory data reveal:

BP	90/60 mm Hg
Heart rate	110/min
Respiratory rate	28/min
24-hour urine output	4,200 ml
24-hour fluid intake	1,800 ml
Serum Values	149 mEq/l
Na	
K	4 mEq/l
Osmolality	305 mOsm/l
Urine Values	
Osmolality	280 mOsm/l
Specific gravity	1.001

2–197. Findings consistent with the diagnosis of diabetes insipidus in this patient include

A. Hypernatremia and polyuria.
B. Tachycardia and hypercapnia.
C. Polydipsia and hypo-osmolality.
D. Hypokalemia and hypertension.

2–198. Appropriate nursing diagnoses for this patient include all of the following *except*

   A. Potential for decreased cardiac output related to hypotension.
   B. Potential for infection related to loss of tissue integrity.
   C. Potential for impaired gas exchange related to multiple rib fractures.
   D. Potential for fluid volume excess related to cerebral edema.

2–199. A patient is admitted to the intensive care unit following a thoracotomy. The patient had intraoperative ECG changes. During surgery the patient received an autologous blood transfusion. Your care of this patient will include

   I. Using universal precautions.
   II. Testing the patient postoperatively for hepatitis.
   III. Monitoring the patient for a transfusion reaction.
   IV. Warming the blood during administration.

   A. I only.
   B. I and III only.
   C. I, II, and IV only.
   D. All of the above.

2–200. A trauma victim is in the intensive care unit immediately after surgery and on a ventilator. There are many family members in the waiting room who wander in and out of the ICU room, despite their being asked to remain in the waiting room. Their behavior is interfering with care. The nurse has identified the problem as ineffective family coping. The most appropriate response at this time would be to

   A. Establish visiting hours acceptable to staff and family.
   B. Allow the family to continue to enter the room.
   C. Ban all visiting until they have calmed down.
   D. Hold a family conference to explain the need for limited visitation.

Answers to Core Review Test 2

2–1. **(B)** ST depression indicates ischemia. T wave inversion is considered nonspecific without other ECG changes. Increased T wave amplitude and tachycardia are normal responses to exercise.

Reference: Reuther, M., and Hansen, C.: Cardiovascular Nursing. Medical Examination Publishing, New York, 1985.

2–2. **(D)** Ventilation, by definition, is the mass movement of gases by bulk flow in and out of the pulmonary system. The majority of ventilation (70%) is accomplished by diaphragmatic contraction.

Reference: West, J.B.: Respiratory Physiology: The Essentials, 3rd ed. Williams & Wilkins, Baltimore, 1990.

2–3. **(B)** Cerebrospinal fluid is reabsorbed into the arachnoid villi, which serve as channels for absorption and are projections from the subarachnoid space into the venous sinuses of the brain.

References: Alspach, J.G. (ed.): AACN Core Curriculum for Critical Care Nursing, 4th ed. W.B. Saunders, Philadelphia, 1991.
Hickey, J.V.: The Clinical Practice of Neurological and Neurosurgical Nursing, 2nd ed. J.B. Lippincott, Philadelphia, 1986.

2–4. **(A)** Intravascular hemolysis from transfusion reaction results in the release of free hemoglobin into the plasma, binding of hemoglobin to haptoglobin, and subsequent removal of the complex through hemoglobinuria. Later, a rise in serum bilirubin and possibly methemalbumin occurs. Renal tubules are susceptible to injury by high urinary levels of pigments (hemoglobinuria and myoglobinuria), especially in the setting of renal hypoperfusion and ischemia. Papillary necrosis and decreased cardiac output are prerenal causes of acute renal failure, and prostatic obstruction is a postrenal cause.

References: Grantham, J.J.: Acute renal failure. In Wyngaarden, J.B., and Smith, L.H. (eds.): Textbook of Medicine, 18th ed. W.B. Saunders, Philadelphia, 1988.
Norris, M.: Acute tubular necrosis: Preventing complications. Dimen Crit Care Nurs, *8*:16–26, 1989.

2–5. **(C)** One liter of fluid weighs approximately 2 pounds. Weight changes readily reflect a patient's fluid status as "ahead" or "behind" relative to fluid needs.

Reference: Swearingen, P.L., Sommers, M.S., and Miller, K.: Manual of Critical Care: Applying Nursing Diagnoses to Adult Critical Illness. C.V. Mosby, St. Louis, 1988.

2–6. **(C)** Systemic vascular resistance is the hemodynamic parameter that measures the resistance to the flow of blood from the left ventricle (afterload). CVP and LVEDP are measures of preload.

Reference: Bustin, D.: Hemodynamic Monitoring for Critical Care. Appleton-Century-Crofts, Norwalk, CT, 1986.

2–7. (**C**) For most near-drowning victims, matching the ventilation to perfusion by increasing the lung volumes and functional residual capacity is sufficient. Occasionally other therapy is indicated, such as barbiturate coma if hypothermia and prolonged submersion occurred. Antibiotic therapy may be needed at some point if pneumonia develops.

Reference: McKinley, M.G.: Near drowning: A nursing challenge. Crit Care Nurs, *9*:52–60, 1989.

2–8. (**A**) Systemic lupus erythematosus is an autoimmune disease affecting connective tissue. Renal "lupus nephritis" results from immune complex deposition and inflammation of glomerular basement membrane, and leads to glomerulosclerosis. Gentamicin, abdominal aortic aneurysm repair, and hemoglobinuria due to intravascular hemolysis may lead to renal failure by causing acute tubular necrosis.

References: Crandall, B.L.: Chronic renal failure. In Ulrich, B.T. (ed.): Nephrology Nursing: Concepts and Strategies. Appleton and Lange, Norwalk, CT, 1989.
Thompson, J., McFarland, G.K., Hirsch, J.E., et al.: Mosby's Manual of Clinical Nursing, 2nd ed. C.V. Mosby, St. Louis, 1989.

2–9. (**C**) A contrecoup effect occurs when a head injury is delivered at high speed. In addition to the contusions and hematomas at the site of the focal injury, the opposite side also becomes injured as a result of intracranial energy dissipation causing diffuse tearing of nerve fibers.

Reference: Hickey, J.V.: The Clinical Practice of Neurological and Neurosurgical Nursing, 2nd ed. J.B. Lippincott, Philadelphia, 1986.

2–10. (**A**) Making a treatment decision is the right of a competent, informed adult patient. The patient must understand the risks and benefits of the recommended treatment and other alternatives for the decision to be an informed one. Coercion may include failure to inform the patient of the available treatment options. Although the patient may wish to discuss the options with family members, he or she has no obligation to do so.

Reference: Douglas, S., and Larson, E.: There's more to informed consent than information. Focus Crit Care, *2*:43–47, 1986.

2–11. (**C**) This patient has carbon monoxide poisoning; carbon monoxide competes with oxygen to bind to hemoglobin. The pulse oximeter measures only how saturated the hemoglobin is, not what it is saturated with. It does not differentiate among oxyhemoglobin, carboxyhemoglobin, and methemoglobin.

Reference: Shapiro, B.A., Harrison, R.A., Cane, R.D., et al.: Clinical Application of Blood Gases, 4th ed. Year Book Medical Publishers, Chicago, 1989.

2–12. (**B**) Hypocalcemia prolongs the duration of both the ST segment and the QT interval.

Reference: Andreoli, K., Fowkes, V., Zipes, D., et al.: Comprehensive Cardiac Care, 6th ed. C.V. Mosby, St. Louis, 1987.

2–13. (**B**) Antacids (such as aluminum-based, magnesium-based, or combination preparations) act by binding with and neutralizing intraluminal hydrogen ions. H_2-receptor antagonists (such as cimetidine, ranitidine, or famotidine) suppress gastric acid secretion. Sucralfate (an anionic, sulfated disaccharide) forms a protective barrier over gastric and duodenal ulcer sites. Prostaglandins are thought to stimulate phospholipid formation in the gastric mucosal barrier.

References: Konopad, E., and Noseworthy, T.: Stress ulceration: A serious complication in critically ill patients. Heart Lung, *17*(4):339–348, 1988.
McEvoy, G.K., and McQuarrie, G.M. (eds.): Drug Information 89. American Society of Hospital Pharmacists, Bethesda, MD, 1989.

2–14. (**C**) Phenytoin, given for status epilepticus, is initially administered at the rate of 15 to 20 mg per kg given no faster than 50 mg per minute in adults and no faster than 3 mg per minute per kg in children. The maximum dose in a 24-hour period is 1 gm. Major side effects associated with phenytoin administration include disturbances in cardiac rhythm. Therefore, the ECG should be assessed particularly for a widening QT segment. If the QT segment widens, the drug should be stopped. Other side effects to observe for include prolonged PR intervals, depression of T waves, and hypotension. Phenytoin typically causes less sedation in large doses than does phenobarbital, another drug that may be administered.

Reference: Kinney, M.R., Packa, D.R., and Dunbar, S.B.: AACN's Clinical Reference for Critical Care Nursing, 2nd ed. McGraw-Hill, New York, 1988.

2–15. (**B**) Dilutional hyponatremia occurs when total body water and sodium are increased, but water is increased more than sodium. Treatment includes diuretics and fluid restriction to decrease the fluid volume.

Reference: Barta, M.: Correcting electrolyte imbalances. RN, *50*(2):30–34, 1987.

2–16. (**B**) The patient has a normal MAP and elevated filling pressures. These findings, associated with a low hematocrit, indicate a hypervolemic state possibly induced by fluid administration during the resuscitation process. Administration of furosemide would reduce the fluid volume by diuresis, thus increasing the hematocrit and lowering the PCWP and CVP. Dopamine infusion at 10 μg/kg/minute and infusion of blood products would increase the PCWP and CVP further.

Reference: Daily, E., and Schroeder, J.: Techniques in Bedside Hemodynamic Monitoring, 3rd ed. C.V. Mosby, St. Louis, 1985.

2–17. (**A**) During the inflammatory response, WBCs are attracted to the site of injury through a process known as chemotaxis. The cells then move through the vascular walls. This is known as emigration. The cells then engulf and destroy, or opsonize, and phagocytize the organism. Agglutination occurs when there are changes in the cell surface that result in the cells' sticking together.

Reference: Alspach, J.G. (ed.): AACN Core Curriculum for Critical Care Nursing, 4th ed. W.B. Saunders, Philadelphia, 1991.

2–18. (**D**) Autoregulation is the brain's ability to maintain a constant rate of blood flow over a wide range of perfusion pressures despite changes in arterial and intracranial pressures. Hyperemia is the perfusion of blood over and above the brain's metabolic needs. Posttraumatic water retention in the neurotrauma patient is a response to injury and stress as the result of hypothalamic stimulation of the antidiuretic hormone (ADH), also known as arginine vasopressin (AVP).

Reference: Cardona, V.D., Hurn, P.D., Mason, P.J.B., et al.: Trauma Nursing: From Resuscitation Through Rehabilitation. W.B. Saunders, Philadelphia, 1988.

2–19. (**B**) Arterial hypoxemia, whether due to cardiac or pulmonary disease, produces widening and thickening of the terminal phalanges of the fingers and toes, as well as convex nails.

Reference: Braunwald, E., Isselbacher, K.J., Petersdorf, R.G., et al. (eds.): Harrison's Principles of Internal Medicine, 11th ed. McGraw-Hill, New York, 1987.

2–20. (**D**) Reperfusion causes CPK levels to peak early and reach higher levels than in acute myocardial infarction where t-PA is not used. The CPK level decreases more quickly after the peak owing to washout during reperfusion.

Reference: Ventura, B.: Thrombolytic therapy for MI. Am J Nurs, *87*:631–640, 1987.

2–21. (**B**) The easiest and most frequently used ventilators are volume-cycled. The others are more complicated and require close monitoring for patient safety.

Reference: Kinney, M.R., Packa, D.R., and Dunbar, S.B.: AACN's Clinical Reference for Critical Care Nursing, 2nd ed. McGraw-Hill, New York, 1988.

2–22. (**B**) Barbiturate coma therapy is used as an adjunctive therapy in the treatment of increased intracranial pressure. A barbiturate such as pentobarbital or thiopental, given by intravenous infusion, is used as a CNS depressant, thus decreasing cerebral metabolic need for oxygen and glucose by as much as 50%. The decreased metabolic rate decreases cerebral blood flow, thus reducing intracranial pressure (ICP). During barbiturate therapy, movement, kreflexes, pupillary response, and smooth muscle tone are absent. The patient must be intubated and on a ventilator.

Reference: Hickey, J.V.: The Clinical Practice of Neurological and Neurosurgical Nursing. J.B. Lippincott, Philadelphia, 1986.

2–23. (**B**) Surgical creation of a temporary ileostomy is indicated in Crohn's disease with regional ileitis and symptomatic fistulas in order to rest the diseased bowel so that tissue healing can occur. This is a high-risk procedure in the critically ill patient. Diverticulitis may be treated with a transverse colostomy. A superior mesenteric artery embolus may be treated with a mesenteric embolectomy. Pyloroplasty and vagotomy are often used to treat a duodenal ulcer.

Reference: Johanson, B.C., Wells, S.J., Hoffmeister, D., et al.: Standards for Critical Care, 3rd ed. C.V. Mosby, St. Louis, 1988.

2–24. (**B**) Atropine is the medication of choice to treat symptomatic bradycardias. The initial dose is 0.5 mg and it may be repeated until a 2.0-mg total has been administered. In this example the QRS duration is 0.12 second and the heart rate is 40, indicating supraventricular origin of the QRS. Atropine improves atrioventricular conduction via its vagolytic action and may restore sinus rhythm. In third degree AV block as demonstrated, temporary pacemaker insertion may be necessary if atropine has been ineffective in restoring the rhythm and the patient remains hypotensive. Isoproterenol is generally infused at a rate of 2 to 10 μg/minute until a temporary pacemaker can be inserted. Lidocaine is not indicated in third degree AV block nor in any bradycardia, since it may suppress the escape rhythm producing asystole.

Reference: American Heart Association: Textbook of Advanced Cardiac Life Support. Dallas, 1987.

2–25. (**C**) DI is an uncommon disease characterized by passage of copious amounts of dilute urine and increased thirst. It is due primarily to impairment of the posterior pituitary or supraoptic pathways that regulate water metabolism. Water metabolism is regulated by the ADH produced in these areas.

Reference: Hartshorn, J., and Hartshorn, E.: Pharmacology update: Vasopressin in the treatment of diabetes insipidus. J Neurosci Nurs, *20*(1):58–59, 1988.

2–26. (**A**) As the concentration of vasopressin increases, there will be an increase in water reabsorption by the distal tubules and collecting systems, causing a decrease in water excretion. Vasopressin causes an increased contraction of smooth muscle of the vasculature, resulting in vasoconstriction and decreased blood flow to the coronary, GI, and splanchnic beds. Blood flow is also decreased to the pancreas, muscles, and skin.

Reference: Hartshorn, J., and Hartshorn, E.: Pharmacology update: Vasopressin in the treatment of diabetes insipidus. J Neurosci Nurs, *20*(1):58–59, 1988.

2–27. (**A**) The sympathomimetics stimulate the adrenergic nerves for adrenal release of epinephrine and norepinephrine. These hormones produce the so-called flight or fight sympathetic response. In addition to relaxing the bronchi, they also cause pupillary dilatation, tachycardia, hypertension, skin pallor, and decreased gastric motility.

Reference: Kersten, L.D.: Comprehensive Respiratory Nursing: A Decision Making Approach. W.B. Saunders, Philadelphia, 1989.

2–28. (**C**) Spontaneous inspiration depresses the waveform and mechanical ventilation elevates the wedge waveform during delivery of a mechanical breath. Discontinuing mechanical ventilation can induce rebound hypervolemia and false elevation of the pulmonary capillary wedge pressure.

Reference: Campbell, M., and Greenberg, C.: Reading pulmonary artery wedge pressures at end expiration. Focus Crit Care, 15:60–63, 1988.

2–29. (**D**) "Myxedema madness" is an acute organic psychosis. It may manifest as paranoia, delusions, schizophrenia, or mania.

Reference: Muthe, N.C.: Endocrinology, A Nursing Approach. Little, Brown, Boston, 1981.

2–30. (**A**) Hypercapnia leads to vasodilation, thereby increasing cerebral blood flow and increasing intracranial pressure. The patient should not be encouraged to cough vigorously because this raises the intracranial pressure. An intact autoregulation mechanism provides compensation for sharp fluctuation in intracranial pressure that might occur during coughing or sneezing. Packing gauze firmly in the nares or ears in the presence of CSF rhinorrhea or CSF otorrhea, respectively, is contraindicated. In addition, suctioning nasotracheally is contraindicated, since suctioning may cause further trauma.

Reference: Cardona, V.D., Hurn, P.D., Mason, P.J.B., et al.: Trauma Nursing: From Resuscitation Through Rehabilitation. W.B. Saunders, Philadelphia, 1988.

2–31. (**B**) Serum albumin, a plasma protein, accounts for a significant amount of calcium binding. The serum albumin level is an indicator of the blood's ionized calcium level. Because 50% of the plasma calcium is a protein-bound fraction, any change in the serum albumin leads to a change in calcium.

Reference: Chambers, J.K.: Metabolic bone disorders: imbalances of calcium and phosphorus. Nurs Clin North Am, 22:861–872, 1987.

2–32. (**C**) Adequate hydration is essential to prevent mucus plugs and secretions from blocking airways.

Reference: Kersten, L.D.: Comprehensive Respiratory Nursing: A Decision Making Approach. W.B. Saunders, Philadelphia, 1989.

2–33. (**A**) Human leukocyte antigens (HLAs) are found on the surface of leukocytes or WBCs. HLA testing is performed to identify tissue compatibility for organ transplants.

Reference: Alspach, J.G. (ed.): AACN Core Curriculum for Critical Care Nursing, 4th ed. W.B. Saunders, Philadelphia, 1991.

2–34. (**D**) Obstructive symptoms are frequently seen in tumors of the left colon, descending colon, and rectum owing to the smaller size of the lumen and firm quality of the feces. Weight loss, anemia, and dyspepsia are more commonly associated with tumors in the right colon, because lesions in the right colon ulcerate rather than obstruct owing to the larger lumen and liquid nature of the feces.

Reference: Luckmann, J., and Sorensen, K.C.: Medical-Surgical Nursing: A Psychophysiologic Approach, 3rd ed. W.B. Saunders, Philadelphia, 1987.

2–35. (**D**) The aminophylline-isoproterenol (Isuprel) regimen, which acts on enzymes active in vasomotor contraction, is used following initial bleeding. Serotonin antagonists such as reserpine (Serpasil) are used to reduce the serotonin levels, which are thought by some to contribute to vasospasm. Calcium channel blockers such as nifedipine reduce the influx of calcium into the cell, thus reducing vasospasm caused by increased intracellular calcium levels. Anticholinesterase drugs are used to treat myasthenia gravis.

Reference: Hickey, J.V.: The Clinical Practice of Neurological and Neurosurgical Nursing, 2nd ed. J.B. Lippincott, Philadelphia, 1986.

2–36. (**D**) Phases 0, 1, and 2 of the action potential together are termed the "absolute refractory period" because the cell cannot be stimulated to produce another action potential. During Phases 3 and 4 the cells may be stimulated to produce another action potential by a very strong stimulus. This period is called the "relative refractory period."

Reference: Kenner, C., Guzzetta, C., and Dossey, B.: Critical Care Nursing: Body—Mind—Spirit. Little, Brown, Boston, 1985.

2–37. (**C**) As the respiratory muscles fatigue, alveolar ventilation decreases. This results in an increased Pa_{CO_2}, dyspnea, increased respiratory rate, and use of accessory muscles.

Reference: Alspach, J.G. (ed.): AACN Core Curriculum for Critical Care Nursing, 4th ed. W.B. Saunders, Philadelphia, 1991.

2–38. (**D**) Hypermagnesemia responds, at least transiently, to IV calcium. Calcium chloride directly antagonizes the effects of hypermagnesemia. Removal of magnesium can be accomplished by other treatments. Patients with adequate urine output and renal function may be treated with IV normal saline infusions and furosemide to promote diuresis of magnesium.

Reference: Janson, C.L.: Fluid and electrolyte balance. In Rosen, P.: Emergency Medicine: Concepts and Practice. C.V. Mosby, St. Louis, 1988.

2–39. (**D**) Cerebellopontine tumors, also called acoustic neuromas, arise from the Schwann cells of the eighth cranial nerve at the junction of the cerebellum and the pons. This tumor affects the function of cranial nerves V, VII, VIII, IX, and X.

Reference: Alspach, J.G. (ed.): AACN Core Curriculum for Critical Care Nursing, 4th ed. W.B. Saunders, Philadelphia, 1991.

2–40. (**B**) The right coronary artery supplies the SA node in 50% to 60% of hearts and the atrioventricular (AV) node in 90% of hearts; 41% to 45% of hearts have a branch of the circumflex that supplies the SA node.

Reference: Kenner, C., Guzzetta, C., and Dossey, B.: Critical Care Nursing: Body—Mind—Spirit. Little, Brown, Boston, 1985.

2–41. (**A**) ECG changes associated with anterior wall myocardial infarction (MI) occur in leads V_1 through V_6 and are caused by occlusion of the left anterior descending artery (LAD) or its tributaries. Occlusion of the circumflex artery causes changes in leads I and aV_L, indicating lateral wall infarction. Occlusion of the right coronary artery causes changes in leads II, III and aV_F, indicating inferior wall MI. The ECG changes that indicate Prinzmetal's angina are ST segment elevations without Q waves.

Reference: Andreoli, K., Fowkes, V., Zipes, D., et al.: Comprehensive Cardiac Care, 6th ed. C.V. Mosby, St. Louis, 1987.

2–42. (**C**) Inflammation is a sequential series of events that results in neutralization of an invading organism and sets the stage for tissue repair and healing. Chemical mediators such as histamine, serotonin, and bradykinins cause changes in capillary permeability. Neutrophils, monocytes, and leukocytes engulf and phagocytize the invading organism at the site of injury.

Reference: Alspach J.G. (ed.): AACN Core Curriculum for Critical Care Nursing, 4th ed. W.B. Saunders, Philadelphia, 1991.

2–43. (**B**) The increasing temperature, decreased Sa_{O_2}, and increased sputum production with a change in color indicates pneumonia. The color change suggests that the pneumonia is probably from Pseudomonas, which is frequently the organism of infection after head injury.

Reference: Kersten, L.D.: Comprehensive Respiratory Nursing: A Decision Making Approach. W.B. Saunders, Philadelphia, 1989.

2–44. (**B**) Sputum cultures should be sent right away so that a broad-spectrum antibiotic can be started.

Reference: Kersten, L.D.: Comprehensive Respiratory Nursing: A Decision Making Approach. W.B. Saunders, Philadelphia, 1989.

2–45. (**B**) There are multiple problems related to sexual functioning in patients with renal failure, including hormonal abnormalities, psychological problems, anemia, hypertension, medications that affect sexual function, and malnutrition. Hemodialysis may result in some improvement; however, the only treatment modality that may result in major improvements or even in normalization of sexual functioning is renal transplantation. In males, testosterone secretion is markedly decreased in renal insufficiency. In addition, there appears to be end-organ resistance to follicle-stimulating hormone, resulting in a marked decrease in spermatogenesis. Psychological factors such as dependency and loss of status within the family contribute to the incidence of impotence.

In females, ovarian hormone secretion is suppressed in renal failure. Although plasma estrogen and progesterone levels may be in the low normal range, they are abnormally low given the high levels of luteinizing hormone in these women. Ovulation is rare, and the incidence of amenorrhea and infertility is high.

Reference: Crandall, B.L.: Chronic renal failure. In Ulrich, B.T. (ed.): Nephrology Nursing: Concepts and Strategies. Appleton and Lange, Norwalk, CT, 1989.

2–46. (**C**) The major goal in protecting the seizure patient against injury is to maintain an adequate airway. Placing the patient in a lateral position assists in preventing aspiration. Current treatment of seizures no longer includes the use of padded tongue blades during a seizure to prevent injury to teeth. Restraints should be loosened during a seizure.

Reference: Kinney, M.R., Packa, D.R., and Dunbar, S.B.: AACN's Clinical Reference for Critical Care Nursing, 2nd ed. McGraw-Hill, New York, 1988.

2–47. (**C**) Concomitant administration of tube feedings with antibiotics exacerbates the problem of diarrhea in these patients. Aplastic anemia is an adverse effect of administration of chloramphenicol. Liver toxicity is associated with erythromycins and antitubercular drugs such as isoniazid (INH). Gentamicin and cefoxitin are associated with nephrotoxicity and neuromuscular blockade. Peripheral neuritis is associated with INH.

References: Farley, J.M.: Current trends in enteral feeding. Crit Care Nurs, 8(4):23–27, 1989.
McEvoy, G.K., and McQuarrie, G.M. (eds.): Drug Information 89. American Society of Hospital Pharmacists, Bethesda, MD, 1989.

2–48. (**D**) In anterior infarction, the onset of second degree AV block is an indication for pacemaker insertion because third degree AV block may follow abruptly. Second degree AV block of the Mobitz II variety is associated with bradycardia and potential significant decreases in cardiac output.

Reference: American Heart Association: Textbook of Advanced Cardiac Life Support. Dallas, 1987.

2–49. (**D**) The patient is in ventricular fibrillation and must be defibrillated before the electrical stimulus of the pacemaker can be effective.

Reference: Kenner, C., Guzzetta, C., and Dossey, B.: Critical Care Nursing: Body—Mind—Spirit. Little, Brown, Boston, 1985.

2–50. (**A**) The A-a gradient indicates how well oxygen diffuses from the alveolus (A) to arterial (a) blood. The smaller the gradient, the more efficient the gas exchange is. Normal values have not been established for an A-a gradient other than at 21% and 100% oxygen. However, the marked increase in the A-a gradient indicates that the lung's ability to exchange gases is being impaired.

Reference: West, J.B.: Respiratory Physiology: The Essentials, 3rd ed. Williams & Wilkins, Baltimore, 1985.

2–51. (**B**) The most forceful drive to breathe is hypercarbia. In COPD, the chronically elevated arterial CO_2 eventually equalizes across to the brain, and this drive becomes ineffective. The primary respiratory drive then is hypoxia. If this drive is also eliminated by elevating the oxygen level, the drive to breathe decreases, and carbon dioxide is retained, resulting in respiratory acidosis.

Reference: Kersten, L.D.: Comprehensive Respiratory Nursing: A Decision Making Approach. W.B. Saunders, Philadelphia, 1989.

2–52. (**D**) Licorice contains an extract of *Glycyrrhiza glabra* root and causes hypokalemia by increasing renal potassium losses.

References: Bigelow, L.A.: Fluids, electrolytes and hemodynamics. In Fincke, M., and Lanros, N.: Emergency Nursing: A Comprehensive Review. Aspen, Rockville, MD, 1986.
Schwartz, M.W.: Potassium imbalances. Am J Nurs, *87*:1292–1299, 1987.

2–53. (**C**) Atropine, an anticholinergic, is the antidote for overdosage of anticholinesterase medications and must be kept in close proximity to the patient. Protamine sulfate is the antagonist for heparin. Neostigmine and Tensilon are anticholinesterase medications used in the treatment of myasthenia gravis.

Reference: Hickey, J.V.: The Clinical Practice of Neurological and Neurosurgical Nursing, 2nd ed. J.B. Lippincott, Philadelphia, 1986.

2–54. (**A**) Medication protocols for the patient with myasthenia gravis are highly individual. However, most patients are treated with anticholinesterase medications and sometimes corticosteroids. Two of the more common anticholinesterase medications are neostigmine (Prostigmin) and pyridostigmine (Mestinon). These drugs enhance cholinergic activity by facilitating transmission of nerve impulses across the myoneural junction. Atropine, an anticholinergic, is the antidote for anticholinesterase medications.

Reference: Hickey, J.V.: The Clinical Practice of Neurological and Neurosurgical Nursing, 2nd ed. J.B. Lippincott, Philadelphia, 1986.

2–55. (**C**) Encouraging the patient to discuss his or her wishes with the physician before an emergency situation arises eliminates the problem of determining whether a person who is critically ill and perhaps receiving mind-altering drugs can make a competent decision. It also gives the person the opportunity to discuss the decision with significant others, if he or she wishes. It would be helpful to know at the time of admission whether a patient had signed a Living Will, but this is probably a poor time to suggest that it be done, if it has not already been discussed. People who are elderly or suffering from a fatal disease should still have the option of receiving advanced care if they desire and if the means are available.

Reference: Younger, S.J.: Do-Not-Resuscitate orders: No longer a secret, but still a problem. Hastings Center Report, *1*:24–33, 1987.

2–56. (**B**) Bile pigments give feces a brown color and their absence produces a clay-colored stool. This is an important assessment finding in cholelithiasis, cholecystitis, and cancer of the biliary tract. Upper GI bleeding usually causes tarry stool. Megadose iron supplementation causes black stool. An eroding pancreatic tumor produces a characteristic silver-colored stool.

Reference: Ganong, W.F.: Review of Medical Physiology, 13th ed. Appleton and Lange, Norwalk, CT, 1987.
Meyers, A.R.: Medicine. John Wiley and Sons, New York, 1986.

2–57. (**B**) D5LR at 200 ml per hour is the most appropriate fluid regime. Although the patient received 4 l of fluid in the operating room, his CVP and PAD are relatively low. Also, as this patient warms, his BP and filling pressures will decrease with vasodilation. The Hct at 28% before a unit of blood can be expected to increase to about 32% after blood administration.

Reference: Fahey, V.: Vascular Nursing. W.B. Saunders, Philadelphia, 1988.

2–58. (**B**) is the most appropriate answer. Furosemide would increase urine output but further decrease BP, PAD, and CVP. The Hct is normal. Elevating the patient's legs would increase BP only slightly and may disrupt the graft. Dopamine would dilate the renal and mesenteric arteries and improve urine output and blood pressure.

Reference: Fahey, V.: Vascular Nursing. W.B. Saunders, Philadelphia, 1988.

2–59. (**D**) Aldosterone increases sodium reabsorption and potassium and hydrogen ion secretion in the distal tubular epithelial cells of the kidney. As a consequence of sodium reabsorption, intravascular volume is expanded. Aldosterone deficiency results in hyponatremia, hyperkalemia, and orthostatic hypotension. Hypoglycemia results from glucocorticoid deficiency. This patient's depression is most likely situational.

Reference: Kohler, P.O., and Jordan, R.M. (eds.): Clinical Endocrinology. John Wiley and Sons, New York, 1986.

2–60. (**B**) Fluid volume deficit related to aldosterone deficiency; impaired physical mobility related to fatigue, weakness, and postural dizziness; and potential for dysrhythmia related to hyperkalemia are appropriate nursing diagnoses for this patient. Weight loss, orthostatic hypotension, tachycardia, and azotemia are associated with fluid volume deficit. Weakness, fatigue, and orthostatic hypotension are associated with impaired physical mobility. Finally, dysrhythmias can be induced by hyperkalemia. Hyperpigmentation is a result of melanocyte stimulation and does not disrupt tissue integrity.

Reference: McLane, A.M. (ed.): Classification of Nursing Diagnoses, Proceedings of the Seventh Conference. C.V. Mosby, St. Louis, 1987.

2–61. **(A)** Calcium is essential for the normal depolarization of nerve, smooth muscle, and myocardial cells. Calcium is also responsible for release of acetylcholine, and magnesium decreases or blocks this release. Magnesium is the fourth most abundant cation in the body and the second most abundant intracellular cation. The magnesium ion functions as a cofactor in almost all aspects of cellular metabolism. It is necessary for DNA and protein synthesis. Nearly all enzymes involved in phosphorus reactions, including membrane ATP, and those in which thiamine pyrophosphate is a cofactor, depend on magnesium for activation. It serves as a stabilizer of RNA, DNA, and ribosomal molecular structures, and is required for glycolysis and oxidative phosphorylation.

Reference: Janson, C.L.: Fluid and electrolyte balance. In Rosen, P.: Emergency Medicine: Concepts and Practice. C.V. Mosby, St. Louis, 1988.

2–62. **(A)** The balloon must remain inflated throughout the respiratory cycle to obtain a correct value. The wedge readings are generally taken a minimum of once in each 8 hours as part of the assessment of the patient and more frequently with changes in the patient's condition.

Reference: Weeks, L.: Advanced Cardiovascular Nursing. Blackwell, Boston, 1986.

2–63. **(B)** The high level of oxygen therapy for this patient will increase the Pa_{O_2}, thus eliminating the hypoxic drive. This will further depress her respirations, leading to respiratory acidosis and decreased pH.

Reference: West, J.B.: Respiratory Physiology: The Essentials, 4th ed. Williams & Wilkins, Baltimore, 1990.

2–64. **(B)** Low flow devices do not deliver the total inspired gas, so the FI_{O_2} will change with tidal volume, respiratory rate, and ventilatory pattern. High flow systems are generally more complicated to use and can deliver both high and low FI_{O_2} levels.

Reference: Alspach, J.G. (ed.): AACN Core Curriculum for Critical Care Nursing, 4th ed. W.B. Saunders, Philadelphia, 1991.

2–65. **(B)** Cholesterol is the precursor hormone for the biosynthesis of all gonadal and adrenal hormones. It is a sterol containing 27 carbon atoms.

Reference: Hadley, M.E.: Endocrinology, 2nd ed. Prentice-Hall, Englewood Cliffs, NJ, 1988.

2–66. **(B)** Coumadin acts on the extrinsic clotting system. PT is used to evaluate the effectiveness of a Coumadin dose. PTT is used to monitor the intrinsic clotting system. Fibrin split products are produced as a fibrin clot breaks down; they are useful in identifying excess clot lysis. Fibrinogen levels are used to assess whether adequate amounts of fibrin are present for a clot to form.

Reference: Alspach J.G. (ed.): AACN Core Curriculum for Critical Care Nursing, 4th ed. W.B. Saunders, Philadelphia, 1991.

2–67. **(C)** Paralysis of the abdominal and intercostal muscles leads to an ineffective cough and retention of secretions. Also, hypoventilation, shallow tidal respirations, and decreased vital capacity all predispose GBS patients to respiratory failure.

Reference: Alspach, J. G. (ed.): AACN Core Curriculum for Critical Care Nursing, 4th ed. W.B. Saunders, Philadelphia, 1991.

2–68. **(B)** The five stages of psychological grieving that are usually experienced by a dying or grieving individual, according to Kubler-Ross, are: *denial,* characterized by an attempt to delay the shock and pain of the diagnosis or event until the individual is better able to deal with the reality of the situation; *anger* and *rage* regarding the unfairness of the diagnosis; *bargaining,* in an attempt to postpone dying until certain tasks are complete and to provide a means for the patient to deal with the situation gradually; *depression,* with the realization that many losses are now imminent; and *acceptance*, a time of acknowledgment and recognition that death is inevitable.

Reference: Caine, R.M., and Bufalino, P.M.: Critically Ill Adults: Nursing Care Planning Guides. Williams & Wilkins, Baltimore, 1988.

2–69. (**D**) Phosphate therapy decreases serum calcium by binding calcium and carrying it to excretion, but may result in the deposit of calcium in the kidney, leading to renal calculi. Edetate disodium (EDTA) and plicamycin (Mithramycin) prevent calcium reabsorption from bones into serum. Sodium bicarbonate may lessen the effects of hypercalcemia by creating metabolic alkalosis and restoring membrane potential.

References: Calloway, C.: When the problem involves magnesium, calcium, or phosphate. RN, *50*:30–36, 1987.
Chambers, J.K.: Metabolic bone disorders: imbalances of calcium and phosphorus. Nurs Clin North Am, *22*:861–872, 1987.

2–70. (**B**) Bleeding esophageal varices can lead to dramatic hemorrhage and subsequent loss of circulating blood volume. This is compounded by thrombocytopenia and clotting disorders. Profound hypovolemia with hypoxemia is life-threatening and has negative consequences for all organ systems. Restoration of circulating volume and stopping the bleeding are the primary objectives for these patients.

Reference: Swearingen, P.L., Sommers, M.S., and Miller, K.: Manual of Critical Care: Applying Nursing Diagnoses to Adult Critical Illness. C.V. Mosby, St. Louis, 1988.

2–71. (**D**) Bleeding esophageal varices are usually treated with infusion of intravenous vasopressin (antidiuretic hormone). Vasopressin reduces portal venous pressure by direct stimulation of smooth muscle contraction of small arterioles. This results in reduced blood flow to the splanchnic, coronary, gastrointestinal, pancreatic, skin, and muscular systems. Oxytocin stimulates contraction of uterine smooth muscle and is not used to treat bleeding varices. The similarity of the trade names Pitocin and Pitressin should be noted to avoid error. Corticotropin is also a pituitary hormone but its anti-inflammatory effects are not useful in bleeding varices. Heparin would exacerbate the bleeding.

Reference: DeGroot, K.D., and Damato, M.B.: Critical Care Skills. Appleton and Lange, Norwalk, CT, 1987.

2–72. (**C**) Right ventricular infarction may cause right heart failure with associated symptoms of venous congestion. Right ventricular ejection (stroke volume) is decreased, as is atrial ejection; therefore an S_4 is not heard. Rales are a symptom of left heart failure.

Reference: Sommers, M., and Russel, A.: Location of myocardial infarction: assessing the patients' response. Dimen Crit Care Nurs, *3*:8–15, 1984.

2–73. (**D**) Since the jugular veins empty into the vena cava, they show symptoms of right ventricular failure earlier than veins of the portal and peripheral circulation, which are more distant from the heart. Rales are a sign of left ventricular failure.

Reference: Weeks, L.: Advanced Cardiovascular Nursing. Blackwell, Boston, 1986.

2–74. (**A**) Acidosis, elevated CO_2, elevated temperature, and increased 2,3, DPG cause a shift of the oxyhemoglobin dissociation curve to the right, which results in a lower oxygen content at any given P_{O_2}. The oxygen binds loosely to hemoglobin.

Reference: Shapiro, B.A., Harrison, R.A., Cane, R.D., et al.: Clinical Application of Blood Gases, 4th ed. Year Book Medical Publishers, Chicago, 1989.

2–75. (**C**) Steroids decrease the mobility of monocytes, decreasing their function and predisposing the patient to infection.

Reference: Alspach, J.G. (ed.): AACN Core Curriculum for Critical Care Nursing, 4th ed. W.B. Saunders, Philadelphia, 1991.

2–76. (**D**) With decreased venous return to the thorax, stretch receptors in the left atrium sense a decrease in volume and send stimulatory impulses up the vagus nerve to the reticular formation of the midbrain, and, finally, to the supraoptic nuclei. The result is an increase in the release of ADH.

Reference: Kohler, P.O., and Jordan, R.M. (eds.): Clinical Endocrinology. John Wiley and Sons, New York, 1986.

2–77. (**C**) Normal serum ammonia is less than 50 µg/dl. Neomycin is a nonabsorbable antibiotic that is administered orally, by nasogastric tube, or by rectal enema to reduce intestinal bacteria that produce ammonia. It is reserved for acute situations owing to its nephrotoxicity and ototoxicity. Chloramphenicol, hydrochlorothiazide, and rifampin would not be indicated because these drugs are hepatotoxic.

Reference: Swearingen, P.L., Sommers, M.S., and Miller, K.: Manual of Critical Care: Application of Nursing Diagnoses to Adult Critical Illness. C.V. Mosby, St. Louis, 1988.

2–78. (**C**) In the patient with subarachnoid hemorrhage, fluids are generally limited; however, it must be emphasized that dehydration should also be avoided. If she is experiencing vasospasm associated with the SAH, it will be treated with hypervolemia. The patient should be placed in a controlled environment, which includes a single quiet, nonstimulating room to keep the patient calm and the BP from rising related to sensory overload. The patient should avoid direct or harsh artificial light particularly if she is experiencing photophobia. While it is important to protect her against injury, restraints are to be avoided.

Reference: Alspach, J.G. (ed.): AACN Core Curriculum for Critical Care Nursing, 4th ed. W.B. Saunders, Philadelphia, 1991.

2–79. (**C**) Enemas are contraindicated for patients with subarachnoid hemorrhage because they increase intraabdominal pressure, thus increasing intracranial pressure. Patients must be cautioned against the Valsalva maneuver, which also increases intracranial pressure. Television, radio, and reading are prohibited. Because the patient is on strict bedrest, antiembolic stockings are indicated. The head of the bed is elevated to promote venous outflow.

Reference: Hickey, J.V.: The Clinical Practice of Neurological and Neurosurgical Nursing, 2nd ed. J.B. Lippincott, Philadelphia, 1986.

2–80. (**A**) With the exception of calcium, the electrolyte composition of the ultrafiltrate equals the electrolyte composition of the blood. Because 41% of calcium is bound to plasma proteins and does not pass across the hemofilter membrane, lower levels of calcium will be found in the ultrafiltrate. As a result of minimal calcium loss in the ultrafiltrate, hypocalcemia occurs infrequently with continuous arteriovenous hemofiltration.

References: Kiely, M.: Continuous arteriovenous hemofiltration. Crit Care Nurs, *4*:39–49, 1984.
Palmer, C., Koorejian, K., London, J., et al.: Nursing management of continuous arteriovenous hemofiltration for acute renal failure. Focus Crit Care, *13*:21–30, 1986.
Price, C.: Continuous arteriovenous ultrafiltration: A monitoring guide for ICU nurses. Crit Care Nurs, *9*:12–19, 1989.

2–81. (**C**) This patient has been receiving toxic levels of nitroprusside for 3 days. A metabolite of nitroprusside is thiocyanate, a form of cyanide, which causes cellular hypoxia when oxygen is bound to hemoglobin molecules and not released to tissues. One of the early symptoms is altered mental status from cerebral hypoxia. Placing the patient in restraints may increase his agitation. Arterial blood gas studies would not show cerebral hypoxia in thiocyanate toxicity.

Reference: Weeks, L.: Advanced Cardiovascular Nursing. Blackwell, Boston, 1986.

2–82. (**C**) Papilledema, sclerosis, hemorrhages, and exudates are common with malignant hypertension and hypertensive encephalopathy, which may occur when the diastolic BP rises above 140 mm Hg. The integrity of the retinal vessels and the optic nerve may not be known until acute changes and edema resolve.

Reference: Underhill, S., Woods, S., Froelicher, E., et al.: Cardiac Nursing, 2nd ed. J.B. Lippincott, Philadelphia, 1989.

2–83. **(B)** There is a risk of damaging or destroying the parathyroid glands during a thyroidectomy. In the absence of parathyroid hormone, osteoclastic activity is not activated and serum calcium regulation is lost. As a result, hypocalcemia develops.

Reference: Kohler, P.O., and Jordan, R.M. (eds.): Clinical Endocrinology. John Wiley and Sons, New York, 1986.

2–84. **(A)** The erythrocyte sedimentation rate (ESR) or "sed rate" is a nonspecific, general test which measures how rapidly RBCs settle to the bottom of a container in 1 hour. The ESR is elevated in acute or chronic inflammation, malignancy, myocardial infarction, or end-stage renal disease.

Reference: Alspach J.G. (ed.): AACN Core Curriculum for Critical Care Nursing, 4th ed. W.B. Saunders, Philadelphia, 1991.

2–85. **(B)** The weight loss, smoking history, and hemoptysis are indicative of lung cancer.

Reference: Kersten, L.D.: Comprehensive Respiratory Nursing: A Decision Making Approach. W.B. Saunders, Philadelphia, 1989.

2–86. **(D)** He will most likely have a lobectomy to resect the tumor, unless it is determined to be unresectable by scalene node biopsy.

Reference: Kersten, L.D.: Comprehensive Respiratory Nursing: A Decision Making Approach. W.B. Saunders, Philadelphia, 1989.

2–87. **(C)** The hypothalamus forms the ventral portion of the diencephalon. Overall control of the autonomic nervous system rests with the hypothalamus. Its functions include rgulation of temperature, food and water intake, behavior, autonomic response, and secretion of the pituitary gland. The posterior pituitary is the neurohypophysis, and the anterior pituitary is the adenohypophysis. The thalamus forms the lateral walls of the third ventricle, receives sensory input, and participates in the affective portion of brain function.

Reference: Alspach J.G. (ed.): AACN Core Curriculum for Critical Care Nursing, 4th ed. W.B. Saunders, Philadelphia, 1991.

2–88. **(D)** As *respondeat superior*, the nurse's employer can be held liable for his or her negligence even though the institution has met its own obligation to hire qualified personnel, write proper policies, provide adequate staffing, and maintain appropriate supervision. This allows a plaintiff the opportunity to seek compensation for injury from a "deep pocket" and perhaps receive a more generous settlement.

Reference: Rahn, J.G.: General theories of hospital liability for negligence. Focus Crit Care, 2:48–49, 1986.

2–89. **(A)** Epigastric pain is the first and most prominent symptom in 95% of cases of acute pancreatitis. Nausea with vomiting is the second most common symptom. The most common cause of acute pancreatitis is a biliary tract disorder such as partial bile duct obstruction from gallstones. The diagnosis is confirmed by elevated serum amylase and lipase levels. Pancreatitis may be associated with hepatic failure, but the patient has no signs of liver disease. Acute pancreatitis is often mistaken for myocardial infarction in cardiac patients until amylase and lipase levels are known. Amylase and lipase elevations are considered direct evidence of pancreatitis.

Reference: Fain, J.A., and Amato-Vealey, E.: Acute pancreatitis: A gastrointestinal emergency. Crit Care Nurs, 8(5):47–64, 1989.

2–90. **(C)** COPD results in increased pulmonary artery pressures. These increased pressures over time produce right heart failure (cor pulmonale), which is manifested by the clinical signs described above.

Reference: Kersten, L.D.: Comprehensive Respiratory Nursing: A Decision Making Approach. W.B. Saunders, Philadelphia, 1989.

2–91. **(D)** The QT interval is rate-dependent and reflects the amount of time required for complete depolarization and repolarization of the ventricles. Its duration should be less than one-half of that for the R-R interval.

Reference: Wharton, J., and Goldschlager, N.: Guide to Interpreting 12-Lead ECGs. Medical Economics, Oradell, NJ, 1984.

2–92. (**A**) This rhythm strip shows the characteristic lengthening of the PR interval followed by a blocked beat, which is characteristic of Wenckebach rhythms.

Reference: Andreoli, K., Fowkes, V., Zipes, D., et al.: Comprehensive Cardiac Care, 6th ed. C.V. Mosby, St. Louis, 1987.

2–93. (**D**) All of these interventions are used in the emergency treatment of hyperkalemia. Insulin increases the permeability of the cell membrane, resulting in a shift of potassium into the intracellular space. Dextrose is necessary to prevent hypoglycemia. $NaHCO_3$ corrects acidosis and aids in movement of potassium by exchanging potassium for hydrogen ions. Although it does not reduce serum potassium, calcium antagonizes the effect of potassium on the heart. Dialysis removes potassium rapidly and efficiently from the serum.

References: Chambers, J.K.: Fluid and electrolyte problems in renal and urologic disorders. Nurs Clin North Am, 22:815–825, 1987.
Lancaster, L.: ESRD: Pathophysiology, assessment and intervention. In Lancaster, L.: The Patient with End Stage Renal Disease, 2nd ed. John Wiley and Sons, New York, 1984.
Schwartz, M.W.: Potassium imbalances. Am J Nurs, 87:1292–1299, 1987.

2–94. (**B**) In correction of hyperkalemia, care should be taken to avoid hypokalemia resulting from the administration of cation exchange resin enemas. Monitoring the patient closely during treatment for normalization of ECG findings and disappearance of other presenting symptoms (lethargy, weakness, etc.) provides information about the potassium level, which can be confirmed with serum values. Close monitoring may prevent resultant hypokalemia.

References: Lancaster, L.: ESRD: Pathophysiology, assessment and intervention. In Lancaster, L.: The Patient with End Stage Renal Disease, 2nd ed. John Wiley and Sons, New York, 1984.
Schwartz, M.W.: Potassium imbalances. Am J Nurs, 87:1292–1299, 1987.

2–95. (**A**) The economic impact of chronic renal failure is significant, with continuous medical expenses and perhaps loss of income if the patient is unable to work. Chronic illness can affect families in different ways. Family relationships, even when strong prior to the discovery of the illness, can deteriorate owing to the stress of the illness and its effects. It is also difficult if the "breadwinner" and manager of household finances is the one who becomes ill. The previously dependent spouse may then become the responsible party.

Reference: Ulrich, B.T.: Psychological aspects of nephrology nursing. In Ulrich, B.T.: Nephrology Nursing: Concepts and Strategies. Appleton and Lange, Norwalk, CT, 1989.

2–96. (**B**) Cortisol is released in a diurnal (24-hour) cycle. The adrenocorticotropic hormone (ACTH) and cortisol blood levels peak at 8 a.m., fall slowly around 12 noon, and reach a low point at midnight. People who are awake at night and sleep during the day may have a different diurnal pattern.

Reference: Muthe, N.C.: Endocrinology, A Nursing Approach. Little, Brown, Boston, 1981.

2–97. (**D**) In the presence of grossly increased intracranial pressure, a lumbar puncture is contraindicated because of the risk of brain stem herniation.

Reference: Hickey, J.V.: The Clinical Practice of Neurological and Neurosurgical Nursing, 2nd ed. J.B. Lippincott, Philadelphia, 1986.

2–98. **(A)** Evaluation criteria for the patient with alteration in cerebral perfusion include maintaining an ICP between 0 and 15 mm Hg with a CPP above 50 mm Hg and maintaining or improving neurologic status. Cerebral perfusion pressure is the amount of pressure necessary in the cerebral vasculature to supply oxygen and nutrients to the brain. A CPP above 50 mm Hg is the minimum for adequate perfusion. An ICP above 15 mm Hg is considered elevated.

References: Caine, R.M., and Bufalino, P.M.: Critically Ill Adults: Nursing Care Planning Guides. Williams & Wilkins, Baltimore, 1988.
Holloway, N.M.: Nursing the Critically Ill Adult, 3rd ed. Addison-Wesley, Menlo Park, CA, 1988.

2–99. **(C)** This response demonstrates that you have heard the patient express a concern about dying. This response permits the patient to clarify the message and allows the individual to respond with their feelings.

Reference: Doenges, M., and Moorhouse, M.: Nursing Diagnosis with Interventions. F.A. Davis, Philadelphia, 1988.

2–100. **(B)** Patients remain in the hyperdynamic (warm) phase of septic shock phase for 6 to 72 hours before developing the hypodynamic (cold) phase of septic shock. Cold shock is characterized by a subnormal temperature, decreased blood pressure, a decrease in cardiac output, and increased systemic vascular resistance. Another indicator of septic shock is the increased $S\bar{v}O_2$, which indicates the cells are not effectively utilizing oxygen at the cellular level and much of the oxygen is returning to the right side of the heart in the venous blood. With a normal platelet count and fibrin split products, a coagulopathy is unlikely. The patient is not immunosuppressed, because she has an elevated WBC count. A systemic vascular resistance (SVR) of 1,600 dynes/sec/cm^{-5} indicates peripheral vasoconstriction and poor circulation.

Reference: Wall, S.C.: Septic shock. Nursing '89, *19*:52–60, 1989.

2–101. **(B)** Respiratory muscle fatigue is caused by increased demand for ventilation or increased work of breathing. Other factors that can increase respiratory muscle fatigue are hypokalemia, hypophosphatemia, hyperthermia, increased bronchospasm, and others.

Reference: Kersten, L.D.: Comprehensive Respiratory Nursing: A Decision Making Approach. W.B. Saunders, Philadelphia, 1989.

2–102. **(B)** Muffled heart tones and pulsus paradoxus are not specific for aneurysm, but are findings also in cardiac tamponade. A heave along the left sternal border is a symptom of right ventricular hypertrophy. The pulsation of a ventricular aneurysm is palpated as an entity separate from the apical impulse. It is a sustained impulse that lasts longer than the apical impulse (ripple effect).

Reference: Underhill, S., Woods, S., Froelicher, E., et al.: Cardiac Nursing, 2nd ed. J.B. Lippincott, Philadelphia, 1989.

2–103. **(D)** Left ventricular hypertrophy and arterial hypertension tend to shift the apical impulse laterally, to the left of the midclavicular line. Pregnancy increases the height of the diaphragm and shifts the PMI lateral to the midclavicular line. The normal apical impulse is felt at the fifth intercostal space at the midclavicular line. COPD causes the apical impulse to move medially because of downward displacement of the diaphragm.

Reference: Andreoli, K., Fowkes, V., Zipes, D., et al.: Comprehensive Cardiac Care, 6th ed. C.V. Mosby, St. Louis, 1987.

2–104. **(B)** The cellular functions of the liver include detoxifying drugs and hormones, producing bile, glycogenesis, glycogenolysis, lipid metabolism, and protein metabolism.

Reference: Luckmann, J., and Sorensen, K.C.: Medical-Surgical Nursing: A Psychophysiologic Approach, 3rd ed. W.B. Saunders, Philadelphia, 1987.

2–105. (**B**) In primary hypernatremia the body absorbs a large volume of sodium-containing fluids. Excess aldosterone results in increased sodium reabsorption, increased total body sodium, and hypervolemia. Hyperglycemia, mannitol, and watery diarrhea all cause free fluid loss. As the body's fluid levels fall and its sodium content remains roughly the same, sodium concentration rises.

References: Barta, M.: Correcting electrolyte imbalances. RN, *50*(2):30–34, 1987.
Thompson, J., McFarland, G.K., Hirsch, J.E., et al.: Mosby's Manual of Clinical Nursing, 2nd ed. C.V. Mosby, St. Louis, 1989.

2–106. (**D**) Nurse/patient exchanges must utilize sound therapeutic communication techniques. They include focusing on the patient's feelings, listening actively, accepting the patient, responding to patient cues, and being direct and honest. Complete cord transsection is an irreversible condition. Statements that the patient *will* gain more control may give the patient false hope and usually are not therapeutic.

Reference: Alspach, J.G. (ed.): AACN Core Curriculum for Critical Care Nursing, 4th ed. W.B. Saunders, Philadelphia, 1991.

2–107. (**D**) When the patient is warmed, vasodilation lowers the wedge pressure. Patients who return from surgery are hypothermic and vasoconstricted. Slightly higher wedge pressures are acceptable in patients after bypass until they begin to mobilize the fluid load accumulated during surgery.

Reference: Weeks, L.: Advanced Cardiovascular Nursing. Blackwell, Boston, 1986.

2–108. (**C**) The right coronary artery is generally easy to reach with balloon angioplasty, and surgery would be considered if the angioplasty was unsuccessful. In patients with isolated occlusions, particularly those patients who have had bypass surgery, angioplasty is preferred to subjecting the patient to reoperation. Thrombolytic agents are generally used in acute events associated with acute myocardial infarction.

Reference: Underhill, S., Woods, S., Froelicher, E., et al.: Cardiac Nursing, 2nd ed. J.B. Lippincott, Philadelphia, 1989.

2–109. (**A**) Restrictive disease shows a pulmonary function pattern with decreased lung volumes and capacities. The FVC is markedly decreased despite rapid exhalation of air.

Reference: West, J.B.: Pulmonary Pathophysiology: The Essentials, 3rd ed. Williams & Wilkins, Baltimore, 1987.

2–110. (**B**) Static compliance is measured under conditions of no flow and is affected by pathologic changes within the lung and chest wall. Dynamic compliance is measured with flow and is affected by changes in the airways and ventilator circuitry. Comparison of the two pressures is useful to identify where changes are occurring in the pulmonary system and to correct problems.

Reference: West, J.B.: Respiratory Physiology: The Essentials, 4th ed. Williams & Wilkins, Baltimore, 1990.

2–111. **(C)** The syndrome of inappropriate secretion of antidiuretic hormone (SIADH) occurs when there is continuous synthesis and release of ADH in the presence of serum hypo-osmolarity. This results in a urine osmolarity that is greater than that of serum. Dilutional hyponatremia occurs in SIADH from an increase in tubular reabsorption of water. The retention of water causes an expansion of plasma volume. This increase in intravascular fluid causes an increase in the glomerular filtration rate and inhibits the reabsorption of sodium and water in the renal tubules. The expansion of the plasma volume also inhibits the release of renin and aldosterone, which further intensifies the hyponatremia. Because SIADH results in the retention of free water and not salt, edema is not a feature of this disorder.

References: German, K.: Fluid and electrolyte problems associated with diabetes insipidus and syndrome of inappropriate ADH. Nurs Clin North Am, 22:785–796, 1987.
Thompson, J., McFarland, G.K., Hirsch, J.E., et al.: Mosby's Manual of Clinical Nursing, 2nd ed. C.V. Mosby, St. Louis, 1989.

2–112. **(C)** The four major complications associated with balloon tamponade of bleeding esophageal varices are: (1) asphyxia secondary to pharyngeal obstruction; (2) pulmonary problems secondary to aspiration; (3) ruptured esophagus; (4) erosion of the esophageal or gastric wall. Rhythm changes are due to hypovolemia, with tachycardia expected until near death. The balloon does not enter the bowel or affect peristalsis, so bowel obstruction is not a complication of this therapy. Portal hypertension is an etiology of esophageal bleeding unaffected by balloon tamponade.

References: DeGroot, K.D., and Damato, M.B.: Critical Care Skills. Appleton and Lange, Norwalk, CT, 1987.
Kinney, M.R., Packa, D., and Dunbar, S.B. (eds.): AACN's Clinical Reference for Critical-Care Nursing. McGraw-Hill, New York, 1988.

2–113. **(D)** The ascending reticular activating system, a cellular network, is responsible for arousal from sleep, alert wakefulness, focusing of attention, and perceptual association. The descending reticular activating system may facilitate or inhibit activity of the motor neurons controlling skeletal musculature.

Reference: Alspach, J.G. (ed.): AACN Core Curriculum for Critical Care Nursing, 4th ed. W.B. Saunders, Philadelphia, 1991.

2–114. **(B)** The patient has an elevated WBC. In addition, the shift to the left is indicative of an increased number of circulating immature neutrophils, also known as bands. The result does not have any implications related to coagulation.

Reference: Alspach J.G. (ed.): AACN Core Curriculum for Critical Care Nursing, 4th ed. W.B. Saunders, Philadelphia, 1991.

2–115. **(C)** Bradydysrhythmias are common with inferior wall infarcts. Papillary muscle rupture may occur with extensive inferior wall infarcts. Damage to the left ventricle from anterior wall necrosis may result in pump failure and cardiogenic shock.

Reference: Kenner, C., Guzzetta, C., and Dossey, B.: Critical Care Nursing: Body—Mind—Spirit. Little, Brown, Boston, 1985.

2–116. **(D)** Right ventricular oxygen saturation is normally 40% to 70%. Left-to-right shunting in septal rupture increases the right ventricular pressure. A loud systolic murmur or palpable thrill may be felt at the left sternal border from the left-to-right movement of blood through the septal defect.

Reference: Daily, E., and Schroeder, J.: Techniques in Bedside Hemodynamic Monitoring, 3rd ed. C.V. Mosby, St. Louis, 1985.

2–117. (**B**) Although the patient may weigh the implications of his or her age, diagnosis, risk-to-benefit ratio, and other considerations, it is the autonomous wish of the patient, expressed personally or through individuals who are well acquainted with the patient, that is the ethical basis of a decision to withhold or withdraw treatment. The physician may share his or her personal values with the patient or family during their discussions, but the decision is implemented according to the patient's wishes. Hospital policies are legal devices that are not directly relevant to ethical decision-making.

References: Meisel, A., Grenvik, A., Pinkus, R.L., et al.: Hospital guidelines for deciding about life-sustaining treatment: Dealing with health "limbo." Crit Care Med, 3:239–246, 1986.
Smith, D.H., and Veatch, R.M. (eds.): Hastings Center Guidelines on the Termination of Life-Sustaining Treatment and Care of the Dying. Indiana University Press, Indianapolis, 1987.

2–118. (**C**) An increase in the arterial-venous oxygen content difference indicates that the oxygen delivery has decreased, resulting in an increased extraction of oxygen to meet metabolic demand. It can also mean that the metabolic rate has increased, resulting in increased extraction. Oxygen delivery is determined by oxygen loading (hemoglobin, Sa_{O_2}, Ca_{O_2}) and cardiac output.

Reference: Snyder, J.V., and Pinsky, M.R.: Oxygen Transport in the Critically Ill. Year Book Medical Publishers, Chicago, 1987.

2–119. (**B**) The ali nasi are considered to be inspiratory muscles and are utilized as accessory muscles when a patient experiences air hunger. Nasal flaring is related to the patient's sensation of "breathlessness," not necessarily to arterial blood gases.

Reference: Slonim, N.B., and Hamilton, L.H.: Respiratory Physiology, 5th ed. C.V. Mosby, St. Louis, 1987.

2–120. (**C**) Air hunger can be relieved only by providing enough flow rate with each breath to provide a fast enough breath to meet the patient's need. This is accomplished by increasing the liter flow per minute for each breath. Sedation, increasing the Fi_{O_2}, and increasing the tidal volume will not eliminate the sensation of air hunger.

Reference: Shapiro, B.A., Harrison, R.A., Cane, R.D., et al.: Clinical Application of Blood Gases, 4th ed. Year Book Medical Publishers, Chicago, 1989.

2–121. (**A**) Complications associated with fulminating meningococcal meningitis include Waterhouse-Friderichsen syndrome (an adrenal hemorrhage) resulting in shock states, DIC, brain abscess, subdural effusions, encephalitis, hydrocephalus, and cerebral edema.

Reference: Alspach, J.G. (ed.): AACN Core Curriculum for Critical Care Nursing, 4th ed. W.B. Saunders, Philadelphia, 1991.

2–122. (**A**) The elevated serum uremic toxins associated with uremia cause inflammation and ulceration of the mucosa along the entire GI tract. Ammonia is a result of urea breakdown by the intestinal bacteria and is an irritant to intestinal mucosa.

References: Crandall, B.L.: Acute renal failure. In Ulrich, T.: Nephrology Nursing. Appleton and Lange, Norwalk, CT, 1989.
Lancaster, L.: ESRD: Pathophysiology, assessment and intervention. In Lancaster, L.: The Patient with End Stage Renal Disease, 2nd ed. John Wiley and Sons, New York, 1984.

2–123. (**A**) Aluminum hydroxide gel (Mylanta) is a magnesium-containing antacid that can cause hypermagnesemia when used in patients with severe renal failure. The kidney plays a major role in regulating serum magnesium levels. In the normal kidney, plasma magnesium is freely filtered by the renal glomerulus and is 92% to 95% conserved by active tubular reabsorption.

Reference: Gerard, S., Hernandez, C., and Khayam-Bashi, H.: Extreme hypermagnesemia caused by an overdose of magnesium-containing cathartics. Ann Emerg Med, 17:728–731, 1988.

2–124. (**A**) Cardiac catheterization should be performed to determine the severity of the ventricular aneurysm demonstrated by persistent ST elevation and ventricular dysrhythmias.

Reference: Kenner, C., Guzzetta, C., and Dossey, B.: Critical Care Nursing: Body—Mind—Spirit. Little, Brown, Boston, 1985.

2–125. (**D**) Allergic reactions may occur with streptokinase use. Frequently, antihistamines and corticosteroids are utilized in mild to moderate allergic reactions. Arterial punctures are contraindicated in the 24-hour period following thrombolytic therapy.

Reference: Underhill, S., Woods, S., Froelicher, E., et al.: Cardiac Nursing, 2nd ed. J.B. Lippincott, Philadelphia, 1989.

2–126. (**C**) The stomach normally secretes 1500 to 3000 ml of gastric juice per day.

Reference: Luckmann, J., and Sorensen, K.C.: Medical-Surgical Nursing: A Psychophysiologic Approach, 3rd ed. W.B. Saunders, Philadelphia, 1987.

2–127. (**A**) Maintenance of gastric pH above 3.5 with antacids is widely accepted to prevent stress ulcerations. Above pH 3.5, acute stress bleeding and gastric perforation are very unlikely. Sucralfate (carafate), an anionic, sulfated disaccharide, forms a protective barrier over ulcer site(s) but does not affect gastric pH. The relationship between gastric pH and nausea is unpredictable, so further data would be required before administering an antiemetic. Histamine is a potent stimulator of gastric acid secretion, but antihistamines do not block the effect of histamine on gastric acid secretion, which is mediated by H_2 receptors of the parietal cells. H_2 receptor antagonists such as cimetidine or ranitidine are the drugs of choice.

Reference: Konopad, E., and Noseworthy, T.: Stress ulceration: A serious complication in critically ill patients. Heart Lung, 17(4):339–348, 1988.

2–128. (**C**) The lungs provide a large surface area for gas exchange to occur across the alveolar-capillary membrane. They also serve as a reservoir for blood and WBCs, and they filter toxins and metabolize compounds. Humidification occurs in the upper airway and oronasopharynx.

Reference: West, J.B.: Respiratory Physiology: The Essentials, 4th ed. Williams & Wilkins, Baltimore, 1990.

2–129. (**D**) The pulmonary artery pressures are elevated but the pulmonary capillary wedge pressure is normal. This eliminates the possibilities of pulmonary edema or congestive heart failure, because the wedge pressure would also be elevated in those conditions. Blood loss would produce a picture of low pulmonary artery and wedge pressures. The hypoxic vasoconstriction is probably due to pulmonary emboli or beginning ARDS.

Reference: Kersten, L.D.: Comprehensive Respiratory Nursing: A Decision Making Approach. W.B. Saunders, Philadelphia, 1989.

2–130. (**D**) All are causes of hypoxemia, yet the most likely cause is $\dot{V}/\dot{Q}$ mismatch. A diffusion defect is caused by fibrotic tissue in the alveolar-capillary membrane and will also cause an elevated Pa_{CO_2}. Alveolar hypoventilation is caused by neurologic deficits or sedation and also shows an elevated Pa_{CO_2}. A low PI_{O_2}/FI_{O_2} is very uncommon and is usually found at high elevations or in areas where air must be rebreathed. This patient is presenting with early adult respiratory distress syndrome (ARDS), which initially manifests as $\dot{V}/\dot{Q}$ mismatch and then progresses to a right-to-left shunt. One of the hallmarks of ARDS is a high right-to-left shunt fraction.

Reference: West, J.B.: Respiratory Physiology: The Essentials, 3rd ed. Williams & Wilkins, Baltimore, 1985.

2–131. **(C)** The level of the collection device is important in determining the rate of ultrafiltration. Lowering the collection device increases the negative pressure and rate of ultrafiltration. For the process to work successfully, the mean arterial pressure (MAP) must be 60 mm Hg and the hematocrit less than 40%. Increased systemic blood flow increases the ultrafiltration rate. Because blood viscosity is inversely related to blood flow and filtration, patients with hematocrits less than 45% are candidates for continuous arteriovenous hemofiltration. If the hematocrit is too high, the blood may sludge and clot in the filter. The tubing should be kept as short as possible to decrease resistance to flow in the system. Lengthening the tubing decreases ultrafiltration rates.

References: Kiely, M.: Continuous arteriovenous hemofiltration. Crit Care Nurs, *4:*39–49, 1984.
Palmer, C., Koorejian, K., London, J., et al.: Nursing management of continuous arteriovenous hemofiltration for acute renal failure. Focus Crit Care, *13:*21–30, 1986.
Thompson, J., McFarland, G.K., Hirsch, J.E., et al.: Mosby's Manual of Clinical Nursing, 2nd ed. C.V. Mosby, St. Louis, 1989.

2–132. **(A)** On physical examination, patients with frontal lobe tumors demonstrate inappropriate behavior, inattention, inability to concentrate, alterations in social behavior, impaired recent memory, difficulty with abstraction, flattened affect, expressive aphasia if the tumor is in the dominant hemisphere, and motor changes. Visual hallucinations are seen with occipital lobe tumors, and paresthesias and loss of left-right discrimination are seen with parietal lobe tumors.

Reference: Alspach J.G. (ed.): AACN Core Curriculum for Critical Care Nursing, 4th ed. W.B. Saunders, Philadelphia, 1991.

2–133. **(B)** A crisis is a state of emotional disequilibrium characterized by the absence of one or more balancing factors. Balancing factors include an accurate perception of the event, ability to utilize usual coping mechanisms, and adequate situational supports. The patient may have a distorted perception of the problem and may be unable to deal with it. This patient may have a distorted perception of the diagnosis, and his usual coping mechanisms may not be present or are insufficient to deal with the stressor. The inability to deal with the stressor causes disequilibrium. The goal of treatment in a crisis is to restore the patient to his pre-crisis state.

Reference: Caine, R.M., and Bufalino, P.M.: Critically Ill Adults: Nursing Care Planning Guides. Williams & Wilkins, Baltimore, 1988.

2–134. **(A)** According to Kubler-Ross, the five stages of psychological grieving that are usually experienced by a dying or grieving individual are: *denial,* characterized by an attempt to delay the shock and pain of the diagnosis or event until the individual is better able to deal with the reality of the situation; *anger* and *rage* regarding the unfairness of the diagnosis; *bargaining* as an attempt to postpone dying until certain tasks are complete and to provide a means for the patient to deal with the situation incrementally; *depression,* with the realization that many losses are now imminent; and *acceptance,* a time of acknowledgment and recognition that death is inevitable.

Reference: Caine, R.M., and Bufalino, P.M.: Critically Ill Adults: Nursing Care Planning Guides. Williams & Wilkins, Baltimore, 1988.

2–135. (**C**) SRS-A, kinins, and histamine cause vasodilation and increased capillary permeability, which in turn allow the loss of fluids and plasma proteins into the interstitial tissue. These, in turn, contribute to the development of hypotension. These substances also cause constriction of bronchial smooth muscle with subsequent respiratory complications seen in anaphylaxis.

Reference: Dickerson, M.A.: Anaphylaxis and anaphylactic shock. Crit Care Nurs Q, *11*:68–74, 1988.

2–136. (**D**) According to the American Heart Association, first check the responsiveness of the patient (he may have dislodged his electrodes in his sleep), then check the integrity of the leads, initiate a precordial thump, then defibrillation at 200 joules.

Reference: American Heart Association: Textbook of Advanced Cardiac Life Support. Dallas, 1987.

2–137. (**A**) A chest x-ray is immediately indicated to check the position of the pacing electrode and to check for mediastinal widening, which would be seen if the pacing electrode had punctured the myocardium and caused the pericardial friction rub.

Reference: Underhill, S., Woods, S., Froelicher, E., et al.: Cardiac Nursing, 2nd ed. J.B. Lippincott, Philadelphia, 1989.

2–138. (**D**) The frontal lobe, in addition to the motor cortex, which controls motor function, is responsible for memory and storage of information, abstract thinking, judgement, personality, and affect.

Reference: Hickey, J.V.: The Clinical Practice of Neurological and Neurosurgical Nursing, 2nd ed. J.B. Lippincott, Philadelphia, 1986.

2–139. (**B**) "Central neurogenic hyperventilation" is the term used to describe the sustained, rapid, regular, deep hyperpnea associated with lesions of the midbrain, often secondary to transtentorial herniation and midpontine lesions. A Cheyne-Stokes respiratory pattern is associated with lesions of the basal ganglia, ataxic breathing is associated with lesions of the posterior fossa, and cluster breathing is associated with lesions of the rostral medulla.

Reference: Alspach J.G. (ed.): AACN Core Curriculum for Critical Care Nursing, 4th ed. W.B. Saunders, Philadelphia, 1991.

2–140. (**C**) When otorrhea—the escape of fluid from the ear—follows head injury, the drainage is likely to be cerebrospinal fluid (CSF). Because CSF contains glucose, it would be appropriate for the nurse to assess the drainage for the presence of glucose. In neurotrauma, pressure is never directly applied to the area of injury because compression of bone fragments into brain tissue may result. Meningitis, an infectious process, can result from packing the draining ear of a patient. Dressings are loosely applied to the external ear to allow for absorption of the drainage.

Reference: Caine, R.M., and Bufalino, P.M.: Critically Ill Adults: Nursing Care Planning Guides. Williams & Wilkins, Baltimore, 1988.

2–141. (**C**) The frothy pink sputum is produced by alteration in the Starling forces. Damage to the alveolar-capillary membrane allows fluid, debris, and proteins (including RBCs) to diffuse down a pressure gradient into the alveoli. The Starling forces are primarily comprised of the hydrostatic and colloid osmotic pressures. The colloid pressure is the major force in the capillaries and is due to proteins in the blood attracting and holding fluid in the vascular space.

Reference: Kinney, M.R., Packa, D.R., and Dunbar, S.F.: AACN's Clinical Reference for Critical Care Nursing, 2nd ed. McGraw-Hill, New York, 1988.

2–142. (**B**) Cold or acidic dialysate, rapid infusion, and air under the diaphragm all cause abdominal pain, but they are not associated with rebound tenderness or a cloudy effluent. A peritoneal infection causes severe diffuse pain, with rebound tenderness secondary to peritonitis, and cloudy effluent.

References: Jett, M., Lancaster, L., and Small, S.: Renal disorders. In Renal and Urologic Disorders. Springhouse, Springhouse, PA, 1984.
Parker, J., and Ulrich, B.T.: Peritoneal dialysis therapy. In Ulrich, B.T.: Nephrology Nursing: Concepts and Strategies. Appleton and Lange, Norwalk, CT, 1989.

2–143. (**C**) With peritonitis there are WBCs and fibrin present in the effluent. The fibrin can accumulate in the catheter and obstruct outflow of the dialysate.

References: Jett, M., Lancaster, L., and Small, S.: Renal disorders. In Renal and Urologic Disorders. Springhouse, Springhouse, PA, 1984.
Parker, J., and Ulrich, B.T.: Peritoneal dialysis therapy. In Ulrich, B.T. (ed.): Nephrology Nursing: Concepts and Strategies. Appleton and Lange, Norwalk, CT, 1989.

2–144. (**A**) Leakage from the anastomosis may follow pancreatectomy due to residual pancreatic exudate, undue tension, poor healing ability, or impaired blood supply. Pseudocyst, mesenteric thrombosis, and coagulopathy are common complications of acute pancreatitis.

Reference: Kinney, M.R., Packa, D.R., and Dunbar, S.B.: AACN's Clinical Reference for Critical Care Nursing, 2nd ed. McGraw-Hill, New York, 1988.

2–145. (**A**) Patients with intracranial aneurysms associated with high arterial pressures are more susceptible to aneurysmal rupture causing a subarachnoid hemorrhage. The subarachnoid hemorrhage increases the patient's intracranial pressure. Level-of-consciousness changes are the earliest and most reliable indicator of increased intracranial pressure.

Reference: Alspach, J.G. (ed.): AACN Core Curriculum for Critical Care Nursing, 4th ed. W.B. Saunders, Philadelphia, 1991.

2–146. (**D**) Patients with grade IV aneurysms present with unresponsiveness, hemiplegia, and nuchal rigidity and may or may not have vasospasm.

Reference: Alspach, J.G. (ed.): AACN Core Curriculum for Critical Care Nursing, 4th ed. W.B. Saunders, Philadelphia, 1991.

2–147. (**C**) Aminocaproic acid (Amicar), an antifibrinolytic, delays the lysis of clots by preventing dissolution of fibrin that forms the basis for the clot. The drug is losing popularity because of risks associated with its administration. The drug is generally considered contraindicated in patients with uremia, cardiac disease, or hepatorenal disease. Side effects include hypotension, bradycardia, dysrhythmias, and deep vein thrombosis. Pulmonary embolus may also occur.

Reference: Hickey, J.V.: The Clinical Practice of Neurological and Neurosurgical Nursing, 2nd ed. J.B. Lippincott, Philadelphia, 1986.

2–148. (**A**) DIC is the result of a precipitating event that activates excess intravascular clotting. Excess thrombin is produced, which enhances clot formation and platelet aggregation. Plasmin inactivates naturally occurring antithrombins, and clots are lysed and clotting factors are consumed. With decreased amounts of clotting factors, the blood loses the ability to form a stable clot. This predisposes a patient to hemorrhage.

Reference: Alspach, J.G. (ed.): AACN Core Curriculum for Critical Care Nursing, 4th ed. W.B. Saunders, Philadelphia, 1991.

2–149. **(D)** When selecting blood components or products, the choice is made to replace the specific deficiency. Therefore, whole blood is not frequently used. The patient with DIC has an unusually rapid consumption of clotting factors. Fresh frozen plasma contains all clotting factors except platelets, which are administered separately. Packed RBCs would supply only erythrocytes and no clotting factors. Cryoprecipitate contains only factors V, VIII, and XIII. Albumin and Plasmanate are used to increase colloidal oncotic pressure and do not provide the necessary clotting factors.

Reference: Von Rueden, K.T., and Walleck, C.A.: Advanced Critical Care Nursing. Aspen, Rockville, MD, 1989.

2–150. **(B)** Chemotherapy itself does not predispose patients to a pulmonary embolus, although the malignancy does.

Reference: Kersten, L.D.: Comprehensive Respiratory Nursing: A Decision Making Approach. W.B. Saunders, Philadelphia, 1989.

2–151. **(C)** When the pulmonary circulation is obstructed by a pulmonary embolus, the pulmonary vascular resistance (PVR) increases. The increased PVR produces right ventricular failure, and that leads to decreased preload to the left ventricle. Vasodilator therapy to decrease the PVR, along with inotropic therapy, is needed. Mini-dose heparin at this point is not indicated because either urokinase or a continuous heparin drip will be started.

Reference: West, J.B.: Pulmonary Pathophysiology: The Essentials. 3rd ed. Williams & Wilkins, Baltimore, 1987.

2–152. **(D)** Characteristic symptoms of myxedema include: (1) cool, yellow or pale, coarse, dry, thick skin; (2) edematous lower extremities that are nonpitting; (3) decreased sweat and oil production; and (4) brittle, thin, and cracked nails.

Reference: Muthe, N.C.: Endocrinology, A Nursing Approach. Little, Brown, Boston, 1981.

2–153. **(C)** Excess levels of T_3 and T_4 may precipitate tachycardia, increased pulse pressure, increased myocardial contractility, tremor, heat intolerance, diaphoresis, and diarrhea. The reason for the heightened adrenergic state is unclear. There may be an increase in the number of beta-adrenergic receptors or an increased sensitization of beta receptors, or thyroid hormone may act directly on sympathetic end-organ receptors.

Reference: Kohler, P.O., and Jordan, R.M. (eds.): Clinical Endocrinology. John Wiley and Sons, New York, 1986.

2–154. **(C)** With increased beta-adrenergic activity, this patient is at risk for dysrhythmias. The patient is tachycardic and has an occasional PVC. Oxygen demand outweighing supply can precipitate ischemia and electrical irritability. Thyroid hormone excess may cause increased GI motility, but this is not life-threatening. The patient's current clinical picture does not warrant continuous reorientation and hand restraints.

Reference: Holloway, N.M.: Nursing the Critically Ill Adult, 3rd ed. Addison-Wesley, Menlo Park, CA, 1988.

2–155. **(B)** Calcitonin inhibits bone reabsorption and increases bone deposition of calcium. Immobilization increases bone reabsorption of calcium and increases urinary calcium and phosphorus excretion. Other treatments decrease calcium, but not by bone reabsorption of calcium. Sodium infusions cause an increased renal excretion of calcium, and corticosteroids inhibit the GI absorption of calcium.

References: Calloway, C.: When the problem involves magnesium, calcium, or phosphate. RN, 50:30–36, 1987.
Chambers, J.K.: Metabolic bone disorders: imbalances of calcium and phosphorus. Nurs Clin North Am, 22:861–872, 1987.

2–156. (**B**) Focusing on postoperative routines reassures the patient that he will survive. Although it is true that the aspirin needed to be discontinued at least 7 days prior to surgery, the patient's fear is the issue now. Telling the patient he will do just fine or to stop worrying are empty reassurances.

Reference: Underhill, S., Woods, S., Froelicher, E., et al.: Cardiac Nursing, 2nd ed. J.B. Lippincott, Philadelphia, 1989.

2–157. (**D**) Pulsus paradoxus occurs in constrictive pericarditis because of the increase in venous pressure, pooling of blood in the pulmonary vasculature, and decreased left ventricular filling. During inspiration there is normally a slight decrease in blood return to the left heart. In pericarditis, this normal response is exaggerated, causing a drop of over 10 mm Hg in the systolic blood pressure during inspiration.

Reference: Kenner, C., Guzzetta, C., and Dossey, B.: Critical Care Nursing: Body—Mind—Spirit. Little, Brown, Boston, 1985.

2–158. (**B**) Clinical symptoms of myocarditis vary widely and are nonspecific. Definitive diagnosis can be made only by endomyocardial biopsy.

Reference: Grady, K., and Constanzo-Nordin, M.: Myocarditis: review of a clinical enigma. Heart Lung, 18:347–353, 1989.

2–159. (**C**) The short duration of the chest pain and conclusive ECG criteria for acute myocardial infarction make this patient a good candidate for tissue plasminogen activator (t-PA) infusion.

Reference: Greco, A.: Treatment protocols: practical considerations for hospital implementation of thrombolytic therapy with tissue plasminogen activator. Heart Lung, 17:787–792, 1988.

2–160. (**A**) Hyperventilation in the head-injured patient causes cerebral vasoconstriction and decreased cerebral blood flow. Hyperventilation raises mean intrathoracic pressure, decreases venous return, and decreases cardiac output.

Reference: Hickey, J.V.: The Clinical Practice of Neurological and Neurosurgical Nursing, 2nd ed. J.B. Lippincott, Philadelphia, 1986.

2–161. (**A**) There are three distinct waves associated with intracranial pressure monitoring—A, B, and C waves. A waves are the most significant from a clinical perspective when cerebral ischemia and brain damage have occurred as a result of the sustained elevation in intracranial pressure for between 5 and 20 minutes. A waves are accompanied by intracranial pressures between 50 to 100 mm Hg and are seen in the advanced stages of increased intracranial pressure. B waves are sharp, rhythmic oscillations and are usually associated with Cheyne-Stokes respiratory patterns and decreased wakefulness. C waves are related to the normal arterial pressure and have no clinical significance. F waves are not associated with intracranial pressure monitoring.

Reference: Hickey, J.V.: The Clinical Practice of Neurological and Neurosurgical Nursing, 2nd ed. J.B. Lippincott, Philadelphia, 1986.

2–162. (**A**) A low platelet count dramatically increases the risk of intraperitoneal hemorrhage from percutaneous liver biopsy. Signs of intraperitoneal bleeding include tachycardia, pallor, and abdominal distention. The patient should be positioned on the right side to tamponade the puncture site. Bedrest should be enforced for 8 to 12 hours after biopsy to minimize risk of site hemorrhage. Although diminished breath sounds on the right are indicative of hemo- or pneumothorax, hemorrhage from the liver flows into the peritoneum without selective displacement of the lungs.

Reference: Swearingen, P.L., Sommers, M.S., and Miller, K.: Manual of Critical Care: Applying Nursing Diagnoses to Adult Critical Illness. C.V. Mosby, St. Louis, 1988.

2–163. (**A**) In hepatic failure, total bilirubin is elevated as a result of the inability of the liver to metabolize bilirubin. This is due to failure in hepatocyte metabolism from severe inflammation, necrosis, or fibrosis. Transaminases (SGOT and SGPT) are usually elevated to more than 300 units/l in acute hepatic failure. Serum albumin is reduced, because the liver is unable to synthesize it while dysfunctional. Normal total bilirubin is less than 1.1 mg/dl. SGOT is normally 7 to 40 units/l. Serum albumin is normally 3.5 to 5.5 gm/dl.

References: Luckmann, J., and Sorensen, K.C.: Medical-Surgical Nursing: A Psychophysiologic Approach, 3rd ed. W.B. Saunders, Philadelphia, 1987.
Swearingen, P.L., Sommers, M.S., and Miller, K.: Manual of Critical Care: Applying Nursing Diagnosis to Adult Critical Illness. C.V. Mosby, St. Louis, 1988.

2–164. (**B**) When the intra-aortic balloon inflates early, aortic root pressure is increased and may force the aortic valve closed. These increased pressures increase the left ventricular work and afterload. Late inflation and early deflation decrease coronary artery filling.

Reference: Weeks, L.: Advanced Cardiovascular Nursing. Blackwell, Boston, 1986.

2–165. (**B**) This rhythm strip demonstrates the classic features of 3:1 second degree AV block, referred to as Mobitz type II or high-grade second degree AV block. For each three P waves there is one normal QRS with a normal and constant PR interval.

Reference: Kenner, C., Guzzetta, C., and Dossey, B.: Critical Care Nursing: Body—Mind—Spirit. Little, Brown, Boston, 1985.

2–166. (**A**) Serum calcium concentrations can fall because of hemodilution following cardiopulmonary bypass. The ionized fraction, which is the free, diffusible, and physiologically active form, decreases with administration of citrated blood and alkalosis. The citrates in blood products all cause hypocalcemia. In alkalosis, bicarbonate complexes combine with calcium to reduce ionized available calcium.

References: Calloway, C.: When the problem involves magnesium, calcium, or phosphate. RN, 50:30–36, 1987.
Chambers, J.K.: Metabolic bone disorders: imbalances of calcium and phosphorus. Nurs Clin North Am, 22:861–872, 1987.

2–167. (**D**) Symptomatic hypocalcemia requires administration of soluble intravenous calcium salts, which immediately increases the serum's calcium ion concentration. Subsequent calcium needs can be met with IV infusions of calcium or oral calcium supplements.

References: Calloway, C.: When the problem involves magnesium, calcium, or phosphate. RN, 50:30–36, 1987.
Thompson, J., McFarland, G.K., Hirsch, J.E., et al.: Mosby's Manual of Clinical Nursing, 2nd ed. C.V. Mosby, St. Louis, 1989.

2–168. (**C**) This is the classic picture of pure emphysema, the "pink puffer." Destruction of the lung parenchyma results in a compensatory rise in the minute ventilation so that the $\dot{V}/\dot{Q}$ ratio remains normal. This accounts for the pink (noncyanotic) appearance of the emphysema patient. The puffing refers to the increased work of breathing that is required to maintain the high minute ventilation.

Reference: West, J.B.: Pulmonary Pathophysiology: The Essentials, 3rd ed. Williams & Wilkins, Baltimore, 1987.

2–169. (**A**) Increasing the pressure within the lungs will decrease the venous return; the level of PEEP at which this happens varies according to the patient, intravascular volume, and cardiac function.

Reference: Shapiro, B.A., Harrison, R.A., Cane, R.D., et al.: Clinical Application of Blood Gases, 4th ed. Year Book Medical Publishers, Chicago, 1989.

2–170. (**A**) If one believes in the sanctity of human life above all else, one may also believe that an individual who is willing to accept death as an alternative to treatment is unable to act in his or her own best interest. The input of the patient's niece would be valuable if she were able to provide insight into his personal beliefs and values throughout life, but she would not be an appropriate person to decide the issue for her uncle. The fact that the patient was willing to undergo surgery for his cancer is inconsistent with the idea that he is suicidal. Discontinuation of futile treatment is not murder.

References: Beresford, H.R.: Legal aspects of terminating care. Semin Neurol, *1*:23–29, 1984.
Younger, S.J.: Do-Not-Resuscitate orders: No longer a secret, but still a problem. Hastings Center Report, *1*:24–33, 1987.

2–171. (**B**) The nurse should act as the patient's advocate by documenting the situation, discussing the matter with the physician and working within the system to effect change. Seeking the intervention of the court would interfere with the physician-patient relationship and should not be pursued unless all resources to resolve the dilemma within the institution have been exhausted.

Reference: Younger, S.J.: Do-Not-Resuscitate orders: No longer a secret, but still a problem. Hastings Center Report, *1*:24–33, 1987.

2–172. (**B**) Radionuclide imaging shows changes in wall motion and ejection fraction, which are more helpful than the alternatives in the prediction of complications in myocardial contusion. Friction rubs commonly occur in myocardial contusion. CPK fractions may be positive. Patients may have an absence of ECG changes or, more commonly, may have PVCs and tachydysrhythmias.

Reference: Chyun, D.: Myocardial contusion: the hidden menace in blunt chest trauma. Am J Nurs, *87*:1459–1462H, 1987.

2–173. (**D**) Glucose constitutes 90% of energy substrate for brain metabolism. The brain has little carbohydrate reserve and metabolism is dependent on a constant supply of glucose. When serum glucose falls below 50 mg/dl, adrenergic signs and central nervous system depression occur. Failure to recognize neuroglucopenia can result in irreversible neural cell damage. Therefore, glucose should be administered. An additional short-term increase in serum glucose during a hyperglycemia-induced coma has less damaging consequences.

Reference: Hamburger, S., Rush, D.R., and Bosker, G.: Endocrine and Metabolic Emergencies. Robert J. Brady, Bowie, MD, 1984.

2–174. (**C**) Hyperosmolality is the major cause of CNS depression. The more rapidly the hyperosmolality develops, the greater the degree of CNS depression.

Reference: Kohler, P.O., and Jordan, R.M. (eds.): Clinical Endocrinology. John Wiley and Sons, New York, 1986.

2–175. (**D**) Beta-adrenergic blockade decreases heart rate and improves ventricular filling by decreasing sympathetic stimulation of the heart. Digoxin is contraindicated because the increased inotropism forces blood against the outflow obstruction and increases backward flow. Vasodilators decrease ventricular volumes and may cause reflex increases in heart rate, which further stress the myocardium in obstructive cardiomyopathy. Propranolol, a beta blocker, is therefore the medication of choice.

Reference: Underhill, S., Woods, S., Froelicher, E., et al.: Cardiac Nursing, 2nd ed. J.B. Lippincott, Philadelphia, 1989.

2–176. (**A**) The development of ring abscesses and myocardial abscesses will cause conduction defects. Congestive failure generally causes tachycardia. CNS complications such as meningitis and cerebral infarct do not affect the PR interval.

Reference: Weeks, L.: Advanced Cardiovascular Nursing. Blackwell, Boston, 1986.

2–177. (**C**) The most common signs of acute subdural hematoma are headache, drowsiness, some agitation, slow cerebration, and confusion. The ipsilateral pupil dilates and eventually becomes fixed. While hemiparesis may occur early, it is usually a late finding.

Reference: Hickey, J.V.: The Clinical Practice of Neurological and Neurosurgical Nursing, 2nd ed. J.B. Lippincott, Philadelphia, 1986.

2–178. (**D**) Basilar skull fractures extend into the anterior, middle, or posterior fossae at the base of the skull. This may cause injury to cranial nerves as well as a tearing of the dura mater, which may result in a CSF otorrhea or rhinorrhea that leads to meningitis. Anterior fossa fractures may result in bilateral periorbital ecchymoses from bleeding into the sinuses and rhinorrhea if the dura is torn. Middle fossa fractures cause otorrhea if the dura is torn and the tympanic membrane ruptured. Posterior fossa fractures result in epidural hematomas with resultant medullary failure and death if left untreated.

Reference: Alspach, J.G. (ed.): AACN Core Curriculum for Critical Care Nursing, 4th ed. W.B. Saunders, Philadelphia, 1991.

2–179. (**B**) The positive results of the ELISA and western blot tests indicate the presence of HIV infection. Therefore, the patient should be given information about safe sex practices to protect sexual partners.

Reference: Gee, G., and Moran, T.A.: AIDS—Concepts in Nursing Practice. Williams & Wilkins, Baltimore, 1988.

2–180. (**D**) Universal precautions provide for using appropriate barriers to protect oneself from possible contact with infectious organisms. Handling blood and blood-contaminated specimens with gloved hands is one of those recommendations. Other recommendations include disposal of needles and syringes as a unit in a puncture-proof container; wearing goggles during procedures that may involve aerosolization of secretions, such as suctioning or endotracheal intubation; and disposal of contaminated items, such as dressings, paper gowns, or paper cups, as contaminated waste products. Procedures such as bathing a patient with intact skin do not require the use of barriers; barriers are used to protect oneself from contact with blood or body secretion.

Reference: Dickerson, M.A.: Protecting yourself from AIDS: Infection control measures for the critical care practitioner. Crit Care Nurs, 9:26–28, 1989.

2-181. (**A**) The mixed venous blood gas is obtained from the distal port of the pulmonary artery catheter. The tip of the catheter should be in the main pulmonary artery where the venous blood is completely mixed.

Reference: Snyder, J.V., and Pinsky, M.R.: Oxygen Transport in the Critically Ill. Year Book Medical Publishers, Chicago, 1987.

2-182. (**B**) The clinical presentation is classic for signs of air hunger and fighting the ventilator. The most common cause is decreased flow during inspiration, which gives the sensation of smothering.

Reference: Alspach, J.G. (ed.): AACN Core Curriculum for Critical Care Nursing, 4th ed. W.B. Saunders, Philadelphia, 1991.

2-183. (**C**) A potential complication associated with the insertion of a peritoneal dialysis catheter is bowel perforation. The classic symptoms of this complication are diarrhea and reduced or fecal-colored peritoneal drainage. Abdominal pain may or may not be present initially, depending in part on the extent of the perforation and the amount of pain medication administered prior to the procedure. Dialysis disequilibrium syndrome is a complication associated with hemodialysis. Pseudomembranous colitis is associated with copious watery diarrhea with an infectious etiology, but the patient's history of catheter insertion make this diagnosis very unlikely. Dumping syndrome is characterized by nausea, vomiting, diarrhea, and weakness occurring shortly after a meal. Although not totally understood, dumping syndrome is believed to be caused by a combination of rapid gastric emptying compounded by intraluminal hyperosmolarity and rapid fluid shifts.

References: Holloway, N.M.: Nursing the Critically Ill Adult, 3rd ed. Addison-Wesley, New York, 1988.
Sleisenger, M.H., and Fordtran, J.S. (eds.): Gastrointestinal Disease: Pathophysiology, Diagnosis, Management, 4th ed. W.B. Saunders, Philadelphia, 1989.

2-184. (**A**) Hyperglycemia, hypernatremia, and protein loss are complications of peritoneal dialysis, but not complications of hemodialysis. Dialysis disequilibrium syndrome is related to the osmotic gradient produced across the blood-brain barrier by the efficient removal of urea from the blood. The urea located in brain tissue draws in water from the extracellular fluid and causes cerebral edema.

References: Crandall, B.L.: Chronic renal failure. In Ulrich, B.T. (ed.): Nephrology Nursing: Concepts and Strategies. Appleton and Lange, Norwalk, CT, 1989.
Thompson, J., McFarland, G.K., Hirsch, J.E., et al.: Mosby's Manual of Clinical Nursing, 2nd ed. C.V. Mosby, St. Louis, 1989.

2-185. (**B**) The independent patient often reacts negatively to the dependent role, as demonstrated by acting out in the form of nonadherence to the medical regimen and anger toward others, as well as denial of symptoms. Patients placed on dialysis need a great deal of emotional support and have many fears and questions.

References: Norris, M.: Acute tubular necrosis: Preventing complications. Dimen Crit Care Nurs, 8:16–26, 1989.
Ulrich, B.T.: Psychological aspects of nephrology nursing. In Ulrich, B.T. (ed.): Nephrology Nursing: Concepts and Strategies. Appleton and Lange, Norwalk, CT, 1989.

2-186. (**D**) Laceration, a more severe sequela of closed head injury, occurs as the brain tissue moves across the uneven base of the skull in contusion. Typically, contusion causes cerebral dysfunction with resultant bruising of the brain. Concussion causes transient loss of consciousness and retrograde amnesia and is generally reversible.

Reference: Alspach, J.G. (ed.): AACN Core Curriculum for Critical Care Nursing, 4th ed. W.B. Saunders, Philadelphia, 1991.

2–187. (**B**) Dilutional hyponatremia occurs during syndrome of inappropriate secretion of ADH (SIADH) as free water is reabsorbed, despite a low serum osmolality. Extracellular fluid osmolality falls as the water-to-sodium ratio increases. Osmosis occurs into the cells where osmolality is higher. Cerebral edema is a consequence of cellular swelling.

Reference: Holloway, N.M.: Nursing the Critically Ill Adult, 3rd ed. Addison-Wesley, Menlo Park, CA, 1988.

2–188. (**D**) Loud, high-pitched bowel sounds accompanied by nausea, vomiting, or cramping abdominal pain usually indicate an intestinal obstruction. Bowel sounds are usually absent in paralytic ileus. Ascites is a collection of fluid in the abdominal cavity that will muffle bowel sounds. Mesenteric thrombosis can be detected by the cessation of bowel sounds accompanied by intense abdominal pain.

Reference: Luckmann, J., and Sorensen, K.C.: Medical-Surgical Nursing: A Psychophysiologic Approach, 3rd ed. W.B. Saunders, Philadelphia, 1987.

2–189. (**B**) Minimizing the extent of spinal cord injury is the highest priority of patient management upon arrival at the facility. All patients with spinal cord injury should be suspected of having cervical spinal injury until this is ruled out by x-ray. Patients with spinal cord injuries must be protected against unnecessary further injury caused by improper handling such as that which might occur in transfers from stretcher to bed. When patients are transported, they must be maintained in a supine position on a flat surface with the head in a neutral position.

Reference: Kinney, M.R., Packa, D.R., and Dunbar, S.B.: AACN's Clinical Reference for Critical Care Nursing, 2nd ed. McGraw-Hill, New York, 1988.

2–190. (**D**) Meningitis occurs as a result of infecting organisms invading the subarachnoid spaces and the meninges. It often follows neurosurgical procedures. *Staphylococcus aureus* or *Staphylococcus epidermidis* is most often the infecting organism. Contamination following neurosurgery results from intraoperative contamination, local wound infection from irrigation systems, drains, or intracranial pressure monitors. Signs and symptoms include fever, tachycardia, chills, petechiae or purpura, headache, nuchal rigidity, and positive Brudzinski's and Kernig's signs.

Reference: Alspach, J.G. (ed.): AACN Core Curriculum for Critical Care Nursing, 4th ed. W.B. Saunders, Philadelphia, 1991.

2–191. (**D**) When perfusion is restored to ischemic muscle, myoglobin is released into circulation. The elevated CPK totals reflect the extent of muscle ischemia present, and serial studies demonstrate the effectiveness of therapy.

Reference: Fahey, V.: Vascular Nursing. W.B. Saunders, Philadelphia, 1988.

2–192. (**A**) To prevent myoglobin released from ischemic muscle from precipitating acute tubular necrosis (ATN), it must be flushed from renal circulation. Fluid therapy with sodium bicarbonate at rates of greater than 150 ml per hour corrects lactic acidosis and clears myoglobin through the renal system. Osmotic diuretics such as mannitol may also be used; however, diuretics such as acetazolamide and furosemide in early phases of treatment may increase the risk of ATN by promoting hypovolemia.

Reference: Fahey, V.: Vascular Nursing. W.B. Saunders, Philadelphia, 1988.

2–193. (**D**) A bowel training program begins with a regular time for elimination based on the patient's normal bowel habit. Vigorous stimulation of the anal sphincter is contraindicated because it could precipitate autonomic dysreflexia. Bulk-building additives are encouraged in order to maintain stool consistency and bowel contractions. Strenuous exercise is contraindicated because it can exacerbate the demyelinating process.

Reference: Swearingen, P.L., Sommers, M.S., and Miller, K.: Manual of Critical Care: Applying Nursing Diagnoses to Critical Illness. C.V. Mosby, St. Louis, 1988.

2–194. (**D**) The serum glucose value during HHNK is usually greater than 600 mg/dl, and the serum osmolality is greater than 320 mOsm/l. The osmotic diuresis can be insidious and prolonged, resulting in profound volume depletion and hyperglycemia. Hyperglycemia worsens when glomerular filtration and renal glucose excretion decrease.

Reference: Hamburger, S., Rush, D.R., and Bosker, G.: Endocrine and Metabolic Emergencies. Robert J. Brady, Bowie, MD, 1984.

2–195. (**C**) The nurse should immediately cover the wound with a dressing and then administer sedation and/or restraints. The positive-pressure ventilation prevents the lung from collapsing. Increasing the suction does not help.

Reference: Kinney, M.R., Packa, D.R., and Dunbar, S.B.: AACN's Clinical Reference for Critical Care Nursing, 2nd ed. McGraw-Hill, New York, 1988.

2–196. (**C**) Stopping the infusion of the contrast agent and changing the IV bag and tubing eliminate any further infusion of the substance. Application of a tourniquet above the IV site can delay circulation and absorption of the antigen. Deterioration of the patient's cardiovascular status may require administration of IV fluids or other medications. The absorption of medications administered intramuscularly would be delayed as a result of poor circulation.

Reference: Dickerson, M.A.: Anaphylaxis and anaphylactic shock. Crit Care Nurs Q, *11*:68–74, 1988.

2–197. (**A**) Arginine vasopressin (antidiuretic hormone, ADH, AVP) increases free water permeability in the renal collecting tubules. This results in an osmotically induced movement of water from the tubular lumen to the medullary interstitium. In the absence of ADH, water reabsorption is impaired. Polyuria occurs, resulting in dehydration and hypernatremia.

Reference: Kohler, P.O., and Jordan, R.M. (eds.): Clinical Endocrinology. John Wiley and Sons, New York, 1986.

2–198. (**D**) Fluid volume deficit related to output exceeding intake is an appropriate nursing diagnosis. Defining characteristics that are present and associated with this nursing diagnosis include: decreased blood pressure, increased heart rate, and output exceeding input. Elevated serum sodium and osmolality, and decreased urine osmolality and specific gravity are associated with free water loss (dehydration).

Reference: Holloway, N.M.: Nursing the Critically Ill Adult, 3rd ed. Addison-Wesley, Menlo Park, CA, 1988.

2–199. **(B)** Prior to elective surgery, the patient who wants to receive an autologous transfusion donates a prescribed number of units of blood, which can then be used during or after surgery. The blood must be typed and cross-matched for identification. The blood is also tested for the presence of HIV and hepatitis B virus. Even though these tests may be negative, the blood may be infectious. Infected blood does present a risk to the health care provider who is not using appropriate infection control precautions. There is no reason to test the patient for hepatitis when he or she is receiving autologous blood. Transfusion reactions, such as a bacterial reaction, can also occur. Blood is not warmed unless the patient has cold agglutinins present.

Reference: Bonato, J.: Blood transfusions: Are they safe? Crit Care Nurs, *9:*40–46, 1989.

2–200. **(A)** The family is unable to cope at this point and needs information and support to help them gain control. The other strategies will not help them gain control and may anger them, making the situation worse.

Reference: Meijs, C.A.: Care of the family of the ICU patient. Crit Care Nurs, *9:*42–44, 1989.

3-1. Myocardial wall tension is determined by which of the following factors?

    A. The contractile state of the myocardium and the heart rate.
    B. Peripheral resistance and ventricular volume.
    C. Ventricular volume and systolic pressure.
    D. Heart rate and systolic blood pressure.

3-2. The major muscle(s) of inspiration is (are) the

    A. Sternocleidomastoid.
    B. Diaphragm.
    C. External intercostals.
    D. Abdominals.

3-3. The blood-brain barrier has several functions. One is to

    A. Limit transfer of certain substances into the extracellular fluid (ECF) or cerebrospinal fluid (CSF) in the brain.
    B. Drain blood from the cavernous sinus of the brain.
    C. Permit selective transport from the blood to the ventricular system.
    D. Allow drugs to diffuse freely into the CSF.

3-4. The best clinical indicator of the glomerular filtration rate is

    A. Creatinine clearance.
    B. Blood urea nitrogen.
    C. Serum creatinine.
    D. Urea clearance.

3–5. Which of the following electrolytes facilitates carbohydrate absorption by increasing cellular permeability to glucose?

   A. Calcium.
   B. Sodium.
   C. Magnesium.
   D. Sulfate.

3–6. A large (32-mm) v wave appears on the pulmonary capillary wedge pressure tracing of a patient unstable after an extensive inferior wall myocardial infarction. This finding is consistent with which of the following clinical states?

   A. Cardiogenic shock.
   B. Congestive heart failure.
   C. Mitral regurgitation.
   D. Pericarditis.

3–7. Aspiration of gastric contents results in

   A. Chemical pneumonitis.
   B. Viral pneumonitis.
   C. Radiation pneumonitis.
   D. Adult respiratory distress syndrome.

3–8. Metabolic acidosis affects calcium regulation by

   A. Decreasing intestinal absorption of calcium.
   B. Decreasing reabsorption of calcium in the distal nephron.
   C. Decreasing bone reabsorption of calcium.
   D. Decreasing osteoclast activity.

3–9. An appropriate nursing diagnosis following intracranial surgery is "Disturbance in self-concept: body image, self-esteem, role-performance, personal identity related to actual/perceived loss of well-being." A nursing intervention associated with this diagnosis is to

   A. Orient the patient to the environment every 2 hours.
   B. Determine the patient's understanding of his or her condition and anticipated outcomes.
   C. Assist the patient to resolve grief.
   D. Perform all nursing interventions quickly to avoid tiring the patient.

3–10. Which of the following is (are) true regarding the legal declaration of death?

   I. Consent of next of kin is required prior to the declaration of death.
   II. Cessation of cardiopulmonary activity is accepted as a definition of death in all states.
   III. Brain death, according to the criteria of the Uniform Determination of Death Act, is accepted as a legal definition of death in all states.
   IV. Declaration of death is sufficient reason to cease care unless organ donation is anticipated or the patient is pregnant and efforts are under way to save the life of the fetus.

   A. II and IV.
   B. I and II.
   C. III and IV.
   D. II and III.

3–11. Serum laboratory values in a near-drowning victim would likely be

   A. Hemodiluted.
   B. Hemoconcentrated.
   C. The same as normal.
   D. Different with salt-water than with fresh-water drowning.

3–12. Which of the following is a normal jugular venous pulse finding in the physical examination?

A. The internal jugular pulse is not visible with the patient supine.
B. The internal jugular pulse is visible to 2 cm above the clavicle with the head of the bed elevated 45°.
C. The internal jugular pulse is visible to 6 cm above the clavicle with the head of the bed elevated 45°.
D. The internal jugular pulse increases in height with deep inspiration.

3–13. A patient has been NPO and comatose for 5 days after a craniotomy for a brain tumor. Full strength tube feeding at 80 ml per hour is now ordered. The patient has a serum albumin of 1.5 gm/dl. The nurse will monitor the patient for development of

A. Hyperglycemia.
B. Hypervolemia.
C. Osmotic diarrhea.
D. Elevated SGOT and SGPT.

3–14. In planning for nursing care of the patient with Guillain-Barré syndrome (GBS), the critical care nurse knows that

A. Only proximal muscles are involved in this disease.
B. Paresthesias associated with the disease cause decreased sensation to pain.
C. Remyelinization and axonal regeneration may take up to 2 years.
D. The patient's level of consciousness may be affected as the disease progresses.

3–15. Renal phosphate excretion is decreased in all of the following *except*

A. Renal failure.
B. Hypomagnesemia.
C. Hypoparathyroid states.
D. Hypokalemia.

3–16. The slow response action potential is characteristic of

A. Purkinje fiber cells.
B. Atrial cells.
C. Ventricular cells.
D. SA and AV nodal cells.

3–17. A patient had an estimated blood loss of 1,500 ml during surgery 3 days ago. You would now expect this patient's reticulocyte count to be

A. Below normal.
B. Normal.
C. Above normal.
D. The same as it was preoperatively.

3–18. A 54-year-old female is admitted with an acoustic neuroma. When assessing this patient, the critical care nurse knows that this tumor generally affects the function of which cranial nerves?

A. III and VII.
B. IV and VIII.
C. IV and IX.
D. VII and VIII.

3–19. A patient is on the ventilator with settings of V_T 800, rate 10 per minute, FI_{O_2} 0.4, and PEEP 0, and his ventilator pressures are at a peak of 40 cm H_2O and a plateau of 36 cm H_2O. His nursing diagnosis is "Impaired gas exchange related to alveolar-capillary membrane changes." Weaning is instituted and his ventilator rate is decreased to 6. Half an hour later, his arterial blood gases show pH 7.32, Pa_{CO_2} 60 mm Hg, HCO_3 20 mEq/l, Pa_{O_2} 85 mm Hg, and Sa_{O_2} 92%.
The acidosis is probably due to

A. Lactic acidosis.
B. Tissue hypoxia.
C. Reduced hypoxic drive.
D. Reduced alveolar ventilation.

3–20. Right atrial hypertrophy is indicated on the 12-lead ECG by P waves that are

A. Greater than 3 mm in amplitude in any lead.
B. Notched in limb leads V_5 and V_6.
C. Negatively deflected in V_1 and V_2.
D. Tall and peaked in leads II and III.

3–21. A 22-year-old male who was involved in a motor vehicle accident 3 days ago develops respiratory failure and is placed on a ventilator. His arterial blood gases are as follows: pH 7.32, Pa_{CO_2} 30 mm Hg, HCO_3 14 mEq/l, Pa_{O_2} 60 mm Hg, Sa_{O_2} 89%, Ca_{O_2} 17.5 ml/dl; he is on FI_{O_2} 0.35, SIMV 12, V_T 750 ml, and PEEP 0. This patient's acid-base dysfunction is

A. Respiratory alkalosis.
B. Metabolic acidosis.
C. Respiratory acidosis.
D. Metabolic alkalosis.

3–22. An abnormal plantar reflex is suggestive of

A. Upper motor neuron lesions.
B. Diffuse cerebral dysfunction.
C. Lower motor neuron lesions.
D. Cerebellar dysfunction.

3–23. Which of the following conditions predispose a patient to fluid volume deficit?

A. GI secretion loss.
B. Prolonged steroid therapy.
C. Hyperaldosteronism.
D. Decreased renal excretion.

3–24. A patient with a blood pressure of 200/142 mm Hg would have which of the following forms of hypertension?

A. Essential hypertension.
B. Accelerated hypertension.
C. Malignant hypertension.
D. Hypertensive encephalopathy.

3–25. When performing a physical assessment of a patient with a brain tumor, the critical care nurse knows that if the patient exhibits astereognosis and hyperesthesia, the patient most likely has involvement of the

A. Frontal lobe.
B. Parietal lobe.
C. Temporal lobe.
D. Occipital lobe.

3–26. Pituitary tumors may

A. Cause hydrocephalus and increased intracranial pressure.
B. Produce symptoms of renin imbalance.
C. Produce symptoms of Addison's disease.
D. Compress the optic chiasm and cause visual changes.

3–27. A patient's lung compliance has increased from 15 to 25 cm H_2O over the last 2 days. This indicates that

A. He needs suctioning.
B. His lungs are getting stiffer.
C. The ventilator needs adjusting.
D. His lungs are improving.

3–28. A 70-kg patient in the coronary care unit after acute myocardial infarction is currently on a continuous infusion of dopamine, 15 μg/kg/minute, and an infusion of nitroglycerin, 2.0 μg/kg/minute. His pulmonary capillary wedge pressure is 25 mm Hg and his blood pressure is 90/60 mm Hg, with a mean arterial pressure of 70 mm Hg. His skin is warm, dry, and pink. All pulses are palpable at 1+. Although he had been pain-free for 4 hours with the above constant infusions and hemodynamic findings, he is now complaining of a severe headache and chest pain. The nurse should obtain a 12-lead ECG and

A. Increase the dopamine infusion to 20 μg/kg/minute to increase blood pressure and coronary artery perfusion.
B. Increase the nitroglycerin infusion to 2.5 μg/kg/minute to improve coronary artery flow and relieve chest pain.
C. Decrease the nitroglycerin infusion to 1.5 μg/kg/minute and evaluate its effect on the patient's headache and expected increase in blood pressure.
D. Administer nitroglycerin 1/150 grain sublingually and monitor its effect on the patient's blood pressure and chest pain.

3–29. A patient with a plasma glucose level of less than 40 mg/dl would most likely be

A. Diaphoretic and tachycardic.
B. Warm with flushed skin.
C. Dyspneic and bradycardic.
D. Mottled and flaccid.

3–30. Assessment of cranial nerve V includes

A. Shining a light into one eye and noting constriction of the contralateral pupil.
B. Shining a light in one eye and observing constriction of the ipsilateral pupil.
C. Touching the back of the tongue and noting the presence of the gag reflex.
D. Touching the cornea with a cotton wisp and noting a blink reflex.

3–31. The most life-threatening renal injury that is likely to present *without* hematuria is

A. Renal pedicle trauma.
B. Renal fragmentation.
C. Renal contusion.
D. Renal laceration.

3–32. Suctioning of the tracheobronchial tree on intubated patients should be performed

A. When secretions are present.
B. At least every 4 hours.
C. At least every 2 hours.
D. At least once a shift.

3–33. A patient with type B blood is given a transfusion of type AB blood and develops a transfusion reaction. The reaction occurs because

A. The patient's blood contains anti-B antibodies.
B. The infused blood contains both anti-A and anti-B antigens.
C. The patient's blood contains anti-A antibodies.
D. The infused blood contains anti-B antibodies.

3–34. Antacids decrease the absorption of

A. Aspirin.
B. Bishydroxycoumarin.
C. Levodopa.
D. Digoxin.

3–35. The pathogenesis of vasogenic cerebral edema is best described by which of the following statements?

A. An increase of fluid within the intracellular space.
B. Cerebral hypoxia associated with global ischemia.
C. Obstructive hydrocephalus.
D. A defect in the blood-brain barrier.

3–36. Which of the following potential problems is a *priority* in the care of a patient who has *just completed* an infusion of tissue plasminogen activator (t-PA) for acute myocardial infarction?

A. Decreased tissue perfusion related to myocardial necrosis.
B. Alteration in comfort, chest pain.
C. Alteration in cardiac output related to dysrhythmias.
D. Fluid volume deficit related to anticoagulation.

3–37. Which of the following is an alterable risk factor for pneumonia?

A. Length of time intubated.
B. Type of endotracheal tube.
C. Length of operation time.
D. Pre-existing pulmonary problems.

3–38. Hypermagnesemia affects cellular activity by

A. Altering cell membrane permeability.
B. Inhibiting the cellular production of energy.
C. Increasing binding between oxygen and hemoglobin.
D. Causing a curare-like effect on the neuromuscular junction.

3–39. When performing a neurologic assessment, the critical care nurse knows to assess cranial nerve III. This pair of cranial nerves is responsible for

A. Abduction of the eye.
B. Response to light, accommodation, and visual acuity.
C. Pupillary constriction, response to light, and extraocular movements.
D. Pupillary constriction only.

3–40. A patient is suspected of having a right ventricular infarction. Which of the following hemodynamic changes would the nurse expect to see?

	CVP	PCWP	MAP
A.	15 mm Hg	5 mm Hg	66 mm Hg
B.	15 mm Hg	12 mm Hg	90 mm Hg
C.	5 mm Hg	18 mm Hg	90 mm Hg
D.	15 mm Hg	18 mm Hg	62 mm Hg

3–41. Treatment for right ventricular myocardial infarction typically includes

A. Diuretic therapy.
B. Nitroglycerin infusion.
C. Oxygen therapy.
D. Sodium and fluid restriction.

3–42. A 70-year-old patient is admitted to the intensive care unit postoperatively. You know that this patient

A. Will be immunosuppressed.
B. May exhibit anergy when tested.
C. Will be treated with prophylactic antibiotics.
D. Is at no risk for developing a postoperative infection.

Questions 3–43 and 3–44 refer to the following situation.

After intubation, a patient has absent breath sounds on the left, decreased Sa_{O_2} by pulse oximeter, decreased left chest expansion, and high peak pressures on the ventilator.

3–43. The most likely problem is

A. Pneumothorax.
B. Right bronchial intubation.
C. Left pleural effusion.
D. Pulmonary embolus.

3–44. The appropriate treatment for this condition would be

A. Streptokinase.
B. Vena caval umbrella.
C. Pull back endotracheal tube.
D. Chest tube.

3–45. The *quickest* means of antagonizing the cardiac and neuromuscular toxicity of hyperkalemia is by the administration of

A. Sodium bicarbonate.
B. Calcium.
C. Glucose.
D. Sodium polystyrene sulfonate (Kayexalate).

3–46. A 46-year-old construction worker is admitted with the diagnosis of C8 anterior cord syndrome. As the nurse caring for him, you know that nursing care must

A. Support total respiratory function.
B. Inform the patient of position when moving his extremities.
C. Avoid application of heat or cold unless specifically ordered.
D. Provide passive range of motion exercises to upper extremities related to loss of biceps and triceps muscle function.

3–47. Urea is formed by the liver to rid the body of

A. Creatinine.
B. Bicarbonate.
C. Bilirubin.
D. Ammonia.

3–48. A cardiac surgical patient develops the dysrhythmia illustrated below.
Which of the following methods would *best* demonstrate atrial activity if any is present in the dysrhythmia below?

A. Obtain an atrial ECG using the atrial pacing wires.
B. Obtain a 12-lead ECG.
C. Perform carotid massage while running a rhythm strip.
D. Change the lead placement to MCL_1.

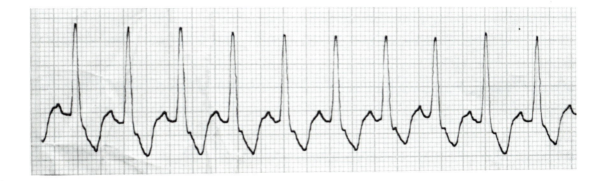

3–49. The rhythm illustrated below is noted in a postoperative coronary artery bypass patient 4 hours after surgery. The patient's arterial blood gases (ABGs) and other laboratory values 1 hour prior were: pH 7.45, P_{O_2} 184 mm Hg, P_{CO_2} 35 mm Hg, O_2 saturation 100%, Hct 32%, sodium 140 mEq/l, potassium 4.5 mEq/l, glucose 140 mg/dl. Respiratory settings on the ventilator remain the same, FI_{O_2} is 40%, and oxygen saturation by pulse oximeter remains 100%. Urine output for the last hour was 80 ml per hour.

The nurse should

A. Increase the FI_{O_2} to 50% and obtain another ABG analysis and serum potassium level.
B. Deliver 10 mEq of KCl over 1 hour and repeat the ABG and potassium determinations.
C. Administer lidocaine, 1 mg/kg by IV push, and obtain a serum potassium determination.
D. Obtain ABG and serum potassium determinations.

3–50. A 68-year-old male has been on a ventilator for 3 weeks. Attempts at weaning have been unsuccessful owing to his anxiety about being off the ventilator. Strategies the nurse can use to help minimize his distress include all of the following *except*

A. Provide sufficient rest periods.
B. Provide sedation.
C. Remain out of the room during weaning.
D. Encourage his participation in decision-making.

3–51. A 76-year-old male has been ventilator-dependent for a week owing to impaired gas exchange related to pneumonia. Attempts to wean have been unsuccessful. He has a history of smoking and a 30-year history of chronic obstructive pulmonary disease (COPD), and has been on oxygen with limited mobility at home. He is 6 feet, 2 inches tall and weighs 150 pounds. A concern at this point would be to maximize and assess

A. Weaning trials.
B. Muscle strength.
C. Activity level.
D. Nutritional status.

3–52. Which of the following is a cause of hyperphosphatemia?

A. Malabsorption syndrome.
B. Thiazide diuretics.
C. Renal failure.
D. Alkalosis.

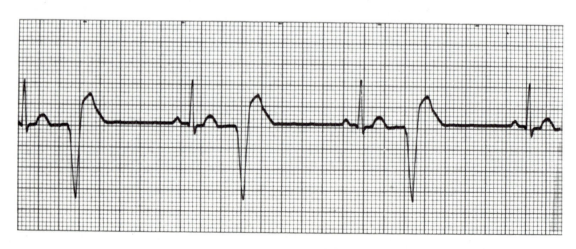

Questions 3–53 and 3–54 refer to the following situation.

A 37-year-old male is admitted following transient episodes of syncope, motor weakness, sensory deficits, and hemianopsia. A diagnosis of possible arteriovenous malformation (AVM) is made.

3–53. Results of a lumbar puncture are:

Intracranial pressure	180 mm H_2O
Color	Xanthochromic
RBCs	Present
WBCs	6 cells/mm^3
Glucose	75 mg/dl

In evaluating these results, the critical care nurse develops a comprehensive nursing care plan for the patient based on

A. Subarachnoid hemorrhage precautions.
B. Meningitis precautions.
C. Profoundly increased intracranial pressure.
D. Herniation precautions.

3–54. The patient undergoes a craniotomy with surgical excision of the AVM. Postoperatively he is on subarachnoid precautions and has a subarachnoid bolt in place. In evaluating care for this patient, the critical care nurse would be most concerned if his laboratory data revealed a

A. Pa_{CO_2} of 32 mm Hg.
B. Pa_{CO_2} of 52 mm Hg.
C. Urine specific gravity of 1.016.
D. Serum sodium of 128 mEq/l.

3–55. The staff of a critical care unit includes a nurse who is rumored to be dependent on narcotics. Her coworkers have noted that her clinical judgements are often questionable, and they have become concerned for patient safety. What is the most reasonable course of action for the nurse's coworkers?

A. Notify the state licensing agency (Board of Nursing).
B. Document the incidents and report their concerns to the supervisor.
C. Inform the narcotics division of the local police force.
D. Protect their colleague by maintaining silence, and protect patients by dividing her assignments among themselves.

3–56. Albumin is synthesized in the

A. Bone marrow.
B. Liver.
C. Spleen.
D. Thymus gland.

3–57. Patients undergoing digital subtraction angiography (DSA) to assess cerebrovascular disease should receive instruction regarding which of the following?

A. The superiority of this technique over conventional angiography techniques.
B. The need for patient cooperation and the potential need for further testing.
C. The potential for nephrotoxicity.
D. The risk of carotid dissection and cerebrovascular embolization.

3–58. After percutaneous arteriography, a patient complains of intense groin pain. Femoral pulses are visibly detected and palpated as 4+ at the puncture site. Distal pulses (dorsalis pedis and posterior tibialis) are 1+. The puncture site is firm and swollen, with minimal discoloration. The etiology of these findings is most likely

A. An embolus.
B. A hematoma.
C. A pseudoaneurysm.
D. Contrast-induced vasospasm.

Questions 3–59 and 3–60 refer to the following situation.

A 17-year-old female was admitted to the intensive care unit 2 days ago, following an automobile accident. Injuries included multiple bruises and lacerations, a left femur fracture, a skull fracture, and multiple rib fractures. She has been unconscious since admission. Vital signs and laboratory data include:

BP	90/60 mm Hg
HR	110/min
RR	28/min
24-hour urine output	4200 ml
24-hour fluid intake	1800 ml

Serum Values

Na	149 mEq/l
K	4 mEq/l
Osmolality	305 mOsm/l

Urine Values

Osmolality	280 mOsm/l
Specific gravity	1.001

3–59. The abnormal elevation in serum osmolality is associated with

A. Cerebral edema.
B. Dehydration.
C. Pneumothorax.
D. Hemorrhage.

3–60. Nursing interventions appropriate for this patient include all of the following *except*

A. Continuous cardiac monitoring.
B. Record daily weights.
C. Place the patient in Trendelenburg's position.
D. Administer IV fluid to replace hourly output.

3–61. A precipitating factor in the development of hyponatremia may be

A. Hypokalemia.
B. Hypercalcemia.
C. Nephrotic syndrome.
D. Osmotic diuretics.

3–62. The rhythm strip below would be classified as

A. Sick sinus syndrome.
B. Junctional escape rhythm.
C. Wolff-Parkinson-White syndrome.
D. Left posterior fascicular block.

Questions 3–63 and 3–64 refer to the following situation.

A 56-year-old male has a well-known history of COPD. He has been in the intensive care unit on a ventilator for 2 weeks following a pneumothorax associated with rib fractures. Weaning is being implemented. Up to this time, he has been cooperative and helpful with his care. Now he is anxious and dependent, refuses treatments and activity, and reacts angrily to any attempt to have him participate in his care.

3–63. The patient's behavior is most likely due to

A. Feelings of dependence.
B. Respiratory muscle fatigue.
C. Alkalosis.
D. Acidosis.

3–64. The most appropriate intervention at this time would be to

A. Eliminate all distractions—i.e., TV, radio.
B. Actively listen to him express doubts and fears.
C. Set limits on his behaviors.
D. Wean at night when he is unaware of it.

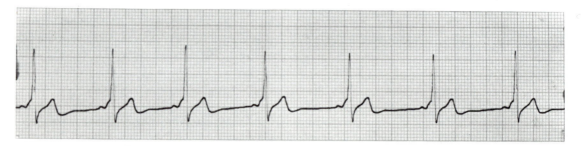

3–65. Drugs that may precipitate hyper-osmolar hyperglycemic nonketotic (HHNK) coma include all of the following *except*

A. Phenytoin (Dilantin).
B. Diazoxide (Proglycem).
C. Triamcinolone (Aristocort).
D. Acetaminophen (Tylenol and others).

3–66. A patient in the intensive care unit has an elevated level of indirect bilirubin. This value indicates that the patient

A. Has increased hemolysis of RBCs.
B. Is developing hepatitis.
C. Has cirrhosis.
D. Has increased erythropoietin production.

3–67. Cerebral blood flow (CBF) is influenced by several factors. Which of the following affects the diameter of the cerebrovascular bed?

A. Autoregulation.
B. Hypoxia.
C. Systolic blood pressure.
D. Diastolic blood pressure.

3–68. The critical care nurse is aware that knowledge of the Monro-Kellie hypothesis is important. This hypothesis states that

A. Increased intracranial pressure is directly proportional to the amount of circulating CSF.
B. Brain tissue water, CSF, and intravascular blood are volumetrically balanced.
C. Cerebral edema is a direct result of orthostatic changes that shift the brain.
D. Brain tissue water, CSF, tumor, and blood are in equal proportions.

3–69. Aluminum hydroxide gels are commonly used in the prevention of renal osteodystrophy (the bone abnormalities that occur with chronic renal failure) because they

A. Increase serum calcium.
B. Decrease serum potassium.
C. Decrease serum phosphate.
D. Increase serum sodium.

3–70. A 69-year-old male is admitted to the intensive care unit for acute upper GI bleeding. He states that he has no next of kin, and there is no one to notify of his illness. He denies a drinking problem but was admitted with a blood alcohol level of 0.25%. A possible nursing diagnosis is

A. Fluid volume excess related to high fluid intake.
B. Unilateral neglect related to poor nutritional intake.
C. Ineffective thermoregulation related to ethanol toxicity.
D. Social isolation related to alcohol abuse.

3–71. The average amount of blood lost during a single bleeding episode from esophageal varices is

A. 1 unit.
B. 5 units.
C. 10 units.
D. 15 units.

3–72. A temporary bipolar pacing catheter that does not sense appropriately may be converted to a unipolar pacemaker by

A. Attaching the positive terminal catheter wire to an ordinary ECG limb electrode.
B. Attaching the negative terminal catheter wire to a suture needle in the skin.
C. Increasing the sensitivity to the maximum level.
D. Disconnecting the negative terminal catheter wire.

3–73. R on T phenomena may be the result of which pacemaker complication?

A. Incomplete capture.
B. Inappropriate sensing.
C. Failure to sense.
D. Failure to pace.

3–74. To what would singed nares and smoke on the face of a firefighter alert the nurse?

A. Plastic surgery may be indicated.
B. Possible damage to teeth.
C. Possible tracheal edema and tracheal burns.
D. Pulmonary edema.

3–75. As you review a patient's laboratory results, you find schistocytes reported on the CBC results. You know that schistocytes

A. Play an important role in clotting.
B. Are the immature form of RBCs.
C. Are platelet precursor cells.
D. Are damaged RBCs.

3–76. An electrocardiographic finding associated with hypercalcemia (serum calcium > 13 mg/dl) is

A. Peaked T waves.
B. Shortened QT interval.
C. Abnormal Q waves.
D. Low-amplitude R waves.

3–77. Which of the following laboratory values suggest the onset of acute pancreatitis?

	Serum Amylase (units/l)	Serum Calcium (mg/dl)	Serum Lipase (units/ml)
A.	25	6	0.2
B.	125	11	0.5
C.	200	13	1.2
D.	300	7	2.2

3–78. The nurse anticipates that a patient with uncomplicated acute spinal cord injury at C7 to C8 will be able to

A. Breathe unassisted.
B. Sit up unsupported.
C. Maintain voluntary bowel function.
D. Coordinate fine hand movements.

3–79. In a patient with spinal shock following a C7 to C8 injury, return of reflex activity may be tested by which of the following reflexes?

A. Oculovestibular.
B. Oculocephalic.
C. Bulbocavernosus.
D. Biceps.

3–80. In assessing an ECG, the findings of bradycardia, ventricular fibrillation, inverted T waves, widening of the QRS complex, and/or prolonged QT interval should alert the nurse to the possibility of a serum potassium level of

A. 2.5 mEq/l.
B. 4.5 mEq/l.
C. 6.5 mEq/l.
D. 8.5 mEq/l.

3–81. A well-informed, well-educated patient who had been on multiple antiarrhythmic medications is to have electrophysiologic studies (EPS) in the morning. The nurse caring for the patient would *best* address the patient's fear and anxiety by

A. Reassuring the patient that his ECG is being continuously monitored and that the staff will respond immediately if needed.
B. Obtaining an order for diazepam and encouraging the patient to take the medication.
C. Encouraging the patient to verbalize his fears.
D. Encouraging the patient to engage in diversionary activities such as reading or TV.

3–82. Which of the following would best describe the dysrhythmia in the rhythm strip shown below?

   A. Sinus exit block.
   B. Wandering atrial pacemaker.
   C. Frequent premature atrial contractions.
   D. Sinus arrhythmia.

3–83. A hormone that stimulates the release of ACTH (adrenocorticotropic hormone) from the anterior pituitary gland is

   A. TRH (thyrotropin releasing hormone).
   B. GnRH (gonadotropin releasing hormone).
   C. PIF (prolactin release inhibiting factor).
   D. CRH (corticotropin releasing hormone).

3–84. A patient has a decreased number of B lymphocytes. This patient is at greatest risk for which of the following?

   A. *Staphylococcus aureus* infection.
   B. Herpes simplex.
   C. *Mycobacterium avium* infection.
   D. *Candida albicans* infection.

Questions 3–85 and 3–86 refer to the following situation.

A 63-year-old female is admitted in respiratory distress. She has a history of lung cancer with treatment consisting of both radiation and chemotherapy. Her nursing diagnosis is "Impaired breathing pattern."

3–85. Upon physical examination, the patient is observed to have deviation of the trachea to the right, decreased breath sounds on the left, diminished vocal fremitus, and dullness on percussion over the left. This is most likely due to

   A. Pneumonia.
   B. Pleural effusion.
   C. Pneumothorax.
   D. Atelectasis.

3–86. This patient also has distended neck veins and edema of the neck, eyelids, and hands. The most likely cause of this is

   A. Superior vena caval syndrome.
   B. Cor pulmonale.
   C. Congestive heart failure.
   D. Right ventricular failure.

3–87. Which of the following is the *least* reliable parameter for assessing increasing intracranial pressure?

   A. Pupillary dilatation.
   B. Change in pulse and blood pressure.
   C. Change in level of consciousness.
   D. Flexor posturing.

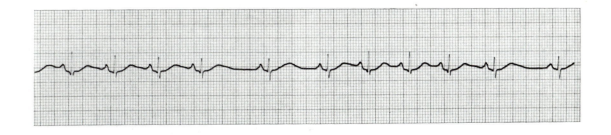

3–88. Three patients await liver transplantation, but only one organ is available. Tissue compatibility is not an issue.

Patient X is an infant with multiple anomalies who will die within days without a liver transplant. With a new liver, the child may live a few weeks.

Patient Y is a 50-year-old executive with adequate insurance and financial resources. His liver disease is the result of continued excessive alcohol intake.

Patient Z is a 24-year-old medical student. Her medical insurance does not cover organ transplantation.

If the committee responsible for the allocation of scarce resources functions under a social justice model, which of the following points might they consider in making their decision?

  I. Patient X will probably die in a short time whether or not a new liver is provided.
  II. Patient Y is responsible for destroying his own liver and therefore does not deserve a transplant.
  III. Patient Z has potential to provide valuable service to society if she survives.
  IV. Provision of service to patients who are unable to pay may lead to the financial ruin of the institution and eventually to an inability to provide any service.

A. I, III, and IV.
B. II.
C. I and II.
D. IV.

3–89. Yesterday, a 43-year-old female had urgent surgical repair of a perforated ulcer of the small intestine. The nurse will make every effort to keep her in which of the following positions?

A. Modified Trendelenburg's.
B. Supine.
C. Semi-Fowler's.
D. Lateral recumbent.

3–90. A head injury patient with a tracheostomy has been on enteral feedings by small-gauge feeding tube at 100 ml per hour. The gastric residuals have been 20 to 50 ml every 2 hours for the shift. Secretions have been small amounts of white thin sputum. The respiratory therapist suctions the patient and reports that sputum obtained this time was a large amount of yellow thick creamy secretions. What has most likely happened?

A. Pneumonia has developed.
B. The tracheal tube cuff has broken.
C. Feedings were aspirated.
D. The patient pulled the feeding tube out.

3–91. A balloon-tipped pacing wire is being inserted in a patient in the intensive care unit. The ECG monitor shows small, inverted P waves. This indicates that the pacing electrode is in the

A. Right atrium.
B. Superior vena cava.
C. Right ventricle.
D. Right ventricle, curled against the tricuspid valve.

3–92. A patient is being paced at 60 beats per minute. At this setting, cardiac output (CO) is 6 liters per minute, pulmonary capillary wedge pressure is 12 mm Hg, and systemic vascular resistance (SVR) is 900 dynes. If the pacemaker rate is increased to 75 beats per minute, which of the following is likely to occur?

A. Systemic vascular resistance will increase.
B. Pulmonary capillary wedge pressure will decrease.
C. Mean arterial pressure will decrease.
D. Cardiac output will increase.

Questions 3–93 through 3–95 refer to the following situation.

A 70-year-old male presents to the coronary care unit with bibasilar crackles, distended neck veins, an S_3 gallop, and marked dependent edema. During the nursing assessment he relates a previous cardiac history. His medications prior to admission include digoxin, furosemide, and potassium. He has been on a 2-gm sodium diet. Laboratory data include the following serum levels:

Sodium	116 mEq/l
Potassium	2.9 mEq/l
Chloride	74 mEq/l
Bicarbonate	28 mEq/l
Magnesium	1.0 mEq/l

3–93. This patient's serum sodium level is most likely the result of

A. Loss of protein.
B. Excessive diuresis.
C. Inappropriate secretion of antidiuretic hormone.
D. Decrease in effective circulatory volume.

3–94. The patient is placed on a cardiac monitor. An ECG change the nurse may expect as a result of his serum magnesium level is

A. Bradycardia.
B. Premature ventricular beats.
C. Shortened QT interval.
D. Complete heart block.

3–95. All of the following may be a contributing factor to this patient's potassium abnormality *except*

A. Furosemide administration.
B. Digitalis.
C. Hypomagnesemia.
D. Hypernatremia.

3–96. Pathologic states that may precipitate the syndrome of inappropriate antidiuretic hormone (SIADH) release include all of the following *except*

A. Ethanol ingestion.
B. Malignant carcinoma.
C. Bacterial pneumonia.
D. Physical and emotional stress.

3–97. Patients with the syndrome of inappropriate antidiuretic hormone (SIADH) release will have a urine specific gravity that is

A. Less than 300 mOsm/l.
B. Greater than 145 mEq/l.
C. Less than 1.005.
D. Greater than 1.020.

3–98. Which one of the following therapies acts *slowest* in reducing cerebral edema?

A. Fluid restriction.
B. Intravenous furosemide.
C. Dexamethasone.
D. Hypertonic solutions.

3–99. Heparin overdose

A. Should be treated with vitamin K.
B. Is diagnosed by monitoring the prothrombin time.
C. Does not occur if the medication is administered using an infusion pump.
D. May result in hematuria, epistaxis, and an acute change in level of consciousness.

3–100. Cryoprecipitate is administered to patients with coagulopathies to

A. Restore clotting factors.
B. Elevate the platelet count.
C. Increase the number of circulating red blood cells.
D. Stimulate production of thrombopoietin.

3–101. Which component of the arterial blood gas survey indicates alveolar ventilation?

A. Pa_{O_2}.
B. Pa_{CO_2}.
C. pH.
D. HCO_3.

3–102. Which of the following electrocardiographic changes occurs in Prinzmetal's angina?

A. Q waves appear greater than 0.03 second in width.
B. Delta waves appear in the initial portion of the R wave.
C. T waves become isoelectric.
D. ST segments elevate.

3–103. Which of the following ECG findings is indicative of left ventricular hypertrophy (LVH)?

A. The S wave in leads I, II, and III is greater than the R wave.
B. The R wave is greater than the S wave in lead V_1.
C. The R wave in lead I is greater than 13 mm.
D. The mean QRS axis is $+30°$ to $+90°$.

3–104. Which of the following problems is a likely cause of posthepatic jaundice?

A. Bile duct obstruction.
B. Cirrhosis.
C. Bacterial toxins.
D. Transfusion-related hemolysis.

3–105. Which of the following treatments for hyperkalemia causes potassium to be shifted from the extracellular to the intracellular fluid?

A. Hypertonic glucose and insulin.
B. Ion exchange resin and normal saline.
C. Calcium gluconate.
D. Dialysis.

3–106. A 19-year-old college student is admitted with headache, nausea and vomiting, seizures, petechiae, and a temperature of 104° F following a myelogram. A diagnosis of meningitis is made. The nurse knows that

A. The causative organism entered the epidural space only.
B. The causative organism entered the subdural space only.
C. The causative organism entered the subarachnoid space.
D. The causative organism entered the falx cerebri.

3–107. Which type of myocardial infarction would be caused by occlusion of the circumflex artery?

A. Inferior wall infarction.
B. Anteroseptal infarction.
C. Anterior wall infarction.
D. Lateral wall infarction.

3–108. A patient with postinfarction ventricular septal defect (VSD) is being stabilized on intra-aortic balloon counterpulsation prior to surgical repair. Which of the following would best decrease the right heart failure associated with this condition?

A. Furosemide (Lasix), 20 mg IV every 12 hours.
B. Proper intra-aortic balloon pump timing.
C. Digoxin, 0.25 mg IV daily.
D. Intravenous infusion of nitroprusside.

3–109. Asthma is characterized by

A. Airway hyper-reactivity.
B. Destruction of alveolar walls.
C. Decreased work of breathing.
D. Decreased airways resistance.

3–110. Bronchodilator therapy may appear to be ineffective in status asthmaticus owing to

A. Mucus plugging.
B. Dilatation of bronchial walls.
C. Increased responsiveness of airways.
D. Hyperinflation of the lungs.

3–111. Which of the following contributing factors make acute renal failure patients at high risk for hemorrhage?

    I. Impaired clotting mechanism.
   II. Capillary fragility.
  III. Decreased production of erythropoietin.

    A. I only.
    B. I and III.
    C. II and III.
    D. III only.

3–112. Vitamin K deficiency may result from

    A. Bile duct obstruction.
    B. Hyperprothrombinemia.
    C. Anticoagulant overdosage.
    D. Lack of intrinsic factor.

3–113. The Glasgow Coma Score (GCS) assesses level of consciousness by determining the patient's best

    A. Sensory response, motor response, and eye opening.
    B. Motor activity, eye movements, and vital signs.
    C. Sensory, motor, and verbal response.
    D. Eye opening, motor response, and verbal response.

3–114. Which of the following substances is found in cells of the immune system?

    A. Epinephrine.
    B. Heparin.
    C. Dopamine.
    D. Insulin.

3–115. The most common complication of intra-aortic balloon counterpulsation is

    A. ICU psychosis.
    B. Limb ischemia.
    C. Dissection of the aorta.
    D. Septicemia.

3–116. Absolute contraindications to intra-aortic balloon counterpulsation include

    A. Mitral insufficiency.
    B. Aortic insufficiency.
    C. Sepsis.
    D. Femoral artery aneurysm.

3–117. An RN who is a Jehovah's Witness believes that the Bible prohibits the transfusion of blood. She receives an order to administer blood to a patient, not a Jehovah's Witness, who consents to the transfusion. The nurse is obligated

    A. Legally to administer the blood.
    B. Ethically to refuse to give the blood.
    C. To arrange for a qualified RN to administer the blood, if she is unwilling to give it herself.
    D. To request that the physician order a nonbiological plasma expander.

Questions 3–118 through 3–120 relate to the following situation.

A 24-year-old male was admitted to the intensive care unit 3 days ago following a motorcycle accident that caused a fractured femur, rib fractures, and multiple lacerations. His chest x-ray now shows a white-out bilaterally in the lungs. Despite intubation and mechanical ventilation with PEEP, the patient's Pa_{O_2} is 62 mm Hg.

3–118. An Oximetrix pulmonary artery catheter is placed in the main pulmonary artery. Initial pressures obtained are pulmonary artery systolic/pulmonary artery diastolic 32/21 mm Hg, pulmonary artery mean 26 mm Hg, pulmonary capillary wedge pressure (PCWP) 7 mm Hg, right atrial pressure (RAP) 5 mm Hg. These results show

    A. Cor pulmonale.
    B. Left-sided heart failure.
    C. Fluid overload.
    D. Hypoxic vasoconstriction.

3–119. The initial S$\bar{v}$O$_2$ upon placement of the Oximetrix pulmonary artery catheter is 64%. The PEEP level on the ventilator is increased to 12 cm H$_2$O with resulting arterial blood gases of pH 7.39, Pa$_{CO_2}$ 43 mm Hg, HCO$_3$ 19 mEq/l, Pa$_{O_2}$ 68 mm Hg, Sa$_{O_2}$ 90%, Ca$_{O_2}$ 17.8 ml/dl. The S$\bar{v}$O$_2$ at this time is 58%. What would be the most likely explanation of the drop in S$\bar{v}$O$_2$?

   A. Drop in cardiac output.
   B. Increase in oxygen consumption.
   C. Drop in arterial oxygen saturation.
   D. Decrease in arterial oxygen content.

3–120. Appropriate therapy to raise the S$\bar{v}$O$_2$ would include

   A. Vasopressors.
   B. Fluid therapy.
   C. Paralysis.
   D. Increase F$_{I_{O_2}}$.

3–121. Which of the following diagnostic tests would the critical care nurse anticipate for the patient with head trauma?

   A. Lumbar puncture.
   B. Cerebral angiography.
   C. Computed tomography.
   D. Myelography.

3–122. In continuous arteriovenous ultrafiltration, the presence of red blood in the ultrafiltrate indicates

   A. Rupture of a capillary fiber.
   B. Clotting within the filter.
   C. Over-heparinization.
   D. Clogging of the filter with plasma proteins.

3–123. If the purpose of continuous arteriovenous hemofiltration is the removal of extracellular fluid and toxic solute clearance, the nurse should anticipate a

   A. Low ultrafiltrate rate with filter replacement fluid.
   B. Low ultrafiltrate rate without filter replacement fluid.
   C. High ultrafiltrate rate with filter replacement fluid.
   D. High ultrafiltrate rate without filter replacement fluid.

3–124. The dysrhythmia shown in the following rhythm strip may be caused by

   A. Increased sympathetic tone.
   B. Decreased parasympathetic tone.
   C. AV node ischemia.
   D. Carotid sinus stimulation.

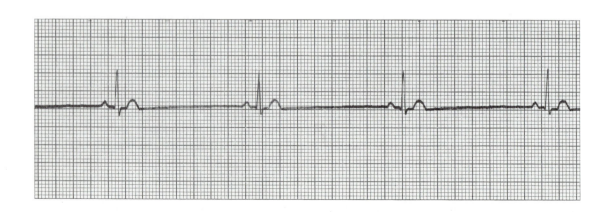

3–125. A patient with significant right ventricular myocardial infarction has hypotension and bradycardia. He would benefit most from

    A. Dopamine infusion at 10 µg/kg/minute.
    B. Atrial pacing at 80 beats per minute and dobutamine (Dobutrex) infusion at 5 µg/kg/minute.
    C. Isoproterenol (Isuprel) infusion at a rate titrated to maintain BP greater than 100 mm Hg systolic and heart rate greater than 60 per minute.
    D. Ventricular pacing at 70 demand and normal saline infusion at 125 ml per hour after a 500 ml bolus.

3–126. Two days ago, a 34-year-old salesman had a partial gastrectomy for a perforated peptic ulcer. He is now stable but has a knowledge deficit about his current health status and prescribed therapies. Which of the following approaches will his nurse use to resolve his knowledge deficit?

    A. Establish with the patient short-term and long-term goals to maintain adequate nutrition.
    B. Instruct family members to avoid discussing food or medications with the patient at this time.
    C. Provide one comprehensive explanation of peptic ulcer prognosis and treatment.
    D. Provide nutrition and medication information only in response to patient questions.

3–127. Which of the following needs is likely to be most important to the family of the alert esophagogastrectomy patient?

    A. A calm intensive care unit environment.
    B. To have realistic hope.
    C. To have chaplains available.
    D. To know names of the caregivers.

3–128. Hypoxia is defined as

    A. Decreased tissue oxygenation.
    B. Decreased arterial blood oxygen tension.
    C. Decreased arterial blood oxygen saturation.
    D. Decreased oxygen extraction.

3–129. Pulse oximetry monitoring is limited by

    A. Skin oxygen consumption.
    B. Arterial oxygen tension.
    C. Thickness of the skin.
    D. Poor tissue perfusion.

3–130. Cyanosis is an unreliable indicator of hypoxemia because

    A. Abnormal hemoglobin (Hgb) will mask it.
    B. Cyanosis depends on at least 5 gm of reduced Hgb.
    C. Carbon monoxide will produce cyanosis.
    D. Anemia alone will produce cyanosis.

Questions 3–131 and 3–132 refer to the following situation.

A 47-year-old chronic alcoholic is admitted to the intensive care unit with a diagnosis of subarachnoid hemorrhage. During an assessment the nurse observes muscle twitching, tremors, and choreiform movements. On further examination the nurse notes positive Chvostek's and Babinski signs. The cardiac monitor reveals a supraventricular tachycardia and ventricular premature contractions.

3–131. Which of the following metabolic alterations would most likely contribute to an alcoholic patient's clinical findings of positive Babinski and Chvostek's signs and arrhythmias?

    I. Hypocalcemia.
    II. Hypomagnesemia.
    III. Hyponatremia.

    A. I and III.
    B. I and II.
    C. II and III.
    D. I, II, and III.

3–132. The patient is rehydrated and hyperalimentation is initiated. Which of the following serum electrolytes can now decrease to dangerous levels?

   A. Phosphorus.
   B. Calcium.
   C. Magnesium.
   D. Potassium.

3–133. Signs associated with a myxedematous state include

   A. Hyperventilation and hypercalcemia.
   B. Hypercapnia and hypoglycemia.
   C. Seizures and hypernatremia.
   D. Coma and hypokalemia.

Questions 3–134 through 3–137 refer to the following situation.

A 16-year-old male is admitted with head trauma following a fall. When he was admitted, his pulse was 88 and his blood pressure was 122/74 mm Hg. Now his pulse is 56 and his blood pressure is 156/78 mm Hg.

3–134. In planning care for this patient, which of the following is true in relation to his intracranial pressure?

   A. His intracranial pressure is 10 mm Hg.
   B. His cerebral perfusion pressure is remaining stable.
   C. He is beginning the decompensation phase.
   D. He is in the compensation phase.

3–135. The patient has a subarachnoid screw inserted to monitor his intracranial pressure (ICP) and cerebral perfusion pressure (CPP). Now his ICP and CPP are both 40 mm Hg. This means that this patient's

   A. Central venous pressure is decreased.
   B. Condition is improving.
   C. Mean systemic arterial pressure is elevated.
   D. Cerebral blood flow has markedly decreased.

3–136. Which of the following statements is *false* regarding nursing care related to intracranial pressure monitoring?

   A. Maintain a closed system with tight connections to prevent infection.
   B. Report A waves of 50 to 100 mm Hg lasting 5 to 20 minutes.
   C. Drain the intraventricular catheter according to physician's order.
   D. Flush the system every hour and whenever necessary if the pressure becomes damped.

3–137. The patient's arterial blood gases return from the laboratory. His pH is less than 7.3, his Pa_{CO_2} is elevated above 45 mm Hg, and his Pa_{O_2} is less than 50 mm Hg. Based on these arterial blood gas data, the critical care nurse knows that

   A. Cytotoxic cerebral edema will result from the hypoxemia.
   B. Acidosis will cause vasoconstriction of cerebral arterioles.
   C. Vasogenic edema results from the hypoxia.
   D. Cerebral blood flow will fall.

3–138. A 62-year-old female patient with a history of diabetes mellitus is admitted to the intensive care unit following a bowel resection for a large, benign tumor. Admitting vital signs and laboratory data reveal the following:

HR	110 beats/min
RR	24/min
T	102° F
BP	90/60 mm Hg
Cardiac output	7.5 l/min
SVR	750 dynes/sec/cm^{-5}
RBC	4.0 million/μl
Hct	35%
Hgb	11.6 mg/dl
WBC	13,200/μl
Platelets	180,000/μl
Fibrin split products	0

After you administer meperidine (Demerol) to the patient, she complains of "feeling cold" and is shivering. She is breathing normally and her vital signs are unchanged. Blood cultures are done and a Gram stain reveals gram-negative organisms in her blood.

Which of the following drug combinations would you expect to use in treating this patient?

A. ASA, dopamine, penicillin.
B. Acetaminophen, naloxone, gentamicin.
C. Erythromycin, ibuprofen, dopamine.
D. Septra, regitine, heparin.

3–139. A patient with an anteroseptal myocardial infarction suddenly complains of severe chest pain and shortness of breath. His extremities are cyanotic and do not become pink with administration of 100% oxygen. The patient also becomes bradycardic at this time with evidence of AV dissociation. A pacing pulmonary artery catheter is inserted and pacing is initiated at 80 beats per minute. The values obtained during catheter insertion are: right atrial pressure 5 mm Hg; right ventricular pressure 40/12 mm Hg; pulmonary artery pressure 20/10 mm Hg; pulmonary capillary wedge pressure 8 mm Hg. The complication associated with these findings is

A. Acute pulmonary edema.
B. Acute pulmonary embolism.
C. Ventricular septal rupture.
D. Cardiogenic shock.

3–140. A patient with a temporary transvenous pacemaker is sitting up eating his lunch when the nurse sees the rhythm shown below suddenly appear on the monitor.

The nurse should *immediately*

A. Place the patient flat in bed on his side.
B. Increase the sensitivity of the pacemaker.
C. Turn off the pacemaker and initiate cardiopulmonary resuscitation (CPR).
D. Administer atropine, 0.5 mg IV push.

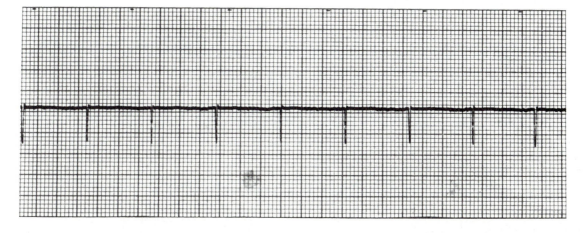

3–141. Nosocomial infectious pneumonias are especially difficult to treat because

 A. The causative organisms are often antibiotic-resistant strains.
 B. They cause fibrosis of the lungs.
 C. They are asymptomatic until late in the disease process.
 D. Sepsis is a common complication.

Questions 3–142 and 3–143 refer to the following situation.

A 70-year-old man with a diagnosis of metastatic carcinoma with osteolytic lesions is transferred to the intensive care unit from an orthopedic unit after developing congestive heart failure (CHF). He has been maintained on digoxin and furosemide prior to and since admission, and he now complains of muscle weakness, fatigue, nausea, and vomiting. The transferring nurse reports that the patient's serum calcium level is 15 mg/dl.

3–142. In addition to digitalis and diuretic therapy, this patient should receive which of the following?

 A. 0.9% sodium chloride IV.
 B. Phosphate IV.
 C. Calcitonin.
 D. Indomethacin.

3–143. Within the next 2 hours, the patient's ECG shows AV conduction delays and widening of the QRS complex. The nurse should be aware that factors contributing to these ECG changes may include

 I. Hypercalcemia.
 II. Hypervolemia.
 III. Digitalis toxicity.

 A. I and II only.
 B. I, II, III.
 C. II and III only.
 D. I and III only.

3–144. In the hepatitis patient, the nursing diagnosis "Altered nutrition, less than body requirements" is most likely related to

 A. Decreased vitamin synthesis and storage in the liver.
 B. Dietary restrictions.
 C. Nitrogen malabsorption.
 D. Hypermetabolic state.

3–145. An 86-year-old male was admitted with subacute subdural hematoma. The nurse knows that this diagnosis is more prevalent in the elderly owing to

 A. Cerebral atrophy from the normal aging process.
 B. Alterations in the blood-brain barrier.
 C. Age-related coagulopathy.
 D. A vitamin C deficit that leads to altered tissue building.

3–146. A 36-year-old male is admitted to your facility with a subdural hematoma sustained following an auto accident. As the nurse caring for this patient, you know that subdural hematomas are

 A. Usually arterial in origin.
 B. Usually venous in origin.
 C. Only acute, requiring immediate attention.
 D. The result of a tear in the internal carotid or middle meningeal artery.

3–147. The physician orders a dehydrating regimen to reduce the cerebral edema in a patient with subdural hematoma to increase fluid loss from the edematous brain tissue. The critical care nurse anticipates administering

 A. D5W.
 B. D10W.
 C. D10W with furosemide.
 D. Mannitol.

3–148. A primary chemical mediator in an anaphylactic reaction is

    A. Myocardial depressant factor.
    B. Histamine.
    C. Complement.
    D. Interferon.

3–149. A 32-year-old patient is having a cerebral angiogram. Shortly after the administration of the contrast agent through the IV, the patient develops shortness of breath and becomes hypotensive. The patient is experiencing

    A. An IgA-mediated reaction.
    B. An anaphylactoid reaction.
    C. A vasovagal reaction.
    D. A type IV hypersensitivity reaction.

Questions 3–150 and 3–151 refer to the following situation.

A 42-year-old female has been on the ventilator for 3 days after thoracotomy. The nursing assessment determines that she has increased rales posteriorly, generalized 2+ pitting edema, decreased hematocrit (Hct) and sodium, a weight gain of 7 kg over the past 3 days, and decreasing lung compliance. The nursing diagnosis based on the assessment is fluid volume excess.

3–150. This clinical picture is most consistent with

    A. Inappropriate IV fluid rates.
    B. Inaccurate weights.
    C. Inappropriate release of ADH.
    D. Loss of RBCs and plasma proteins.

3–151. Appropriate therapy for this patient would be to

    A. Administer a diuretic and limit saline solutions.
    B. Reweigh and recalculate intake and output.
    C. Administer packed RBCs and saline.
    D. Institute PEEP.

Questions 3–152 and 3–153 refer to the following situation.

A 60-year-old female complaining of dyspnea, nausea, and vomiting was admitted to the intensive care unit with a diagnosis of thyroid storm. She had a history of angina and hyperthyroidism and underwent cardiac catheterization 3 weeks ago. The family stated that she had become increasingly agitated and inattentive in the last few weeks. She was restless, tremulous, and diaphoretic with flushed skin, and had bibasilar crackles. Her heart rate was 150 beats per minute and her ECG showed normal sinus rhythm with an occasional PVC.

Vital signs and laboratory data:

BP	170/80 mm Hg
T	104° F
RR	32/min
Cardiac index	4.7 l/min/m²
Serum glucose	320 mg/dl
WBC	6,000/mm³
Neutrophils	50%
Band cells	3%

3–152. The most likely precipitating cause for this patient's development of thyroid storm is

    A. Hyperglycemia.
    B. Acute infection.
    C. Congestive heart failure.
    D. Exposure to iodine dye.

3–153. The drug of choice to reduce fever in this patient is

    A. Ibuprofen (Motrin, Advil, Medipren).
    B. Dexamethasone (Decadron).
    C. Acetaminophen (Tylenol).
    D. Acetylsalicylic acid (aspirin).

3–154. Impulses for voluntary movement are found in which of the following descending tracts of the spinal cord?

    A. Rubrospinal and tectospinal tracts.
    B. Ventral and lateral corticospinal tracts.
    C. Spinocerebellar tracts.
    D. Spinothalamic tracts.

3–155. Which of the following causes of acute renal failure following trauma is intrarenal?

    A. Shock state with low cardiac output.
    B. Rupture of the bladder.
    C. Pressure from hematomas.
    D. Rhabdomyolysis.

3–156. The most accurate method to determine if pulsus paradoxus is present in an alert patient with pericarditis would be to

    A. Instruct the patient to take deep breaths while the nurse auscultates the blood pressure.
    B. Instruct the patient to take normal breaths while the nurse auscultates the blood pressure.
    C. Instruct the patient to hold his breath while the nurse auscultates the blood pressure.
    D. Instruct the patient to tap the nurse's shoulder when he exhales, because pulsus paradoxus is heard only upon exhalation.

3–157. The following routine orders are written for a patient admitted for a transmural myocardial infarction:
    Electrocardiogram Q 8 hours times 3, then daily.
    Oxygen 2–6 liters via nasal cannula.
    NTG 1/150 sublingually p.r.n. chest pain.
    Morphine sulfate 2 mg IV p.r.n. for severe pain.
    Heparin 5,000 units subcutaneously BID.
    On the *third day after admission,* the patient complains of stabbing pain when he breathes and you note that the patient has a pericardial friction rub. Which of the following interventions is most appropriate?

    A. Discontinue heparin.
    B. Obtain 12-lead ECG each 8 hours for 24 hours.
    C. Increase oxygen to 6 liters by nasal cannula.
    D. Give nitroglycerin 1/150 sublingually.

3–158. A 65-year-old male is admitted for evacuation of a subdural hematoma resulting from a fall. On physical examination, the nurse notes ascites and visible blood vessels radiating from the umbilicus to the sternum and ribs. Bruits are audible in the right upper quadrant of the abdomen. He has large hemorrhoids. The nurse suspects that the patient has

    A. Liver abscess.
    B. Portal hypertension.
    C. Perforated ulcer.
    D. Chronic pancreatitis.

3–159. Cardiovascular effects of hypothyroidism may include

    A. Bradycardia and pericardial effusions.
    B. Decreased cardiac index and tachycardia.
    C. Elevated cardiac index and hypotension.
    D. Prominent apical pulse and systolic murmur.

3–160. A 17-year-old female is receiving a combination of neostigmine (Prostigmin) and pyridostigmine (Mestinon) for maintenance therapy following a myasthenic crisis. In determining the effectiveness of these drugs, the critical care nurse knows to assess for

    A. Cholinergic crisis, which is treated with atropine sulfate.
    B. Cholinergic crisis, which is treated with anticholinesterase drugs.
    C. Myasthenic crisis, which is treated with corticosteroids.
    D. Myasthenic crisis, which is treated with thymectomy.

3–161. Patients with myasthenia gravis must be taught to be alert for symptoms of cholinergic crisis. These symptoms include all of the following *except*

    A. Motor weakness and gastrointestinal hyperirritability.
    B. Acute motor weakness, nausea, and vomiting.
    C. Acute respiratory distress, severe cramps, and bradycardia.
    D. Restlessness and tachycardia.

Questions 3–162 through 3–164 refer to the following situation.

A 73-year-old widower developed multiple complications after pneumonectomy. He is now stable but his gastric pH is 2.5, despite antacid therapy. He suddenly complains of sharp, severe, midepigastric pain. His abdomen is tender to palpation. His bowel sounds are hypoactive.

3–162. The nurse suspects that the patient has developed

    A. Acute pancreatitis.
    B. Bile duct obstruction.
    C. Small bowel obstruction.
    D. Perforated ulcer.

3–163. Which of the following assessment findings is this patient likely to exhibit?

    A. Hyperactive bowel sounds.
    B. Shallow respirations.
    C. Hyperglycemia.
    D. Jaundice.

3–164. Which of the following positions will be most comfortable for this patient?

    A. Sims.
    B. Semi-Fowler's.
    C. Prone.
    D. Supine.

3–165. In formulating a care plan for a patient with dilated cardiomyopathy, interventions for the nursing diagnosis "Decreased cardiac output related to altered ventricular function" should include

    I. Administer laxative of choice.
    II. Maintain bedrest in high Fowler's position.
    III. Administer antiarrhythmic medications as ordered.

    A. I and II only.
    B. II and III only.
    C. I and III only.
    D. I, II, and III.

3–166. Psychosocial interventions for a patient with cerebral aneurysm are most important because

    A. Fear and anxiety related to unknown factors and surgical intervention may be present.
    B. Alteration in tissue perfusion may be causing increased intracranial pressure and changes in level of consciousness.
    C. Sensory deficits may be present, resulting in altered perception of the environment.
    D. Potential for injury exists.

3–167. Heparin may be administered to patients with disseminated intravascular coagulation. The rationale for using this drug is that

    A. Heparin inhibits clotting by delaying the production of platelets.
    B. Heparin combines with plasminogen to prevent thrombolysis.
    C. Heparin inhibits the production of fibrin split products, which inhibit clot formation.
    D. Heparin interferes with thrombin generation to interrupt clotting.

3–168. A 60-year-old widow has a history of alteration in gas exchange related to chronic obstructive pulmonary disease (COPD). She was previously able to care for herself alone at home. She has now been on a ventilator for 2 weeks, and when weaning has been attempted she becomes anxious, dyspneic, diaphoretic, and tachycardic. The nurse should suspect that the patient's problem is

    A. Carbon monoxide retention.
    B. Hypoxemia.
    C. Ineffective coping.
    D. Exhaustion.

3–169. Lung compliance increases with

    A. Pleural effusion.
    B. Flail chest.
    C. Age.
    D. Kyphoscoliosis.

Questions 3–170 and 3–171 refer to the following situation.

A Jehovah's Witness has given written consent to coronary artery bypass surgery under the condition that he not be given blood or blood products. Postoperatively, the patient experiences excessive blood loss and becomes hypotensive. The physician orders an infusion of 5% albumin. When the nurse reminds the physician of the patient's religious belief, he answers, "I can't allow a patient to die because of an irrational belief. Albumin doesn't even look like blood . . . the patient and his family won't know the difference."

3–170. If the nurse administers albumin to this patient, the nurse would

 I. Violate the principles of veracity and fidelity.
 II. Uphold the sanctity of life over the patient's right to self-determination.
 III. Be immune from litigation because of acting in the best interest of the patient and society.
 IV. Possibly be sued for causing mental anguish and spiritual distress, even if the patient's life were saved.

 A. I, II, and IV.
 B. I, II, and III.
 C. I and II.
 D. III.

3–171. If the nurse refuses to administer albumin to the patient, the nurse would be

 I. Upholding the value of autonomy over sanctity of life.
 II. Fulfilling the role of patient advocate.
 III. Required to immediately notify the nursing supervisor and document the situation and the action taken.
 IV. Legally justified only if he or she were a Jehovah's Witness.

 A. II, III, and IV.
 B. III and IV.
 C. I, II, and III.
 D. I, II, III, and IV.

3–172. A patient with malignant hypertension is extremely restless and has multiple complaints including headache, blurred vision, chest pain, and a "funny feeling" in the arms. After receiving nitroglycerin 1/150 grain sublingually, the patient screams that he feels like he is being stabbed. The nurse should

 A. Assist the patient with relaxation exercises because he is obviously becoming hysterical.
 B. Palpate upper extremity pulses for strength and equality.
 C. Medicate the patient with morphine to relieve the pain.
 D. Encourage the patient to breathe into a paper bag to increase his carbon dioxide levels and relieve the tingling in his hands.

Questions 3–173 through 3–175 refer to the following situation.

A patient admitted to the intensive care unit is disoriented and complaining of weakness, leg cramps, and polyuria. He is lethargic with dry, cracked lips; poor skin turgor; a weak rapid pulse; decreased bowel sounds; and rapid, deep respirations.

Laboratory and physical assessment findings are:

T	97° F
BP	70/60 mm Hg
RR	22/min
Hct	47%
pH	7.29
K	5.1 mEq/l
Na	132 mEq/l
Osmolality	310 mOsm/l
Glucose	400 mg/dl
Cl	95 mEq/l
HCO_3	15 mEq/l
WBC	9,000/mm³
Neutrophils	50%
Band cells	3%
Urine nitroprusside test (Acetest)	Negative

3–173. The most likely reason the nitroprusside reagent (Acetest) tested negative is because there is an absence of

    A. Lactate.
    B. Bicarbonate.
    C. Acetoacetate.
    D. 3-Hydroxybutyrate.

3–174. As the acidosis is corrected, the serum potassium level will

    A. Decrease.
    B. Increase.
    C. Remain unchanged.
    D. Increase and then decrease.

3–175. An arterial blood gas value that would be anticipated for this patient is

    A. P_{CO_2} <40 mm Hg.
    B. P_{O_2} <90 mm Hg.
    C. P_{CO_2} >50 mm Hg.
    D. P_{O_2} >150 mm Hg.

3–176. A patient with aortic valve regurgitation is admitted for treatment of endocarditis. Which of the following symptoms are associated with the complications of this condition?

    I. Hemoptysis.
    II. Hematuria.
    III. Left upper quadrant pain.
    IV. Tachycardia.

    A. I and IV only.
    B. I, II, III.
    C. II, III, IV.
    D. I, II, III, IV.

3–177. Symptoms of cocaine intoxication include

    A. Hypotension.
    B. Tachycardia.
    C. Tinnitus.
    D. Bradycardia.

3–178. A brief sensory experience that occurs prior to the onset of some seizures is called a(an)

    A. Prodromal phase.
    B. Aura.
    C. Epileptic cry.
    D. Ictus.

Questions 3–179 and 3–180 refer to the following situation.

A patient is admitted to the intensive care unit with a history of enlarged lymph nodes, weight loss of 30 pounds over the last 6 weeks, complaints of feeling tired, and persistent diarrhea. The following laboratory results are obtained:

RBC	5.2 million/µl
WBC	4000/µl
T cells	140 (normal 1,800)
T4:T8	1:2 (normal 2:1)
Platelets	200,000/µl

3–179. Based on the history and laboratory information, you anticipate that the patient may be at risk for

    A. Anemia.
    B. Bleeding.
    C. Infection.
    D. Polycythemia.

3–180. What other test would you expect to be ordered for this patient?

    A. Western blot test.
    B. Coombs test.
    C. Bleeding time.
    D. Immunoglobulin assays.

3–181. A 30-year-old victim of a motor vehicle accident is on a ventilator at FI_{O_2} 0.60, V_T 750 ml, rate of 20 per minute, PEEP 12 cm H_2O. The pressure limit alarm on the ventilator sounds. Upon assessing the patient, the nurse finds her in respiratory distress, with a rapid pulse, asymmetric chest expansion with the left side slightly larger, and bulging of intercostal spaces on the left. This picture is most probably an indication that

    A. A pleural effusion has developed.
    B. A mucous plug has developed.
    C. A pneumothorax has occurred.
    D. Atelectasis has developed.

3–182. A postsurgical intervention that can affect morbidity and mortality is

A. Early ambulation.
B. Change smoking habits.
C. Administer antibiotics prophylactically.
D. Pulmonary function testing.

3–183. Postoperative bradycardia and hypotension after carotid endarterectomy are most often caused by

A. Increased intracranial pressure.
B. Vagal nerve stimulation.
C. Cerebral ischemia.
D. Blood loss during surgery.

Questions 3–184 and 3–185 refer to the following situation.

A 29-year-old mother of two small children has recently been started on hemodialysis. During a treatment she tells the nurse that whenever she thinks she is getting better, she feels ill again. She is angry and frustrated that she cannot take care of herself and her family.

3–184. The best response from the nurse would be to

A. Explain to the patient that after she gets used to the dialysis she will feel perfectly well.
B. Tell the patient and family that she will soon return to normal activities.
C. Explore the patient's feelings and recognize the stressors she is experiencing.
D. Set goals for the patient's recovery.

3–185. In formulating a plan of care for this patient, the nursing diagnosis *best* explaining her reaction is

A. Disturbance of self-concept related to physical effects of renal disease and presence of a shunt.
B. Sexual dysfunction related to effects of renal disease and its treatment.
C. Alteration in thought process related to the effects of renal failure on the nervous system.
D. Ineffective patient coping related to the effects of renal failure and its treatment on lifestyle.

3–186. Following aortic aneurysm repair, a patient has the following hemodynamic and hematologic findings:

BP	80/60 mm Hg
HR	120/min
PAP	20/8 mm Hg
PCWP	6 mm Hg
Hct	28%

The most appropriate therapy would be

A. Transfusion with one unit of packed RBCs.
B. Intravenous fluid bolus with 250 ml of normal saline.
C. Dopamine infusion at 5 to 10 μg/kg/minute.
D. Verapamil, 5 mg slow IV push.

3–187. On postoperative day 2, a coronary artery bypass graft patient has his left atrial line discontinued by the surgeon. The chest tube drains 175 ml per hour for the first hour and 20 ml over the second hour. The amount and pattern of drainage are

A. A normal finding after invasive cardiac lines are discontinued.
B. An acceptable finding only if future drainage remains below 20 ml/hour.
C. An abnormal finding; the nurse should obtain an order for a complete blood count.
D. An abnormal finding that may signify development of pericardial tamponade.

Questions 3–188 and 3–189 refer to the following situation.

A 52-year-old male was admitted to the intensive care unit complaining of weight loss, fatigue, weakness, muscle cramps, postural dizziness, and diarrhea. He had a history of adrenal insufficiency and was on maintenance hydrocortisone, 30 mg per day. His wife died unexpectedly 2 weeks ago, and since then he has been severely depressed. Physical examination revealed hyperpigmented palms and buccal mucosa.

Vital signs and serum laboratory data:

BP	110/64 mm Hg flat
	90/60 mm Hg sitting
HR	100/min flat
	120/min sitting
RR	16/min
K	5.7 mEq/l
Na	128 mEq/l
BUN	22 mg/dl
Glucose	88 mg/dl

3–188. Orthostatic hypotension in this patient is a result of decreased renal reabsorption of

    A. Urea.
    B. Sodium.
    C. Glucose.
    D. Potassium.

3–189. Discharge planning for this patient should include

    A. Transfer to a tertiary care facility.
    B. Obtaining a Medic-Alert bracelet.
    C. Obtaining informed consent for a future adrenalectomy.
    D. Instruction to medicate himself with higher steroid doses.

3–190. Patients with acute complete transsection of the cord above T5 will most likely have

    A. A blood pressure of 78/56 mm Hg.
    B. A pulse of 138/minute.
    C. A vital capacity of 25 ml/kg.
    D. An intracranial pressure of 21 mm Hg.

3–191. A patient is in the coronary care unit after removal of his automatic implanted cardioverter-defibrillator (AICD). The nurse notes the dysrhythmia illustrated below.
The nurse should first

    A. Perform a precordial thump.
    B. Administer verapamil, 5 mg IV push.
    C. Perform synchronous cardioversion at 75 joules.
    D. Check the patient's level of consciousness and blood pressure.

3–192. The following patients are in the intensive care unit:

    I. A 26-year-old man who has a crush injury to the left leg.
    II. A 40-year-old woman who has leukemia.
    III. A 16-year-old girl who is a fresh-water near-drowning victim.
    IV. A 65-year-old man who has developed a gram-negative septicemia following a bowel resection.

Which of the patients are at risk for developing disseminated intravascular coagulation (DIC)?

    A. I and IV only.
    B. I, II, and IV only.
    C. III and IV only.
    D. All of the above.

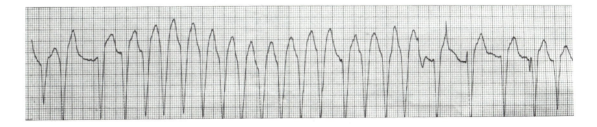

3–193. A 53-year-old woman is admitted to the intensive care unit with hypoxemia and reduced tidal volume related to liver failure and ascites. She was irritable but alert and oriented at admission. Six hours later, her pulmonary status has improved but she is now confused and difficult to arouse. This sensory-perceptual alteration is probably related to

A. Shortened prothrombin time.
B. Elevated plasma ammonia level.
C. Elevated RBC count.
D. Elevated SGOT and SGPT.

3–194. A patient undergoing treatment for cardiogenic shock is on the intra-aortic balloon pump at 1:4 augmentation. The patient's hemodynamic findings include a heart rate of 74 beats per minute, blood pressure (systemic) of 120/64 mm Hg, and a pulmonary capillary wedge pressure of 12 mm Hg. These findings indicate that the patient is

A. Intra-aortic balloon pump–dependent.
B. In a state of continued failure and the augmentation should be increased to 1:2.
C. Successfully being weaned from intra-aortic balloon support.
D. Demonstrating early symptoms of sepsis.

3–195. Transsection of the spinal cord at T4 results in dysfunction of what inspiratory muscle(s)?

A. Abdominals.
B. Diaphragm.
C. External intercostals.
D. Scalenes.

3–196. Preventive therapy for pulmonary emboli includes all of the following *except*

A. Minidose heparin.
B. Intermittent calf muscle compression stockings (sequential).
C. Graded elastic compression (TED) hose.
D. Early ambulation.

3–197. A 26-year-old male is complaining of a severe headache. On assessment he has nuchal rigidity and a positive Kernig's sign. Which of the following conditions is most likely present?

A. Epidural hematoma.
B. Subdural hematoma.
C. Subarachnoid hemorrhage.
D. Increased intracranial pressure.

3–198. When planning care for a patient with an epidural hematoma, the nurse knows that it

A. Results from venous bleeding.
B. Results from arterial bleeding.
C. Always causes unconsciousness.
D. Has the highest mortality of all head injuries.

3–199. The best initial approach to helping the renal failure patient deal with the loss of self-esteem is to

A. Find out how he or she behaved in healthy times with a life change.
B. Provide the patient with reading material on the disease and treatment modalities.
C. Encourage verbalization and reinforce the notion that everything will be OK.
D. Introduce the patient to another with renal failure who has adjusted to the disease.

3–200. The following lead II rhythm strip demonstrates which dysrhythmia?

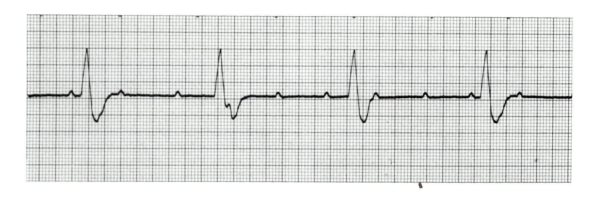

     A. Mobitz type I (Wenckebach) second degree heart block.
     B. Mobitz type II second degree heart block.
     C. Third degree heart block.
     D. Junctional rhythm.

Answers to Core Review Test 3

3–1. (**C**) Myocardial wall tension is determined by the volume or size of the ventricular cavity and the pressure generated during contraction to eject the volume of blood.

Reference: Daily, E., and Schroeder, J.: Techniques in Bedside Hemodynamic Monitoring, 3rd ed. C.V. Mosby, St. Louis, 1985.

3–2. (**B**) The diaphragm is the major muscle of inspiration and provides 70% of the inspiratory effort. The external intercostals provide some inspiratory effort, but the sternocleidomastoid muscles are used only during increased respiratory effort. The abdominal muscles are used for active expiration.

Reference: West, J.B.: Respiratory Physiology: The Essentials, 4th ed. Williams & Wilkins, Baltimore, 1990.

3–3. (**A**) The blood-brain barrier provides a measure of stability or homeostasis to the nervous system. The blood-brain barrier is a network of endothelial cells and astroglial membranes adjacent to the neurons. The barrier prevents certain substances from selectively crossing the barrier (e.g., sodium, potassium, and glutamic acid) while permitting others increased permeability (e.g., water, O_2, CO_2, glucose, and lipid-soluble compounds). In addition, it prevents most drugs from affecting the brain and the spinal cord. The blood-cerebrospinal fluid barrier, not the blood-brain barrier, permits selective transport from the blood to the ventricular system.

References: Alspach, J.G. (ed.): AACN Core Curriculum for Critical Care Nursing, 4th ed. W.B. Saunders, Philadelphia, 1991.
Hickey, J.V.: The Clinical Practice of Neurological and Neurosurgical Nursing, 2nd ed. J.B. Lippincott, Philadelphia, 1986.

3–4. (**A**) BUN provides only a rough determination of renal function, since it is also affected by intake of protein and extracellular fluid volume. Measures of serum creatinine must be used in combination with other diagnostic tests because the level varies with muscle mass. Because the glomerular filtration rate indicates the volume of plasma of a given substance cleared in a specific period of time, clearance tests are closely related to glomerular filtration rate. Urea clearance assesses overall renal function. The creatinine clearance test provides a more accurate evaluation of glomerular filtration rate.

References: Lancaster, L.: ESRD: Pathophysiology, assessment and intervention. In Lancaster, L. (ed.): The Patient with End Stage Renal Disease, 2nd ed. John Wiley and Sons, New York, 1984.
Ulrich, B.: Renal anatomy and physiology. In Ulrich, B. (ed.): Nephrology Nursing: Concepts and Strategies. Appleton and Lange, Norwalk, CT, 1989.

3–5. (**B**) Sodium increases cellular permeability to glucose, thereby facilitating carbohydrate absorption. Calcium, magnesium, and sulfate are not easily absorbed and they do not have a known role in carbohydrate absorption.

Reference: Ganong, W.F.: Review of Medical Physiology, 13th ed. Appleton and Lange, Norwalk, CT, 1987.

3–6. (**C**) The v wave is caused by bulging of the mitral valve back into the left atrium during ventricular contraction. The presence of a large v wave after inferior infarction signals papillary muscle dysfunction and mitral regurgitation.

Reference: Kenner, C., Guzzetta, C., and Dossey, B.: Critical Care Nursing: Body—Mind—Spirit. Little, Brown, Boston, 1985.

3–7. (**A**) The aspiration of gastric contents including hydrochloric acid results in a widespread severe chemical pneumonitis with diffuse alveolar filling.

Reference: Kersten, L.D.: Comprehensive Respiratory Nursing: A Decision Making Approach. W.B. Saunders, Philadelphia, 1989.

3–8. (**B**) Metabolic acidosis promotes renal calcium losses, reducing the amount of plasma calcium that is protein-bound and thereby unfilterable. Tubular reabsorption of calcium is enhanced by parathyroid hormone, metabolic alkalosis, and thiazide diuretics.

Reference: Janson, C.L.: Fluid and electrolyte balance. In Rosen, P. (ed.): Emergency Medicine: Concepts and Practice. C.V. Mosby, St. Louis, 1988.

3–9. (**B**) The condition that necessitates surgery may be causing either a temporary or permanent alteration in the patient's neurologic status. The uncertainty surrounding the anticipated outcomes of the surgery may be stressing the patient's available coping mechanisms; therefore, determining the patient's understanding of his or her condition and the anticipated outcomes is essential to an effective recovery.

Reference: Caine, R.M., and Bufalino, P.M.: Critically Ill Adults: Nursing Care Planning Guides. Williams & Wilkins, Baltimore, 1988.

3–10. (**A**) The Uniform Determination of Death Act has not been accepted in all states, although all states do recognize cardiopulmonary criteria for death. Death of the patient terminates the obligation to provide care, except in the case of anticipated organ donation or when a viable fetus may be salvaged. Declaration of death does not require consent of kin.

Reference: Smith, D.H., and Veatch, R.M. (eds.): Hastings Center Guidelines on the Termination of Life-Sustaining Treatment and Care of the Dying. Indiana University Press, Indianapolis, 1987.

3–11. (**C**) There is essentially no change in serum electrolyte and hemoglobin values in the near-drowning victim, despite the drowning medium. The primary pathologic changes occur in the lungs.

Reference: Kinney, M.R., Packa, D.R., and Dunbar, S.B.: AACN's Clinical Reference for Critical Care Nursing, 2nd ed. McGraw-Hill, New York, 1988.

3–12. (**B**) Neck veins are normally distended in the supine position. When pulsations occur at more than 3 cm above the clavicle, it indicates jugular venous distention. Pulsations usually decrease with deep inspiration. Increases in pulsations with deep inspiration may indicate tamponade or congestive heart failure.

Reference: Kenner, C., Guzzetta, C., and Dossey, B.: Critical Care Nursing: Body—Mind—Spirit. Little, Brown, Boston, 1985.

3–13. (**C**) Normal serum albumin is 3.5 to 5.0 gm/dl. Low serum proteins can cause malabsorption owing to a gap between the low intravascular osmolarity and high intraluminal osmolarity. Osmotic diarrhea then occurs when substances in the intestine that are not absorbed accumulate fluid and electrolytes. Osmolarity intolerance is treated by reducing the osmolarity of the enteral formula. Hyperglycemia is unlikely to be due to the osmotic gap in this patient. Hypervolemia is unlikely to be due to the osmotic gap. In fact, hypovolemia is very likely, and careful attention must be paid to providing adequate free water with enteral feeding. Liver function tests are frequently elevated by total parenteral nutrition (TPN) but not enteral nutrition.

References: Farley, J.M.: Current trends in enteral feeding. Crit Care Nurs, *8*(4):23–27, 1989.
Hennessy, K.: Nutritional support and gastrointestinal disease. Nurs Clin North Am, *24*(2):373–382, 1989.

3–14. (**C**) Guillain-Barré syndrome, or postinfectious polyneuritis, causes segmental demyelinization of the peripheral nerves and secondary damage to the axon. The onset is abrupt and characterized by muscle weakness progressing to flaccid paralysis usually beginning symmetrically in the lower extremities and ascending in a period of hours to weeks. The paresthesia associated with GBS is temporary and may cause a pins-and-needles sensation, pain, or numbness. The myelin sheaths and axons are able to regenerate after injury, but this may take up to 2 years to occur. GBS does not affect a patient's level of consciousness.

Reference: Hickey, J.V.: The Clinical Practice of Neurological and Neurosurgical Nursing, 2nd ed. J.B. Lippincott, Philadelphia, 1986.

3–15. (**D**) Hypokalemia results in a decreased renal phosphate reabsorption and hypophosphatemia from increased losses. Renal phosphate excretion is decreased in renal failure, hypomagnesemia, and hypoparathyroid states and results in a rise in serum phosphorus levels.

Reference: Chambers, J.K.: Metabolic bone disorders: Imbalances of calcium and phosphorus. Nurs Clin North Am, 22:861–872, 1987.

3–16. (**D**) In the pacemaker cells, the threshold for stimulation is -40 mV. These cells are depolarized by a slow influx of sodium and calcium. Purkinje, atrial, and ventricular cells have a characteristic five-phase fast response action potential.

Reference: Kenner, C., Guzzetta, C., and Dossey, B.: Critical Care Nursing: Body—Mind—Spirit. Little, Brown, Boston, 1985.

3–17. (**C**) Reticulocytes are the immediate precursor stage of erythrocytes. The normal reticulocyte count is 0.5% to 1.5%. With blood loss a patient loses RBCs and the secretion of erythropoietin is stimulated. Increased numbers of reticulocytes are released into the circulation as a result of erythropoietin-stimulating bone marrow activity.

Reference: Alspach, J.G. (ed.): AACN Core Curriculum for Critical Care Nursing, 4th ed. W.B. Saunders, Philadelphia, 1991.

3–18. (**D**) An acoustic neuroma, also called a schwannoma or neurofibroma, arises from the sheath of the Schwann cells. Tumors vary in size, are generally benign, and are located in an area that makes access difficult. Smaller, pea-sized tumors confined to the internal auditory canal involve the vestibular branch of cranial nerve VIII, whereas larger tumors displace cranial nerves VII, V, IX, and X. Cranial nerve III is the oculomotor nerve and cranial nerve IV is the trochlear nerve, neither of which is involved in acoustic neuromas.

Reference: Hickey, J.V.: The Clinical Practice of Neurological and Neurosurgical Nursing, 2nd ed. J.B. Lippincott, Philadelphia, 1986.

3–19. (**D**) Alveolar ventilation is made up of the tidal volume times the respiratory rate, minus the dead space. When the rate or volume is decreased, CO_2 is not eliminated as efficiently and acidosis results.

Reference: Shapiro, B.A., Harrison, R.A., Cane, R.D., et al.: Clinical Application of Blood Gases, 4th ed. Year Book Medical Publishers, Chicago, 1989.

3–20. (**D**) In right atrial hypertrophy, P waves are tall and peaked in leads II, III, and aV_F and tall and diphasic in V_1. In left atrial hypertrophy, P waves are wide and notched in leads V_4 to V_6 and biphasic with a broad negative deflection in V_1.

Reference: Andreoli, K., Fowkes, V., Zipes, D., et al.: Comprehensive Cardiac Care, 6th ed. C.V. Mosby, St. Louis, 1987.

3–21. **(B)** The pH shows acidosis. A low Pa_{CO_2} produces alkalosis, so it is not the cause of the acidosis. The low HCO_3 indicates a metabolic acidosis. The hypoxemia is producing a lactic acidosis that causes lactate to bind with bicarbonate.

Reference: Shapiro, B.A., Harrison, R.A., Cane, R.D., et al.: Clinical Application of Blood Gases, 4th ed. Year Book Medical Publishers, Chicago, 1989.

3–22. **(A)** The plantar reflex is elicited by stroking the lateral aspect or sole of the foot with a semisharp object. A normal response is flexion of the great toe, whereas an abnormal response is extension, or the Babinski sign. The Babinski sign indicates pyramidal tract or upper motor neuron lesions. Diffuse cerebral dysfunction is determined by testing the grasp, snout, or glabellar reflex. Cerebellar dysfunction is determined by testing volitional movements such as dystaxia, hypotonia, nystagmus, and dysarthria.

Reference: Alspach, J.G. (ed.): AACN Core Curriculum for Critical Care Nursing, 4th ed. W.B. Saunders, Philadelphia, 1991.

3–23. **(A)** GI secretion loss through vomiting, diarrhea, nasogastric suction, or fistulas predisposes a patient to fluid volume deficit. Prolonged steroid therapy, hyperaldosteronism, and reduced renal excretion predispose a patient to fluid volume excess.

Reference: Holloway, N.M.: Nursing the Critically Ill Adult, 3rd ed. Addison-Wesley, New York, 1988.

3–24. **(C)** Malignant hypertension is associated with a diastolic blood pressure of greater than 140 mm Hg. Accelerated hypertension is associated with diastolic blood pressures of greater than 120 mm Hg. Both can lead to hypertensive encephalopathy if untreated. Hypertensive encephalopathy is associated with dysfunction of cerebral autoregulation leading to stroke or hemorrhage. Essential hypertension is systolic and diastolic blood pressure elevation of unknown etiology.

Reference: Weeks, L.: Advanced Cardiovascular Nursing. Blackwell, Boston, 1986.

3–25. **(B)** Parietal lobe involvement is generally diagnosed when patients exhibit hyperesthesia (excessive sensitivity), paresthesia (altered sensation), loss of two-point discrimination, astereognosis (inability to recognize objects by touch), loss of left-right discrimination, agraphia (inability to express ideas in writing or to recall the hand movements necessary for writing), constructional apraxia (loss of understanding of the use of things), homonymous hemianopsia (loss of sight of the same one-half of the visual fields), and unilateral neglect.

Reference: Alspach, J.G. (ed.): AACN Core Curriculum for Critical Care Nursing, 4th ed. W.B. Saunders, Philadelphia, 1991.

3–26. **(D)** Pituitary tumors are space-occupying tumors that compress the optic chiasm, resulting in visual changes and hypopituitarism. These tumors can be either nonsecreting, which account for approximately 90% of all pituitary tumors, or secreting tumors. There are two types of secreting tumors, those that secrete ACTH (stimulating production of cortisol, resulting in Cushing's syndrome) and growth hormone–secreting tumors (causing giantism in children or acromegaly in adults). Large acoustic neuromas may cause hydrocephalus and increased intracranial pressure.

Reference: Alspach, J.G. (ed.): AACN Core Curriculum for Critical Care Nursing, 4th ed. W.B. Saunders, Philadelphia, 1991.

3–27. **(D)** Lung compliance indicates the distensibility of the lungs and how much pressure it takes to deliver a volume. The smaller the compliance, the stiffer the lungs are and the more pressure it takes to deliver the volume.

Reference: Shapiro, B.A., Harrison, R.A., Cane, R.D., et al.: Clinical Application of Blood Gases, 4th ed. Year Book Medical Publishers, Chicago, 1989.

3–28. (**C**) Normal coronary artery perfusion pressure is 60 to 80 mm Hg and may be derived by subtracting the pulmonary capillary wedge pressure from the mean arterial pressure. Pressures above 80 mm Hg can cause chest pain from coronary artery vasoconstriction. Pressures below 60 mm Hg may cause chest pain from inadequate coronary artery perfusion. In this case, the coronary artery perfusion pressure is 45, indicating hypoperfusion. Increasing the dopamine to vasoconstricting levels may increase both the blood pressure and the wedge pressures, effecting little change in the coronary artery perfusion pressure. Decreasing the dopamine may further decrease the blood pressure and coronary artery perfusion pressure. Increasing the nitroglycerin may also further decrease the blood pressure and impair coronary flow. Decreasing the nitroglycerin infusion to 1.5 µg/kg/minute would still provide the patient with a therapeutic level of nitroglycerin, improve the blood pressure slightly, and thus improve coronary perfusion. The decrease in nitroglycerin may also relieve his headache.

Reference: Bustin, D.: Hemodynamic Monitoring for Critical Care. Appleton-Century-Crofts, Norwalk, CT, 1986.

3–29. (**A**) There is an increase in circulating catecholamines during hypoglycemia. Epinephrine acts in opposition to the hypoglycemic effect of insulin by stimulating glycogenolysis, gluconeogenesis, and lipolysis. Sweating, tachycardia, palpitations, and pallor are manifestations of the adrenergic response.

Reference: Kohler, P.O., and Jordan, R.M. (eds.): Clinical Endocrinology. John Wiley and Sons, New York, 1986.

3–30. (**D**) The examiner approaches the eye from the side and touches the cornea lightly with a wisp of cotton, avoiding the eyelashes. Observing for the presence of a blink reflex tests cranial nerves V (trigeminal) and VII (facial). Cranial nerves II and III (optic and oculomotor, respectively) are tested by shining a light into the eyes and observing the pupil for constriction on the same (ipsilateral) and opposite (contralateral) side. Testing for the gag reflex assesses cranial nerves IX (glossopharyngeal) and X (vagus).

Reference: Holloway, N.M.: Nursing the Critically Ill Adult. Addison-Wesley, Menlo Park, CA, 1988.

3–31. (**A**) Renal pedicle trauma involves tearing of the blood vessels supplying the kidney. The absence of hematuria may be the result of a drastic decrease in renal blood flow due to shock or, more commonly, vascular thrombosis and/or avulsion of the ureter, precluding hematuria. Patients with renal fragmentation and renal laceration have sustained an injury with considerable impact and present with persistent and grossly positive hematuria. Blood in the urine is almost always present, at least in microscopic amounts, with a renal contusion.

Reference: Cook, L.: Genitourinary injuries and renal management. In Cardona, V.D., Hurn, P.D., and Mason, P.J.B., et al. (eds.): Trauma Nursing: From Resuscitation to Rehabilitation. W.B. Saunders, Philadelphia, 1988.

3–32. (**A**) Suctioning should never be performed on a routine basis because unnecessary suctioning can traumatize the trachea. The procedure should be tailored to the needs of the individual patient.

Reference: Kinney, M.R., Packa, D.R., and Dunbar, S.B. (eds.): AACN's Clinical Reference for Critical Care Nursing, 2nd ed. McGraw-Hill, New York, 1988.

3–33. (C) The patient's type B blood contains B antigens on the red blood cells and anti-A antibodies in the serum. The infused type AB blood contains both A and B antigens on the red blood cells and neither anti-A nor anti-B antibodies. The anti-A antibodies in the patient's blood will react with the A antigens in the infused blood, resulting in a transfusion reaction.

Reference: Alspach, J.G. (ed.): AACN Core Curriculum for Critical Care Nursing, 4th ed. W.B. Saunders, Philadelphia, 1991.

3–34. (D) Antacid administration decreases the absorption of digoxin but increases the absorption of aspirin, bishydroxycoumarin, and levodopa.

Reference: Chernow, B.: The Pharmacologic Approach to the Critically Ill Patient, 2nd ed. Williams & Wilkins, Baltimore, 1988.

3–35. (D) Vasogenic edema primarily affects the white matter and is the most commonly occurring type of cerebral edema. The pathogenesis is assumed to be increased capillary permeability of the arterial walls to large molecules from a defect in the blood-brain barrier. As a result, there is leakage into the extracellular space. Cytotoxic edema is an increase of fluid within the intracellular space and is frequently associated with cerebral hypoxia, anoxia, and hypo-osmolar conditions. Interstitial edema, the third type of cerebral edema, occurs with obstructive hydrocephalus.

Reference: Hickey, J.V.: The Clinical Practice of Neurological and Neurosurgical Nursing, 2nd ed. J.B. Lippincott, Philadelphia, 1986.

3–36. (C) Reperfusion dysrhythmias are a sign of successful t-PA administration and are often life-threatening. Treatment of the dysrhythmias by defibrillation, cardioversion, and pharmacologic means is a priority.

Reference: Underhill, S., Woods, S., Froelicher, E., et al.: Cardiac Nursing, 2nd ed. J.B. Lippincott, Philadelphia, 1989.

3–37. (D) Pulmonary problems may predispose a patient to complications such as pneumonia. Pulmonary rehabilitation and maximizing lung function through exercise and medication will help to prevent pneumonia.

Reference: Kersten, L.D.: Comprehensive Respiratory Nursing: A Decision Making Approach. W.B. Saunders, Philadelphia, 1989.

3–38. (D) Calcium alters cell membrane permeability and phosphorus affects cellular production of energy and binding between oxygen and hemoglobin. Magnesium is a cofactor in all transphosphorylation reactions involving ATP. The manifestations of hypermagnesemia are largely in the central nervous system and the cardiovascular system. Ionized magnesium is a sedative that depresses the function of the central nervous system and exerts a curare-like effect on the neuromuscular junction at high concentrations (greater than 10 mEq/l).

References: Calloway, C.: When the problem involves magnesium, calcium, or phosphate. RN, *50:*30–36, 1987.
Smith, L.H.: Disorders of magnesium metabolism. In Wyngaarden, J.B., and Smith, L.H. (eds.): Textbook of Medicine, 18th ed. W.B. Saunders, Philadelphia, 1988.

3–39. (C) The oculomotor nerve (III) innervates the levator palpebrae muscle, which elevates the eyelid and the muscles that control the iris and the ciliary body. Tests of the optic nerve (II) determine visual acuity.

Reference: Hickey, J.V.: The Clinical Practice of Neurological and Neurosurgical Nursing, 2nd ed. J.B. Lippincott, Philadelphia, 1986.

3–40. (A) Right ventricular infarction causes pure right-sided heart failure with elevated CVP, venous congestion, and decreased left ventricular filling pressures (PCWP) and stroke volume. Decreased stroke volume will decrease cardiac output and MAP.

Reference: Sommers, M., and Russell, A.: Location of myocardial infarction: Assessing the patient's response. Dimen Crit Care Nurs, *3:*8–15, 1984.

3–41. **(C)** All patients with myocardial infarction should be placed on oxygen. Patients with right ventricular infarction require higher filling pressures and fluid replacement to maintain cardiac output. Diuretics, nitroglycerin, and sodium and fluid restriction decrease filling pressures and will therefore decrease cardiac output in the patient with right ventricular infarction.

Reference: Sommers, M., and Russell, A.: Location of myocardial infarction: Assessing the patient's response. Dimen Crit Care Nurs, 3:8–15, 1984.

3–42. **(B)** As people age, function of the immune system declines. Testing reveals no response to antigens, a condition that is known an anergy. Anergy occurs in approximately two-thirds of individuals over the age of 70 years. Since the immune system is not fully functional, the patient is more prone to the development of infections.

Reference: Smith, S.: The immune system: Physiologic considerations in the critically ill. In American Association of Critical-Care Nurses: Proceedings of the Sixteenth Annual National Teaching Institute. American Association of Critical-Care Nurses, Newport Beach, CA, 1989.

3–43. **(B)** Even though a pneumothorax may have occurred during CPR from a broken rib lacerating the lung, the most likely problem is right bronchial intubation. This results in lack of airflow and ventilation to the left side and directs all the ventilator flow to the right side. This causes increased ventilator pressures and decreases the Pa_{O_2}, because perfusion to the left lung is not oxygenated.

Reference: Kersten, L.D.: Comprehensive Respiratory Nursing: A Decision Making Approach. W.B. Saunders, Philadelphia, 1989.

3–44. **(C)** Appropriate therapy for a bronchial intubation is to pull the endotracheal tube back past the carina and resecure.

Reference: Kersten, L.D.: Comprehensive Respiratory Nursing: A Decision Making Approach. W.B. Saunders, Philadelphia, 1989.

3–45. **(B)** Calcium, which acts as a gatekeeper for sodium and potassium passing into and out of cells, immediately antagonizes the cardiac and neuromuscular toxicity of hyperkalemia, particularly if hypocalcemia is present. Calcium infusions are only temporary measures, however, with results occurring in 2 to 5 minutes and having a duration of approximately 1 hour. Sodium bicarbonate acts within 15 minutes by correcting any accompanying acidosis and lasts 1 to 2 hours. Glucose, given with insulin, moves potassium into the cells. It acts within 30 to 60 minutes, lasts for several hours, and should not be used for immediate lifesaving results. Sodium polystyrene sulfonate, either orally or rectally, exchanges sodium for potassium in the intestine. It takes longer to act than the other treatments and should be used for moderate hyperkalemia and not when severe cardiac or neuromuscular symptoms are present.

Reference: Calloway, C.: When the problem involves magnesium, calcium, or phosphate. RN, 50:30–36, 1987.

3–46. **(C)** Anterior cord syndrome, an incomplete cord transection, is associated with complete motor loss and loss of pain and temperature sensation below the level of the lesion, with sparing of proprioception and vibratory sensation. Loss of respiratory function is associated with complete cord transsection at C1 to C4 and possibly C5. While C8 lesions cause quadriplegia, biceps and triceps muscles are intact, but patients have no function of intrinsic hand muscles.

Reference: Alspach, J.G. (ed.): AACN Core Curriculum for Critical Care Nursing, 4th ed. W.B. Saunders, Philadelphia, 1991.

3–47. (**D**) The liver removes ammonia from the body fluids through formation of urea. In the absence of this function, plasma ammonia levels rise rapidly, leading to hepatic coma and eventual death. Plasma ammonia levels are probably not the only toxin leading to hepatic coma.

Reference: Guyton, A.C.: Textbook of Medical Physiology, 7th ed. W.B. Saunders, Philadelphia, 1986.

3–48. (**A**) Atrial pacing wires may be used to obtain an atrial ECG. The pacing wire is attached to one of the monitor leads or to the V_1 lead of the 12-lead ECG. It is the best of the above choices, since it addresses the source of atrial activity. Carotid massage may slow the heart rate to allow P waves to become visible, but it is not always effective.

Reference: Kenner, C., Guzzetta, C., and Dossey, B.: Critical Care Nursing: Body—Mind—Spirit. Little, Brown, Boston, 1985.

3–49. (**C**) The rhythm is bigeminy and requires immediate treatment with lidocaine. PVCs occur in the postoperative cardiac patient because of irritable myocardial tissue, hypoxia, and low serum potassium. This patient's oxygen saturation is 100%, and none of the ventilator settings has changed. Serum potassium was 4.5 mEq/l 1 hour prior and there has been no excessive increase in urine output to suggest massive loss of potassium. Many postoperative protocols for coronary artery bypass patients contain sliding scale potassium orders to maintain the serum potassium at 4.5 mEq/l or greater, so it would be acceptable to obtain a serum potassium after delivering the lidocaine to decrease ventricular irritability.

Reference: Kenner, C., Guzzetta, C., and Dossey, B.: Critical Care Nursing: Body—Mind—Spirit. Little, Brown, Boston, 1985.

3–50. (**C**) The psychological dependence on the ventilator is the primary reason for the failure to wean. Mild sedation may help to relieve some of the psychological as well as physical stress. Remaining *in* the room during weaning periods will reassure him that he will be closely monitored, and providing diversionary activities such as TV, games, reading, and music may distract him.

Reference: Handerhan, B., and Allegrezza, N.: Getting your patient off a ventilator. RN, *52*:60–64, 1989.

3–51. (**D**) COPD patients in particular are predisposed to malnutrition. Malnutrition weakens respiratory muscles, and patients with a pre-existing chronic illness are already in a state of malnutrition before the added insult of an acute process.

Reference: Kersten, L.D.: Comprehensive Respiratory Nursing: A Decision Making Approach. W.B. Saunders, Philadelphia, 1989.

3–52. (**C**) Phosphate excretion by the kidneys is directly related to the number of functioning nephrons. In renal failure, the decreased glomerular filtration rate reduces phosphate excretion. Malabsorption syndrome, thiazide diuretics, and alkalosis cause hypophosphatemia.

References: Calloway, C.: When the problem involves magnesium, calcium, or phosphate. RN, *50*:30–36, 1987.
Liddle, V.R.: Nutrition for the patient with end stage renal disease. In Lancaster, L. (ed.): The Patient with End Stage Renal Disease, 2nd ed. John Wiley and Sons, New York, 1984.

3–53. (**A**) The major concern and complication associated with arteriovenous malformations (AVMs) is hemorrhage. Bleeding may be either minor or major. Lumbar puncture, although contraindicated by clinical evidence of increased intracranial pressure, would show the following: pressure would be normal or elevated, and there would be red or xanthochromic cells present with bleeding into the subarachnoid space.

Reference: Hickey, J.V.: The Clinical Practice of Neurological and Neurosurgical Nursing, 2nd ed. J.B. Lippincott, Philadelphia, 1986.

3–54. (**B**) Hypercapnia, defined as a Pa_{CO_2} greater than 45 mm Hg, is a potent vasodilating factor that causes cerebral vasodilation and increased blood volume in the brain, resulting in increased intracranial pressure. Hypercapnia is often associated with hypoxia, and therefore arterial blood gases should be assessed frequently in these patients to prevent decreased oxygen supply to cerebral cells.

Reference: Hickey, J.V.: The Clinical Practice of Neurological and Neurosurgical Nursing, 2nd ed. J.B. Lippincott, Philadelphia, 1986.

3–55. (**B**) Because there is no proof that the nurse is impaired by drugs or that illegal drugs are involved, it would be premature to inform the police or the Board of Nursing. Keeping silent does nothing to correct the problem of questionable clinical judgement. The supervisor should be notified so that the nurse can be evaluated, counseled, and relieved of patient care responsibilities, if appropriate. If the nurse is found to be drug-impaired, the licensing agency should then be notified.

References: Creighton, H.: Legal implications of the impaired nurse—Part I. Nurs Manag, *1*:21–23, 1988. Creighton, H.: Legal implications of the impaired nurse—Part II. Nurs Manag, *2*:20–21, 1988.

3–56. (**B**) The only organ that synthesizes albumin is the liver. Because albumin maintains colloid osmotic pressure, hepatic failure results in dependent edema, ascites, and pleural effusion. The bone marrow, spleen, and thymus gland are blood-forming organs.

Reference: Kinney, M.R., Packa, D.R., Dunbar, S.B. (eds.): AACN's Clinical Reference for Critical Care Nursing, 2nd ed. McGraw-Hill, New York, 1988.

3–57. (**B**) Because motion artifacts, breathing, and swallowing can affect the DSA image, patient cooperation during this procedure is essential. Resolution is limited with DSA, and conventional angiography may be necessary to detect small lesions. Risks associated with this procedure include nephrotoxicity from the contrast medium, but this does not need to be overly emphasized, because it may increase the patient's anxiety. DSA does not involve arterial puncture.

Reference: Fahey, V.: Vascular Nursing. W.B. Saunders, Philadelphia, 1988.

3–58. (**C**) 4+ pulses signify development of an aneurysm or pseudoaneurysm. An embolism, hematoma, or vasospasm would diminish the palpated pulse in the groin over the femoral artery.

Reference: Fahey, V.: Vascular Nursing. W.B. Saunders, Philadelphia, 1988.

3–59. (**B**) A 2% rise in serum osmolality induces the release of antidiuretic hormone (ADH) from the posterior pituitary gland. In the course of diabetes insipidus, free water is lost, the serum osmolality rises, and there is no ADH response. Hemorrhage results in an isotonic loss that does not affect the water-to-solute ratio.

Reference: Kohler, P.O., and Jordan, R.M. (eds.): Clinical Endocrinology. John Wiley and Sons, New York, 1986.

3–60. (**C**) Increased intracranial pressure can result from head trauma. Since elevation of the head of the bed has been found to decrease intracranial pressure, Trendelenburg's position is contraindicated. Cardiac monitoring, daily weights, and administering fluid are interventions done to monitor and correct the fluid volume deficit.

Reference: Holloway, N.M.: Nursing the Critically Ill Adult, 3rd ed. Addison-Wesley, Menlo Park, CA, 1988.

3–61. (**C**) Hyponatremia may occur in edematous conditions such as nephrotic syndrome, wherein there is an impairment of the renal diluting capacity. Hypokalemia, hypercalcemia, and osmotic diuretics are all associated with hypernatremia. There is enhanced proximal tubule reabsorption of sodium and water, leading to delivery of a small fluid volume to the distal nephron, impairing formation of hypotonic urine.

Reference: Janson, C.L.: Fluid and electrolyte balance. In Rosen, P. (ed.): Emergency Medicine: Concepts and Practice. C.V. Mosby, St. Louis, 1988.

3–62. (**C**) Wolff-Parkinson-White syndrome is recognized by the classic delta wave (slurred initial portion of the QRS) and a shortened PR interval.

Reference: Weeks, L.: Advanced Cardiovascular Nursing. Blackwell, Boston, 1986.

3–63. (**A**) This behavior is most likely due to his mixed feelings about the ventilator and being weaned from it. This ambivalence comes from regarding the ventilator as both a friend and an intruder and uncertainty about success of the weaning.

Reference: Kersten, L.D.: Comprehensive Respiratory Nursing: A Decision Making Approach. W.B. Saunders, Philadelphia, 1989.

3–64. (**B**) He needs to be able to express his fears and mixed feelings about the ventilator and his ability to be weaned from it. Weaning should never be done at night and especially when he is unaware of it, since he will then mistrust the staff. He should be allowed to control his environment as much as possible, and distractions should be provided.

Reference: Kersten, L.D.: Comprehensive Respiratory Nursing: A Decision Making Approach. W.B. Saunders, Philadelphia, 1989.

3–65. (**D**) Diazoxide and phenytoin inhibit pancreatic release of insulin, resulting in hyperglycemia. Triamcinolone has glucocorticoid properties that stimulate lipolysis, gluconeogenesis, and glycogenolysis. Acetaminophen does not affect glucose metabolism or insulin release.

Reference: Kohler, P.O., and Jordan, R.M. (eds.): Clinical Endocrinology. John Wiley and Sons, New York, 1986.

3–66. (**A**) When RBCs are hemolyzed, free hemoglobin is released into plasma. This results in an increase in the indirect bilirubin.

Reference: Griffin, J.P.: Hematology and Immunology. Appleton-Century-Crofts, Norwalk, CT, 1986.

3–67. (**A**) The two factors that influence CBF are changes in cerebral perfusion pressure (CPP) and the diameter of the cerebrovascular bed. The diameter of the cerebrovascular bed is affected by autoregulation and hypercapnia. Autoregulation maintains constant blood flow within a range of perfusion pressures. Hypercapnia leads to vasodilation, thereby increasing CBF.

Reference: Alspach, J.G. (ed.): AACN Core Curriculum for Critical Care Nursing, 4th ed. W.B. Saunders, Philadelphia, 1991.

3–68. (**B**) The intracranial cavity is filled to capacity with noncompressible contents, which include CSF, intravascular blood, and brain tissue water (interstitial fluid). The Monro-Kellie hypothesis states that if the volume of one of the components increases, a reciprocal decrease in one or both of the other components must occur or the intracranial pressure will increase.

Reference: Alspach, J.G. (ed.): AACN Core Curriculum for Critical Care Nursing, 4th ed. W.B. Saunders, Philadelphia, 1991.

3–69. (**C**) Osteodystrophies result from abnormalities of calcium, phosphorus, and vitamin D metabolism. Lowering the serum phosphate is the single most important therapeutic modality in the prevention and treatment of renal osteodystrophy and metastatic calcification. The usual method of accomplishing this is the administration of phosphate-binding medications, such as aluminum hydroxide gels.

References: Calloway, C.: When the problem involves magnesium, calcium, or phosphate. RN, *50:*30–36, 1987.
Chambers, J.K.: Metabolic bone disorders: Imbalances of calcium and phosphorus. Nurs Clin North Am, *22:*861–872, 1987.
Crandall, B.L.: Chronic renal failure. In Ulrich, T. (ed.): Nephrology Nursing. Appleton and Lange, Norwalk, CT, 1989.

3–70. (**D**) Because of this patient's disease process and high blood alcohol level, the nurse suspects that alcohol abuse is an etiology for social isolation. Patients who abuse alcohol frequently are socially isolated owing to the diminished support of nonusers. Most or all significant others can be lost. Lack of social support significantly reduces the patient's resources for recovery, both in the intensive care unit and upon discharge. Fluid volume deficit due to blood loss is much more likely than fluid volume excess. Unilateral neglect refers to neglect of one side of the body due to hemiparesis rather than to general self-neglect. Ineffective thermoregulation is unlikely at a blood alcohol level of 0.25%.

Reference: Luckmann, J., and Sorensen, K.C.: Medical-Surgical Nursing: A Psychophysiologic Approach, 3rd ed. W.B. Saunders, Philadelphia, 1987.

3–71. (**C**) Ten units is the average amount of blood lost during a single bleeding episode from esophageal varices. Understandably, patients fear that they are bleeding to death. The amount of blood lost may be underestimated because the hematocrit does not change during the first few hours, since both plasma and red cells are lost proportionately. Patients with an acute bleeding episode require immediate treatment for hypovolemic shock.

References: Sleisenger, M.H., and Fordtran, J.S. (eds.): Gastrointestinal Disease: Pathophysiology, Diagnosis, Management, 4th ed. W.B. Saunders, Philadelphia, 1989.
Swearingen, P.L., Sommers, M.S., and Miller, K.: Manual of Critical Care: Applying Nursing Diagnoses to Adult Critical Illness. C.V. Mosby, St. Louis, 1988.

3–72. (**A**) In a temporary pacemaker, the negative electrode catheter delivers the stimulus and the positive electrode receives the stimulus or "senses." In bipolar pacing, the catheter contains two poles and two electrode wires for attachment to the pacemaker. When the positive wire is attached to an ordinary limb electrode or a suture in the skin, the stimulus must travel to this attachment instead of the positive pole of the pacing catheter near the tip. This is the basis of unipolar pacing. Detaching the negative terminal would discontinue cardiac pacing and merely twitch the muscles at the attachment site. Changing the sensitivity would not change the pacemaker to a unipolar mode.

Reference: Underhill, S., Woods, S., Froelicher, E., et al.: Cardiac Nursing, 2nd ed. J.B. Lippincott, Philadelphia, 1989.

3–73. (**C**) Failure to sense appropriately may allow the pacemaker to fire on the T wave, inducing ventricular fibrillation. In inappropriate sensing, the pacemaker recognizes the T wave as a QRS and may fail to fire appropriately.

Reference: Kenner, C., Guzzetta, C., and Dossey, B.: Critical Care Nursing: Body—Mind—Spirit. Little, Brown, Boston, 1985.

3–74. (**C**) Singed nares and smoke around the nose and mouth indicate possible burns in the trachea. This can lead to edema with total airway obstruction. An emergency tracheotomy kit should be kept at the bedside.

Reference: Kinney, M.R., Packa, D.R., and Dunbar, S.B. (eds.): AACN's Clinical Reference for Critical Care Nursing, 2nd ed. McGraw-Hill, New York, 1988.

3–75. (**D**) Schistocytes are a form of RBC. In some diseases, such as disseminated intravascular coagulopathy (DIC), the clotting cascade is activated and fibrin is deposited in capillaries. Schistocytes result when the RBCs are damaged as they circulate through the capillaries where these fibrin deposits are present. Reticulocytes are the immature form of RBCs.

Reference: Von Rueden, K.T., and Walleck, C.A.: Advanced Critical Care Nursing. Aspen, Rockville, MD, 1989.

3–76. (**B**) Increased extracellular calcium increases myocardial contractility. Shortened ST segments and QT intervals are a reflection of an increase in isometric force and shortened ventricular systole.

Reference: Mountcastle, V.B. (ed.): Medical Physiology, 14th ed. C.V. Mosby, St. Louis, 1980.

3–77. (**D**) As the pancreatic acini and ducts are destroyed, amylase and lipase are released. Serum amylase levels elevate rapidly but return to normal in several hours. Serum lipase levels rise in the first 48 hours but remain elevated for 5 to 7 days. Hypocalcemia occurs because of a reduction in ionized calcium as calcium is deposited in fatty necrotic areas in the abdominal cavity. Serum calcium remains down for 7 to 10 days. Normal serum amylase is 25 to 125 units/l. Normal serum calcium is 9.0 to 11.0 mg/dl. Normal serum lipase is generally below 1.5 units/ml.

References: Fain, J.A., and Amato-Vealey, E.: Acute pancreatitis: A gastrointestinal emergency. Crit Care Nurs, 8(5):47–60, 1989.
Luckmann, J., and Sorensen, K.C.: Medical-Surgical Nursing: A Psychophysiologic Approach, 3rd ed. W.B. Saunders, Philadelphia, 1987.

3–78. (**A**) A spinal cord injury at C7 to C8 usually causes quadriplegia with intact biceps and triceps. There is loss of function of the intrinsic hand muscles. Diaphragmatic breathing is intact in injuries below C4. There are varying amounts of intercostal and abdominal muscle functional loss; therefore, patients require support when in the upright position. Bowel and bladder function is lost.

Reference: Alspach, J.G. (ed.): AACN Core Curriculum for Critical Care Nursing, 4th ed. W.B. Saunders, Philadelphia, 1991.

3–79. (**C**) Spinal shock is a state of transient reflex depression below the level of the lesion. The intensity of the shock varies with the level of the lesion. Reflex return also varies, generally in a rostral direction with anal and bulbocavernosus reflexes and plantar stimulation manifested earlier. The bulbocavernosus reflex is tested by inserting a gloved, lubricated finger into the anus and feeling for anal contraction. The oculovestibular and oculocephalic reflexes would not provide useful information about this patient. Once reflex function has returned, spastic paralysis typical of an upper motor neuron lesion is manifested.

Reference: Alspach, J.G. (ed.): AACN Core Curriculum for Critical Care Nursing, 4th ed. W.B. Saunders, Philadelphia, 1991.

3–80. (**D**) As potassium levels approach 6 mEq/l, tall, peaked T waves develop. At concentrations above 8 or 9 mEq/l, conduction becomes progressively impaired. Conduction through the atrial muscle fails, the PR interval lengthens, and amplitude of the P wave diminishes. The QRS complex widens markedly and the characteristic T waves may disappear or become inverted.

References: Janson, C.L.: Fluid and electrolyte balance. In Rosen, P. (ed.): Emergency Medicine: Concepts and Practice. C.V. Mosby, St. Louis, 1988.
Sweetwood, H.: Clinical Electrocardiography for Nurses, 2nd ed. Aspen, Rockville, MD, 1989.

3–81. (**A**) All patients undergoing EPS testing have their antiarrhythmic medications discontinued prior to the procedure, so their fear of fatal arrhythmias is real. Reassuring patients that they will be continuously monitored and immediately treated will address their safety needs. Encouraging patients to verbalize fears must still be tempered with the reassurance that they are being monitored closely.

Reference: Monticco, L., and Hill, K.: EPS studies: When they're called for, what they reveal. RN, *52*:54–58, 1989.

3–82. (**D**) The variation in heart rate corresponds to a respiratory rate of approximately 12 per minute. Sinus arrhythmia is often caused by respiration. Heart rate increases with inspiration and decreases with expiration as changes in intrathoracic pressure during respiration influence vagal tone. The P-P intervals vary rhythmically without variation in the PR interval. In sinus exit block there is absence of a normally expected P wave with the pause between P waves being a multiple of the usual P-P interval. In wandering atrial pacemaker, the P waves appear to have different morphologies. Although the contour of the atrial premature P wave in atrial premature contractions may resemble the sinus P wave, it is generally different and indicates a focus of different origin.

Reference: Andreoli, K., Fowkes, V., Zipes, D., et al.: Comprehensive Cardiac Care, 6th ed. C.V. Mosby, St. Louis, 1987.

3–83. (**D**) The release of hormones from the anterior pituitary gland (adenohypophysis) is regulated by neurohormones or hypophysiotropic factors. Release of CRH from the hypothalamic neurons into the hypophyseal portal system results in an increase in ACTH release from the anterior pituitary gland.

Reference: Hadley, M.E.: Endocrinology, 2nd ed. Prentice-Hall, Englewood Cliffs, NJ, 1988.

3–84. (**A**) B lymphocytes are responsible for providing protection against bacterial infections, such as infections caused by *Staphylococcus aureus*. T lymphocytes provide primary protection against viral infections such as herpes simplex infections, fungal infections such as *Candida albicans* infections, and mycobacterial infections such as those caused by *Mycobacterium avium*.

Reference: Alspach, J.G. (ed.): AACN Core Curriculum for Critical Care Nursing, 4th ed. W.B. Saunders, Philadelphia, 1991.

3–85. (**B**) Pneumonia and atelectasis would produce deviation of the trachea *toward* the affected side, whereas a pneumothorax would show *increased* vocal fremitus and tympany on percussion. A pleural effusion increases the pressure on the affected side and causes a deviation of the trachea away from the affected side. Fluid within the pleural space causes decreased breath sounds and the additional physical findings.

Reference: Kersten, L.D.: Comprehensive Respiratory Nursing: A Decision Making Approach. W.B. Saunders, Philadelphia, 1989.

3–86. (**A**) Masses in the lungs or neck often impede blood flow through the superior vena cava, producing venous distention. This is manifested by edema in the face, neck, and upper extremities. The other options also are characterized by increased jugular venous distention but without the accompanying edema.

Reference: Braunwald, E., Isselbacher, K.J., Petersdorf, R.G., et al. (eds.): Harrison's Principles of Internal Medicine, 11th ed. McGraw-Hill, New York, 1987.

3–87. (**B**) Whereas vital signs are generally considered a necessary part of any assessment, pulse and blood pressure are notoriously unreliable as parameters of a cerebral disorder. When pulse and blood pressure changes do occur, they arise late in the course of increasing intracranial pressure.

Reference: Alspach, J.G. (ed.): AACN Core Curriculum for Critical Care Nursing, 4th ed. W.B. Saunders, Philadelphia, 1991.

3–88. (**A**) The social justice model is utilitarian in nature, since its purpose is to provide the greatest good or least harm for the greatest number. It does not function to punish individuals for unacceptable behavior. Ability to pay may become a factor to consider if diminished financial resources threaten the ability of society to continue to provide for the greatest good.

References: Thompson, J.B., and Thompson, H.O.: Ethics in Nursing. Macmillan, New York, 1981.
Wlody, G.S., and Smith, S.: Ethical dilemmas in critical care, a proposal for hospital ethics advisory committees. Focus Crit Care, 5:41–46, 1985.

3–89. (**C**) Patients at high risk for peritonitis and intraperitoneal abscess are placed in semi- to high Fowler's position. This encourages fluid to drain into the pelvic area. Pelvic abscesses are easier to treat and have a lower morbidity than subphrenic or hepatic abscesses. This position also enhances respiratory excursion.

Reference: Johanson, B.C., Wells, S.J., Hoffmeister, D., et al. (eds.): Standards for Critical Care, 3rd ed. C.V. Mosby, St. Louis, 1988.

3–90. (**C**) The abrupt change in secretion consistency and color indicates aspiration of the enteral feedings. Aspiration can occur without the cuff's being broken, but it is important to check the cuff pressure when patients are being enterally fed.

Reference: Kersten, L.D.: Comprehensive Respiratory Nursing: A Decision Making Approach. W.B. Saunders, Philadelphia, 1989.

3–91. (**B**) During the insertion of a balloon-tipped pacing electrode, the monitor will show small, inverted P waves in the superior vena cava (the wave of atrial depolarization is away from the vena cava), large biphasic P waves when the electrode is in the right atrium, and progressively smaller P waves when the electrode is in the right ventricle.

Reference: Millar, S., Sampson, L., and Soukup, M.: AACN Procedure Manual for Critical Care, 2nd ed. W.B. Saunders, Philadelphia, 1985.

3–92. (**D**) Increasing a slow heart rate (HR) is one means of increasing cardiac output because $CO = SV \times HR$. SVR decreases because the cardiac output increases.

Reference: Bustin, D.: Hemodynamic Monitoring in Critical Care. Appleton-Century-Crofts, Norwalk, CT, 1986.

3–93. (**D**) Congestive heart failure is associated with generalized vasoconstriction, backup of blood to the venous circuit, and decreased cardiac output. A persistent decrease in effective arterial circulatory volume activates compensatory mechanisms that lead to decreased renal perfusion and increased aldosterone and ADH secretion with sodium and water retention. This results in hemodilution with a subsequent decrease in electrolyte concentrations.

Reference: Janson, C.L.: Fluid and electrolyte balance. In Rosen, P. (ed.): Emergency Medicine: Concepts and Practice. C.V. Mosby, St. Louis, 1988.

3–94. (**B**) A normal range of magnesium is between 1.5 and 2.5 mEq/l. Manifestations of hypomagnesemia include premature atrial and ventricular beats and supraventricular and ventricular tachycardias. Hypomagnesemia is also included in electrolyte disturbances that cause torsades de pointes, possibly as a result of a prolonged QT interval.

References: Janson, C.L.: Fluid and electrolyte balance. In Rosen, P. (ed.): Emergency Medicine: Concepts and Practice. C.V. Mosby, St. Louis, 1988.
Sweetwood, H.: Clinical Electrocardiography for Nurses, 2nd ed. Aspen, Rockville, MD, 1989.

3–95. **(D)** Furosemide blocks renal reabsorption of sodium, yielding a greater sodium load for exchange with potassium. As a result, large amounts of potassium are secreted and excreted. Digitalis inactivates the sodium-potassium pump. Magnesium is needed for the sodium-potassium pump to return potassium to the cell, and hypomagnesemia is associated with hypokalemia.

References: Gilman, A.G., Goodman, L.S., Rall, T.W., et al. (eds.): Goodman & Gilman's The Pharmacologic Basis of Therapeutics, 7th ed. Macmillan, New York, 1985.
Hoffman, B.F., and Bigger, J.: Digitalis and allied cardiac glycosides. In Gilman, A.G., Goodman, L.S., Rall, T.W., et al. (eds.): Goodman & Gilman's The Pharmacologic Basis of Therapeutics, 7th ed. Macmillan, New York, 1985.
Schwartz, M.W.: Potassium imbalances. Am J Nurs, 87:1292–1299, 1987.

3–96. **(A)** Ethanol inhibits vasopressin release, resulting in diuresis. Malignant cells are capable of synthesizing, storing, and releasing ADH. Pulmonary tissue may synthesize ADH, and physical and emotional stress may stimulate the hypothalamic neurohypophysis, resulting in increased ADH release.

Reference: Kohler, P.O., and Jordan, R.M. (eds.): Clinical Endocrinology. John Wiley and Sons, New York, 1986.

3–97. **(D)** A normal specific gravity for urine is 1.010 to 1.020. A patient with SIADH has an elevated specific gravity, whereas a patient with diabetes insipidus has a specific gravity of less than 1.005.

Reference: Cardona, V.D., Hurn, P.D., Mason, P.J.B., et al. (eds.): Trauma Nursing: From Resuscitation Through Rehabilitation. W.B. Saunders, Philadelphia, 1988.

3–98. **(C)** Hypertonic solutions act quickly to reduce intracranial pressure, whereas steroids, such as dexamethasone (Decadron), act more slowly. Steroids are a controversial approach for management of the neurologic or neurosurgical patient. They are an accepted form of therapy for the management of vasogenic edema in patients with brain tumors.

Reference: Hickey, J.V.: The Clinical Practice of Neurological and Neurosurgical Nursing, 2nd ed. J.B. Lippincott, Philadelphia, 1986.

3–99. **(D)** Bleeding related to excessive anticoagulation may lead to blood in the urine (hematuria), nosebleeds (epistaxis), and spontaneous subdural hematomas with a change in level of consciousness. Heparin anticoagulates the blood by acting on the intrinsic system, which is monitored by the partial thromboplastin time (PTT). The antidote for heparin is protamine sulfate. Although the administration of the medication should be carefully monitored, using an infusion pump in no way eliminates the risk of administering an overdose.

Reference: Mathewson, M.K.: Pharmacotherapeutics: A Nursing Process Approach. F.A. Davis, Philadelphia, 1986.

3–100. **(A)** Cryoprecipitate contains factors V, VIII, and XIII. It is administered to restore clotting factors.

Reference: Alspach, J.G. (ed.): AACN Core Curriculum for Critical Care Nursing, 4th ed. W.B. Saunders, Philadelphia, 1991.

3–101. **(B)** Alveolar ventilation (V_A) is inversely indicated by the Pa_{CO_2}. As alveolar ventilation increases, the Pa_{CO_2} will decrease as CO_2 is eliminated through the lungs (i.e., $\downarrow V_A \rightarrow \uparrow CO_2$). The pH will change based upon the changes in the Pa_{CO_2}. HCO_3 is eliminated through the kidneys. The Pa_{O_2} indicates oxygenation, not ventilation.

Reference: Shapiro, B.A., Harrison, R.A., Cane, R.D., et al.: Clinical Application of Blood Gases, 4th ed. Year Book Medical Publishers, Chicago, 1989.

3–102. (**D**) In Prinzmetal's angina, ST elevations occur during periods of coronary artery spasm. Q waves do not appear in Prinzmetal's angina, because myocardial necrosis has not occurred. ST segments elevate during periods of myocardial cellular hypoxia, signifying normal depolarization and rapid repolarization of the tissue. Delta waves are found in Wolff-Parkinson-White syndrome and signify the slowed ventricular conduction occurring from the accessory pathway. T waves generally become tall and peaked during periods of angina.

Reference: Andreoli, K., Fowkes, V., Zipes, D., et al.: Comprehensive Cardiac Care, 6th ed. C.V. Mosby, St. Louis, 1987.

3–103. (**C**) Left ventricular hypertrophy produces the following changes in the ECG: deeper S waves in leads V_1 and V_2, taller R waves in leads I, aV_L, V_5, and V_6. Right ventricular hypertrophy causes tall R waves to appear over the right precordial leads (V_1 and V_2) and deep S waves over left precordial leads (V_5 and V_6). Normal QRS axis is 0° to +90°.

Reference: Andreoli, K., Fowkes, V., Zipes, D., et al.: Comprehensive Cardiac Care, 6th ed. C.V. Mosby, St. Louis, 1987.

3–104. (**A**) Posthepatic jaundice is produced when bile ducts are obstructed. Prehepatic jaundice results from excessive red blood cell destruction due to bacterial toxins, transfusion reactions, severe burns, or hemolytic anemia. Hepatic jaundice is caused by defective management of bilirubin within the liver due to liver cell dysfunction or necrosis, such as that with cirrhosis.

Reference: Luckmann, J., and Sorensen, K.C.: Medical-Surgical Nursing: A Psychophysiologic Approach, 3rd ed. W.B. Saunders, Philadelphia, 1987.

3–105. (**A**) Shifting of potassium into the intracellular compartment occurs by the administration of $NaHCO_3$ or by the infusion of hypertonic glucose solutions and insulin. Insulin increases the permeability of the cell membrane, resulting in the shift of potassium into the intracellular space; dextrose is necessary to prevent hypoglycemia. Other treatments listed work in other ways in the management of hyperkalemia. Ion exchange resins exchange sodium for potassium across the intestinal mucosa. Calcium promotes stabilization of the membranes during depolarization. Dialysis removes potassium ions from the plasma.

References: Chambers, J.K.: Fluid and electrolyte problems in renal and urologic disorders. Nurs Clin North Am, 22:815–825, 1987.
Crandall, B.L.: Chronic renal failure. In Ulrich, T. (ed.): Nephrology Nursing. Appleton and Lange, Norwalk, CT, 1989.

3–106. (**C**) Meningitis occurs as a result of pathologic organisms gaining access to the subarachnoid space and the meninges. Exudate forms and inflammation of the meninges occurs, leading to cortical irritation and possibly increased intracranial pressure as a result of hydrocephalus and cerebral edema.

Reference: Alspach, J.G. (ed.): AACN Core Curriculum for Critical Care Nursing, 4th ed. W.B. Saunders, Philadelphia, 1991.

3–107. (**D**) The left circumflex artery supplies the lateral wall of the left ventricle, the left atrium, and the inferior and diaphragmatic surface of the left ventricle. Inferior infarctions are associated with right coronary artery occlusion. Anterior and anteroseptal infarctions are associated with left anterior descending artery occlusions.

Reference: Kenner, C., Guzzetta, C., and Dossey, B.: Critical Care Nursing: Body—Mind—Spirit. Little, Brown, Boston, 1985.

3–108. (**B**) Afterload reduction is the most effective method to decrease left-to-right shunting of blood through the VSD. Proper intra-aortic balloon pump timing is essential to decrease afterload, which will decrease the left-to-right shunt. Nitroprusside decreases right- and left-sided pressures, making it ineffective in reducing shunting of blood through the VSD. Furosemide and digoxin do not reduce afterload.

Reference: Underhill, S., Woods, S., Froelicher, E., et al.: Cardiac Nursing, 2nd ed. J.B. Lippincott, Philadelphia, 1989.

3–109. (**A**) Asthma is characterized by hyper-reactivity of the airways in response to various stimuli. This presents as narrowing of airways and mucosal edema, which result in increased work of breathing and airway resistance.

Reference: Kersten, L.D.: Comprehensive Respiratory Nursing: A Decision Making Approach. W.B. Saunders, Philadelphia, 1989.

3–110. (**A**) Increased respiratory rate and tidal volume eliminate humidity and water vapor from the respiratory tree. This thickens and increases production of secretions, and also reduces clearance of secretions. The mucus plugging, edema in the mucosal walls, and hardened secretions combine to decrease the responsiveness of the smooth muscle walls to bronchodilator therapy.

Reference: Alspach, J.G. (ed.): AACN Core Curriculum for Critical Care Nursing, 4th ed. W.B. Saunders, Philadelphia, 1991.

3–111. (**A**) Abnormalities in platelet function, specifically a reduction in platelet adhesiveness and platelet aggregation, impair the clotting mechanism in acute renal failure patients. Capillary fragility is due to chronic hypocalcemia associated with chronic renal failure. The platelet count is normal or slightly decreased. Erythropoietin does not affect bleeding but affects red cell production.

References: Calloway, C.: When the problem involves magnesium, calcium, or phosphate. RN, 50:30–36, 1987.
Crandall, B.L.: Acute renal failure. In Ulrich, T. (ed.): Nephrology Nursing. Appleton and Lange, Norwalk, CT, 1989.

3–112. (**A**) Because it is fat-soluble, vitamin K can be absorbed only in the presence of bile. Vitamin K deficiency can also result from inadequate dietary intake, malabsorption syndrome, profound liver damage, and treatment that destroys GI bacteria that synthesize vitamin K. Since vitamin K catalyzes prothrombin synthesis within liver cells, vitamin K deficiency will cause hypoprothrombinemia (deficient amount of circulating prothrombin). Intrinsic factor is required for absorption of vitamin B_{12}.

Reference: Luckmann, J., and Sorensen, K.C.: Medical-Surgical Nursing: A Psychophysiologic Approach, 3rd ed. W.B. Saunders, Philadelphia, 1987.

3–113. (**D**) The Glasgow Coma Score (GCS) is a standardized assessment tool that evaluates level of consciousness. Responses in three areas—eye opening, motor response, and verbal response—are graded and the scores summed. Scores range from a low of 3 to a high of 15, with 15 being normal.

Reference: Alspach, J.G. (ed.): AACN Core Curriculum for Critical Care Nursing, 4th ed. W.B. Saunders, Philadelphia, 1991.

3–114. (**B**) Heparin is found in the mast cells in the lungs. The presence of heparin is important since it results in chest drainage being naturally anticoagulated. In addition, heparin is released during anaphylactic and anaphylactoid reactions and may account in part for the coagulopathies associated with these reactions. Epinephrine is a naturally occurring catecholamine and is released from the adrenal glands. Both dopamine and epinephrine are neurotransmitters. Insulin is required for normal glucose metabolism.

Reference: Mathewson, M.K.: Pharmacotherapeutics: A Nursing Process Approach. F.A. Davis, Philadelphia, 1986.

3–115. (**B**) Limb ischemia may occur from catheter obstruction, arterial injury, and thromboembolism. Symptoms of limb ischemia include diminished or other pulse changes, paresthesias, pain, motor deficits, and decreased extremity temperature. These changes are seen more often than ICU psychosis and septicemia, which are preventable complications, and aortic dissection, which is rare.

Reference: Funk, M., Gleason, J., and Foell, D.: Lower limb ischemia related to the use of the intraaortic balloon pump. Heart Lung, 18:542–552, 1989.

3–116. (**B**) Aortic insufficiency is the only absolute contraindication to intraaortic balloon counterpulsation because balloon inflation in the aorta would cause backward flow of blood into the left ventricle. Femoral artery aneurysm is not an absolute contraindication because the device may be inserted into the abdominal aorta.

Reference: Kinney, M., Packa, D., and Dunbar, S. (eds.): AACN's Clinical Reference for Critical Care Nursing, 2nd ed. McGraw-Hill, New York, 1988.

3–117. (**C**) Although no nurse is required to administer care or treatment that is morally objectionable to him or her, there is an obligation to arrange for the continued care of the patient. This obligation must be met before the nurse may refuse to provide care. There is no justification to ask that a reasonable therapy be discontinued for the benefit of the nurse.

Reference: American Nurses Association: Code for Nurses with Interpretive Statements. American Nurses Association, Kansas City, MO 1976.

3–118. (**D**) Both the RAP and PCWP are low normal, which eliminates cor pulmonale, left heart failure, and fluid overload. The main alteration is in the lungs and is caused by vasoconstriction secondary to regional hypoxia.

Reference: Kersten, L.D.: Comprehensive Respiratory Nursing: A Decision Making Approach. W.B. Saunders, Philadelphia, 1989.

3–119. (**A**) The $S\bar{v}O_2$ is an indication of how well the heart and lung function to meet the tissue oxygen demand. If the $S\bar{v}O_2$ drops, it can be due to a drop in cardiac output, an increase in oxygen consumption, or a drop in oxygen loading in the lungs. In this case, the increase in PEEP to keep the Pa_{O_2} and Sa_{O_2} normal has decreased venous return to the heart and dropped the cardiac output.

Reference: Snyder, J.V., and Pinsky, M.R.: Oxygen Transport in the Critically Ill. Year Book Medical Publishers, Chicago, 1987.

3–120. (**A**) Paralysis would decrease the oxygen consumption, but the problem in this case is inadequate delivery—decreased cardiac output. Increasing the PEEP will decrease the cardiac output further, and increasing the $F_{I_{O_2}}$ will not improve the cardiac output. The best therapy would be to add a low-dose vasopressor drug such as dobutamine or dopamine to improve cardiac function.

Reference: Snyder, J.V., and Pinsky, M.R.: Oxygen Transport in the Critically Ill. Year Book Medical Publishers, Chicago, 1987.

3–121. (**C**) Computed tomography (CT) is a valuable diagnostic aid in almost all intracranial pathology and is of particular value in head injury. Lumbar puncture is generally contraindicated until intracranial pathology is ruled out. Likewise, cerebral angiography is associated with the risk of cerebrovascular accident resulting from a dislodged thrombus; therefore, intracranial hemorrhage is generally ruled out through use of CT or magnetic resonance imaging prior to angiography. Myelography is typically used in patients with intervertebral disc disease or spinal cord injuries.

Reference: Alspach, J.G. (ed.): AACN Core Curriculum for Critical Care Nursing, 4th ed. W.B. Saunders, Philadelphia, 1991.

3–122. (**A**) When a capillary fiber ruptures, blood leaks into the ultrafiltrate and the ultrafiltrate color changes from colorless or yellow to blood-tinged. Clotting in the filter can result in dark blood in the hemofilter and arterial and venous tubings and a decreased ultrafiltration rate. Over-heparinization can result in bleeding, which can be observed in the nasogastric aspirate, incisional lines, insertion sites, and stools. Clogging of the filter results in decreased ultrafiltration rate.

References: Kiely, M.: Continuous arteriovenous hemofiltration. Crit Care Nurs, 4:39–49, 1984.
Palmer, C., Koorejian, K., London, J., et al.: Nursing management of continuous arteriovenous hemofiltration for acute renal failure. Focus Crit Care, 13:21–30, 1986.

3–123. (**C**) If the objective of treatment is both extracellular fluid removal and toxic solute (urea, potassium, creatinine) clearance, high ultrafiltration rates with filter replacement fluid are used. Clearance of small molecular substances, specifically urea, is made possible by allowing a maximal ultrafiltration rate while replacing plasma volume and electrolytes. Ultrafiltration helps to decrease uremic toxin concentrations in the blood while avoiding hypovolemia through fluid replacement.

References: Palmer, C., Koorejian, K., London, J., et al.: Nursing management of continuous arteriovenous hemofiltration for acute renal failure. Focus Crit Care, 13:21–30, 1986.
Williams, V., and Perkins, L.: Continuous ultrafiltration: A new ICU procedure for the treatment of fluid overload. Crit Care Nurs, 4:44–49, 1984.

3–124. (**D**) Carotid sinus stimulation inhibits the vasomotor center and causes reflex parasympathetic stimulation. Parasympathetic stimulation in vagal nerve fibers acts to decrease the firing rate of the SA node. Increased sympathetic tone would increase the heart rate. AV node ischemia would not affect the firing rate of the SA node but would increase the PR interval.

Reference: Andreoli, K., Fowkes, V., Zipes, D., et al.: Comprehensive Cardiac Care, 6th ed. C.V. Mosby, St. Louis, 1987.

3–125. (**D**) Right ventricular infarction is associated with hypovolemia from hepatic and peripheral venous congestion. The patient needs increased preload to maintain perfusion, although diuretic therapy may be indicated when the acute phase is over. Catecholamine infusions are not indicated in hypovolemic situations. Because right ventricular infarctions are also associated with atrioventricular blocks, ventricular pacing should be used.

Reference: Weeks, L.: Advanced Cardiovascular Nursing. Blackwell, Boston, 1986.

3–126. (**A**) Establishing short-term and long-term goals is an initial intervention in knowledge deficits for critically ill patients. Family members should be encouraged to reinforce correct information about diagnosis and therapy. Critically ill patients usually need multiple explanations before information is understood and retained. Frequent patient interaction and exploration are essential because the patient may not even know what to ask.

Reference: Swearingen, P.L., Sommers, M.S., and Miller, K.: Manual of Critical Care: Applying Nursing Diagnoses to Adult Critical Illness. C.V. Mosby, St. Louis, 1988.

3–127. (**B**) Of the many needs and concerns identified by families of critically ill alert surgical patients (and all families across most studies) the need for hope is valued as most important. The intensive care unit environment, availability of counselors or chaplains, and knowledge of names of caregivers are not rated as very important by families of critically ill adults.

Reference: Simpson, T.: Research review: Needs and concerns of families of critically ill adults. Focus Crit Care, *16*(5):388–397, 1989.

3–128. (**A**) Hypoxia is determined by clinical diagnosis. A decrease in arterial blood oxygen tension or saturation is diagnosed by arterial blood gases. Oxygen extraction is assessed by obtaining venous blood gases from a pulmonary artery catheter and comparing the venous oxygen tension to the arterial blood gas.

Reference: Snyder, J.V., and Pinsky, M.R.: Oxygen Transport in the Critically Ill. Year Book Medical Publishers, Chicago, 1987.

3–129. (**D**) Pulse oximetry provides continuous real-time trending of the Sa_{O_2} by sensing arterial pulsations and determining the saturation through dual lightwave lengths. Pulse oximetry is dependent on oxygen delivery to the tissues to determine the arterial pulsations. If there is poor tissue perfusion, the pulsations are not sensed and the Sa_{O_2} is inaccurate. The skin oxygen consumption and thickness do not affect pulse oximetry.

Reference: Schroeder, C.H.: Pulse oximetry: A nursing care plan. Crit Care Nurs, *8*(8):50–68, 1988.

3–130. (**B**) Cyanosis requires that at least 5 gm/dl of hemoglobin be reduced. Carboxyhemoglobinemia produces a cherry-red color and therefore masks cyanosis. Methemoglobin promotes cyanosis because thiocyanate is bound to hemoglobin; anemia masks cyanosis because in anemia the absolute hemoglobin level is very low.

Reference: Shapiro, B.A., Harrison, R.A., Cane, R.D., et al.: Clinical Application of Blood Gases, 4th ed. Year Book Medical Publishers, Chicago, 1989.

3–131. (**B**) Hypomagnesemia commonly occurs in patients with acute or chronic alcoholism, especially during the withdrawal phase. The causes can include poor dietary intake, vomiting, diarrhea, and use of antacids that bind phosphate and reduce its absorption. The serum potassium level may be further reduced by the hyperventilation characteristic of alcohol withdrawal and by the therapeutic infusion of glucose. Hypomagnesemia does not occur alone but is accompanied by metabolic alkalosis, hypocalcemia, and hypokalemia. Hyponatremia is not associated with alcoholism.

References: Johnson, D.: Fluid and electrolyte dysfunction in alcoholism. Crit Care Q, *8*:53–60, 1986.
Smith, L.H.: Phosphorus deficiency and hypophosphatemia. In Wyngaarden, J.B., and Smith, L.H. (eds.): Textbook of Medicine, 18th ed. W.B. Saunders, Philadelphia, 1988.

3–132. (**A**) Phosphorus is decreased in alcoholics because of decreased intake, respiratory alkalosis, vomiting and diarrhea, and increased urinary excretion of phosphorus. As the patient is rehydrated and started on hyperalimentation, serum phosphorus levels can decrease significantly. Refeeding of malnourished patients increases phosphate incorporation into nucleic acids and phosphorylated compounds in the cell. The intracellular shift of phosphate causes the serum phosphate levels to drop.

References: Johnson, D.: Fluid and electrolyte dysfunction in alcoholism. Crit Care Q, 8:53–60, 1986.
Porth, C.M.: Pathophysiology: Concepts and Altered Health States, 2nd ed. J.B. Lippincott, Philadelphia, 1986.

3–133. (**B**) There are several factors that may precipitate carbon dioxide retention. These include: (1) extreme tongue swelling disrupting airway patency; (2) restrictive pulmonary function caused by myxedematous infiltration of the respiratory muscles; (3) low pulmonary surfactant levels; (4) an abnormality in central respiratory regulation; and (5) depressive respiratory effects of drugs. Decreased effects of glucocorticoid hormones (gluconeogenesis and glycogenolysis) due to decreased thyroid hormone may result in hypoglycemia. Hypoglycemia may also be present if there is a pituitary or hypothalamic defect causing the thyroid hormone deficiency.

Reference: Hamburger, S., Rush, D.R., and Bosker, G.: Endocrine and Metabolic Emergencies. Robert J. Brady, Bowie, MD, 1984.

3–134. (**C**) There are four stages associated with the physiologic and clinical signs of increased intracranial pressure. They include stage 1 or the compensation phase, in which there are no changes in vital signs; stage 2, or the end of compensation, during which time there is only a slight change in the patient's vital signs; stage 3, the beginning of decompensation, which includes increased systolic blood pressure, widening of the pulse pressure, bradycardia, and cardiac dysrhythmias. The decompensation phase or stage 4 is a continuation of stage 3. If no treatment is undertaken, death results.

Reference: Hickey, J.V.: The Clinical Practice of Neurological and Neurosurgical Nursing, 2nd ed. J.B. Lippincott, Philadelphia, 1986.

3–135. (**D**) Cerebral perfusion pressure (CPP) is defined as the pressure gradient across the brain and is calculated as the difference between the mean arterial pressure (MAP) and the intracranial pressure (ICP) in the arteries. The calculation is represented by the formula

$$CPP = MAP - ICP$$

The CPP is an estimate of the adequacy of cerebral circulation. The average CPP in the adult is approximately 80 to 100 mm Hg with a range between 60 and 150 mm Hg. When ICP approaches the MAP, autoregulation is impaired and cerebral blood flow diminishes.

Reference: Hickey, J.V.: The Clinical Practice of Neurological and Neurosurgical Nursing, 2nd ed. J.B. Lippincott, Philadelphia, 1986.

3–136. (**D**) An ICP monitoring device system (e.g., subarachnoid screw, intraventricular catheter, or epidural sensor) should be assessed for the presence of air, blood, tissue, or kinks if the waveform becomes damped. Air bubbles can be removed by turning off the stopcock closest to the patient, opening the two-way transducer stopcock, and gently flushing the system with a saline-filled syringe (some physicians permit only 0.1 ml of preservative-free sterile saline). After flushing, the two-way stopcock closest to the patient should be opened to re-establish function of the monitoring device and transducer system. Finally, the nurse should observe the waveform. Catheters should be drained upon a specific physician order and the color, clarity, consistency, and amount of drainage should be recorded and reported.

References: Caine, R.M., and Bufalino, P.M.: Critically Ill Adults: Nursing Care Planning Guides. Williams & Wilkins, Baltimore, 1988.
Holloway, N.M.: Nursing the Critically Ill Adult. Addison-Wesley, Menlo Park, CA, 1988.

3–137. (**A**) Hypoxia causes cytotoxic cerebral edema as a result of space-occupying lesions. It also causes cerebral vasodilatation, particularly when the Pa_{O_2} falls below 60 mm Hg. Vasogenic cerebral edema is caused by a breakdown of the blood-brain barrier, which allows water to leak into the interstitium.

References: Alspach, J.G. (ed.): AACN Core Curriculum for Critical Care Nursing, 4th ed. W.B. Saunders, Philadelphia, 1991.
Hickey, J.V.: The Clinical Practice of Neurological and Neurosurgical Nursing, 2nd ed. J.B. Lippincott, Philadelphia, 1986.

3–138. (**B**) Acetaminophen is used to reduce the elevated temperature. Naloxone blocks the release of endorphins, which helps to reverse peripheral vasodilation and improve myocardial contractility. Aminoglycosides such as gentamicin are used to treat the gram-negative septicemia.

Reference: Wall, S.C.: Septic shock. Nursing '89, *19*:52—60, 1989.

3–139. (**C**) Acute ventricular septal rupture would cause the collective symptoms of cyanosis, AV dissociation, and elevated right ventricular pressures. Pulmonary edema and embolism would elevate pulmonary artery pressures. Cardiogenic shock would elevate the wedge pressure.

Reference: Underhill, S., Woods, S., Froelicher, E., et al.: Cardiac Nursing, 2nd ed. J.B. Lippincott, Philadelphia, 1989.

3–140. (**A**) Since the patient's pacemaker has suddenly lost capture, placing the patient flat in bed on his side may restore pacemaker capture. If the pacemaker capture is not restored and the patient loses consciousness, he will already be flat in bed and CPR may be initiated. The pacemaker need not be turned off during CPR. Advanced life support and pharmacotherapy are initiated after CPR is started.

Reference: Kenner, C., Guzzetta, C., and Dossey, B.: Critical Care Nursing: Body—Mind—Spirit. Little, Brown, Boston, 1985.

3–141. (**A**) Nosocomial pneumonias are especially difficult to treat because of the widespread use of broad-spectrum antibiotics, which produces strains of organisms that are antibiotic-resistant. An example is methacillin-resistant *Staphylococcus aureus* (MRSA) pneumonia.

Reference: Kersten, L.D.: Comprehensive Respiratory Nursing: A Decision Making Approach. W.B. Saunders, Philadelphia, 1989.

3–142. (**A**) Diuretics may enhance the urinary excretion of calcium if renal function is normal. Because of the potential for acute renal failure due to dehydration and the need to maintain high urinary flow rates, adequate volume status and replacement fluids must accompany diuretic therapy. IV normal saline, at a rate of 2 to 5 liters per 24 hours, should be used.

References: Calloway, C.: When the problem involves magnesium, calcium, or phosphate. RN, *50*:30–36, 1987.
Chambers, J.K.: Metabolic bone disorders: Imbalances of calcium and phosphorus. Nurs Clin North Am, *22*:861–872, 1987.

3–143. (**D**) Hypercalcemia causes AV conduction disturbances, and ECG characteristics include widening of the QRS. The ECG manifestations of hypercalcemia are similar to those seen with administration of digitalis, and hypercalcemia predisposes and accentuates digitalis toxicity. AV conduction disturbances can also be a sign of digitalis toxicity. Hypervolemia usually leads to heart chamber stretching, resulting in dysrhythmias of irritability, not heart block.

References: Janson, C.L.: Fluid and electrolyte balance. In Rosen, P. (ed.): Emergency Medicine: Concepts and Practice. C.V. Mosby, St. Louis, 1988.
Sweetwood, H.: Clinical Electrocardiography for Nurses, 2nd ed. Aspen, Rockville, MD, 1989.

3–144. (**A**) The patient with hepatitis is likely to have altered nutrition, less than body requirements, related to decreased vitamin synthesis and storage in the inflamed liver. The hepatitis patient may have any foods as tolerated, with a low fat, high carbohydrate diet usually most appealing if the patient is also anorexic. Nitrogen malabsorption and hypermetabolic state are not commonly present in the hepatitis patient.

Reference: Holloway, N.M.: Nursing the Critically Ill Adult, 3rd ed. Addison-Wesley, New York, 1988.

3–145. (**A**) Subacute subdural hematomas are more prevalent in the elderly as a result of the cerebral atrophy that occurs with the normal aging process. When cerebral trauma occurs, the cortex separates from the dura, and the bridging veins, which have become fragile as a result of age, bleed. Cerebral atrophy may also be seen in the patient with chronic alcohol ingestion.

Reference: Hickey, J.V.: The Clinical Practice of Neurological and Neurosurgical Nursing, 2nd ed. J.B. Lippincott, Philadelphia, 1986.

3–146. (**B**) Subdural hematomas are usually caused by venous bleeding. Epidural hematomas are usually caused by arterial bleeding from the middle meningeal artery.

Reference: Alspach, J.G. (ed.): AACN's Core Curriculum for Critical Care Nursing, 4th ed. W.B. Saunders, Philadelphia, 1991.

3–147. (**D**) Mannitol (Osmitrol) is a hypertonic osmotic diuretic solution that is relatively impermeable to the blood-brain barrier unless high concentrations are present in the plasma or the patient is acidotic. The usual dose is 1.5 to 2 gm/kg of body weight over 30 to 60 minutes. Following administration, water moves rapidly from the cells to the extracellular fluid and from red cells to plasma. Rapid reduction in cerebrospinal fluid pressure is seen approximately 15 minutes after intravenous administration. The goal of administration is to maintain the serum osmolarity between 305 and 315 mOsm/kg.

Reference: Hickey, J.V.: The Clinical Practice of Neurological and Neurosurgical Nursing, 2nd ed. J.B. Lippincott, Philadelphia, 1986.

3–148. (**B**) During the secondary immune response, antigen cross-bridging causes the mast cells to degranulate and release histamine, a primary chemical mediator of anaphylaxis. Myocardial depressant factor is found in the serum of patients with septic shock and is believed to be at least in part responsible for depressed myocardial function and decreased ejection fraction in those patients. Activation of the complement cascade contributes to the activation of both humoral and cell-mediated immune responses. This in turn may result in mast cell degranulation and in neutrophil aggregation and adherence to vascular endothelium, as well as increased production of prostaglandin and leukotrienes. Interferons are produced by cells to block viral replication and growth.

References: Dickerson, M.A.: Anaphylaxis and anaphylactic shock. Crit Care Nurs Q, *11*:68–74, 1988.
Littleton, M.T.: Pathophysiology and assessment of sepsis and septic shock. Crit Care Nurs Q, *11*:30–47, 1988.

3–149. (**B**) Radiologic contrast media may cause an anaphylactic reaction, which does not involve the production of IgE. The reaction, also known as an anaphylactoid reaction, is the result of complement activation of the mast cells with degranulation and the release of histamine. IgA, one of five immunoglobulins, is found on the surfaces of mucous membranes. It prevents antigens from adhering to the mucous membrane. Type IV hypersensitivity reactions are also known as cell-mediated hypersensitivity reactions. Rejection of transplanted tissue and graft-versus-host disease are examples of type IV reactions. A vasovagal reaction occurs when the vagus nerve is stimulated and results in bradycardia, vasoconstriction, and possibly loss of consciousness.

Reference: Dickerson, M.A.: Anaphylaxis and anaphylactic shock. Crit Care Nurs Q, *11*:68–74, 1988.

3–150. (**C**) The positive pressure delivered by a ventilator increases the intrathoracic pressure, which impedes venous return to the right side of the heart. The blood pressure then decreases during inspiration. This results in the inappropriate release of the antidiuretic hormone (ADH) and decreased renal blood flow and glomerular filtration.

Reference: Kersten, L.D.: Comprehensive Respiratory Nursing: A Decision Making Approach. W.B. Saunders, Philadelphia, 1989.

3–151. (**A**) The positive fluid balance indicates a need for diuretic therapy. Saline solutions should be limited because salt causes fluid retention. Once the excess fluid is eliminated, the sodium and hematocrit levels will return to normal and lung compliance should increase.

Reference: Kersten, L.D.: Comprehensive Respiratory Nursing: A Decision Making Approach. W.B. Saunders, Philadelphia, 1989.

3–152. (**D**) Radiopaque dyes used during cardiac catheterization contain iodine, which is actively transported and concentrated in the thyroid gland. Oxidized iodine combines with tyrosine in thyroglobulin to form monoiodotyrosine (MIT) and diiodotyrosine (DIT). The coupling of two DIT molecules forms thyroxine (T_4) and the coupling of one DIT molecule and one MIT molecule forms triiodothyronine (T_3). Lysosomal protease breaks apart thyroglobulin, and T_3 and T_4 are released from the cell. Exposure to an iodine load can precipitate a hyperthyroid state.

Reference: Mountcastle, V.B. (ed.): Medical Physiology, 14th ed. C.V. Mosby, St. Louis, 1980.

3–153. (**C**) More than 99% of circulating thyroid hormone is bound to plasma proteins—thyroxine-binding globulin (TBG) and thyroxine-binding prealbumin (TBPA)—and is biologically inactive. Acetylsalicylic acid displaces T_3 from TBG, making it available to cells in the biologically active form, further increasing T_3 levels. Therefore, acetaminophen is the drug of choice.

Reference: Kohler, P.O., and Jordan R.M. (eds.): Clinical Endocrinology. John Wiley and Sons, New York, 1986.

3–154. (**B**) The descending tracts transmit impulses from the brain to the motor neurons of the spinal cord. The ventral and lateral corticospinal tracts, so named because of the column in which they travel, the location of their cells, and the location of axon termination, originate in the cerebral cortical motor areas and carry impulses responsible for voluntary motor movement. The anterolateral spinothalamic tracts ascend the spinal cord and convey information about temperature, pain, light touch, and pressure sensations. The rubrospinal tract conveys impulses to control muscle tone and synergy, whereas the tectospinal tract mediates optic and auditory reflexes. The ascending dorsal and ventral spinocerebellar tracts convey proprioceptive information.

Reference: Alspach, J.G. (ed.): AACN Core Curriculum for Critical Care Nursing, 4th ed. W.B. Saunders, Philadelphia, 1991.

3–155. (**D**) Rhabdomyolysis is the result of destruction of large muscles that release myoglobin molecules into the circulating blood volume. These molecules filter into the tubules but are too large to pass through the system, resulting in loss of kidney function. Shock with a low cardiac output is a prerenal cause of renal failure due to a decrease in circulating volume. Rupture of the bladder and pressure from hematomas are postrenal causes of renal failure in the trauma patient.

Reference: Cook, L.: Genitourinary injuries and renal management. In Cardona, V.D., Hurn, P.D., and Mason, P.J.B., et al. (eds.): Trauma Nursing: From Resuscitation to Rehabilitation. W.B. Saunders, Philadelphia, 1988.

3–156. (**B**) In patients whose breathing is normal, pulsus paradoxus is recognized by a difference of greater than 10 mm Hg between initial auscultation of Korotkoff sounds (heard only on expiration) and the continuous auscultation of Korotkoff sounds during both inspiration and expiration.

Reference: Kenner, C., Guzzetta, C., and Dossey, B.: Critical Care Nursing: Body—Mind—Spirit. Little, Brown, Boston, 1985.

3–157. (**A**) Patients with pericarditis are at increased risk for developing cardiac tamponade, so heparin should be discontinued. The 12-lead ECG is not indicated each 8 hours as the patient is known to have an acute myocardial infarction. The sharp inspiratory pain is not anginal pain and will not respond to nitroglycerin. Increasing the oxygen will not relieve the pain associated with pericarditis.

Reference: Underhill, S., Woods, S., Froelicher, E., et al: Cardiac Nursing, 2nd ed. J.B. Lippincott, Philadelphia, 1989.

3–158. (**B**) Patients with portal hypertension usually have caput medusae (radiating epigastric vessels between umbilicus and ribs), hemorrhoids, bruits audible in the upper abdominal quadrants, and ascites if there is concurrent liver disease. A suspicious fall causing serious injury is a hallmark sign for alcohol intoxication. Alcohol abuse is a common etiology of portal hypertension secondary to cirrhosis.

Reference: Luckmann, J., and Sorensen, K.C.: Medical-Surgical Nursing: A Psychophysiologic Approach. W.B. Saunders, Philadelphia, 1987.

3–159. (**A**) Hypothyroidism has negative inotropic and chronotropic effects on the heart. Although heart rate and cardiac index are reduced, hypertension may exist. Pericardial effusions are also associated with hypothyroidism in about one-third of patients.

Reference: Hamburger, S., Rush, D.R., and Bosker, G.: Endocrine and Metabolic Emergencies. Robert J. Brady, Bowie, MD, 1984.

3–160. (**A**) Medication protocols are highly individual and based on cooperation of the patient. The treatment plan uses two groups of drugs—anti-cholinesterase drugs, such as neostigmine (Prostigmin) and pyridostigmine (Mestinon), and corticosteroids. Side effects of both neostigmine and pyridostigmine include the muscarinic (epigastric distress, eructation, diarrhea, blurred vision, increased mucus secretion, diaphoresis, and increased salivation) and nicotinic (skeletal muscle fasciculation and muscle cramping) symptoms associated with myasthenia gravis. Myasthenic crisis in the patient known to have myasthenia gravis is frequently associated with underdosage of the prescribed medication, stress, or fatigue. Acute muscle weakness is seen in myasthenic crisis, which must be treated immediately with anticholinesterase medications. Cholinergic crisis is caused by overdosage of the anticholinesterase (cholinergic) medications. In addition to the muscarinic and nicotinic signs, patients may experience bradycardia, hypotension, and acute muscle weakness. Because respiratory distress may occur as a result of the patient's inability to manage secretions, immediate intervention is necessary or the patient will aspirate and experience respiratory arrest. Atropine, an anticholinergic drug, is the antidote for overdosage of anticholinesterase drugs and should be kept in close proximity to the patient. Often, myasthenic and cholinergic crises are difficult to diagnose because respiratory distress is a prominent symptom that must be treated immediately. The Tensilon test is frequently used to differentiate the crises.

Reference: Hickey, J.V.: The Clinical Practice of Neurological and Neurosurgical Nursing, 2nd ed. J.B. Lippincott, Philadelphia, 1986.

3–161. (**D**) Cholinergic crisis is caused by overmedication with anticholinesterase drugs. Signs and symptoms include acute muscle weakness, respiratory distress, nausea, vomiting, miosis, pallor, diaphoresis, increased salivation, gastrointestinal hyperirritability, severe cramps, diarrhea, and bradycardia.

Reference: Hickey, J.V.: The Clinical Practice of Neurological and Neurosurgical Nursing, 2nd ed. J.B. Lippincott, Philadelphia, 1986.

3–162. (**D**) Low gastric pH, history of complicated critical illness, sharp midepigastric pain, tender abdomen, and hypoactive bowel sounds suggest a perforated stress ulcer followed by peritonitis. The hallmark of pancreatitis is severe pain in the left upper quadrant and persistent vomiting. Emesis, mild jaundice, and radiating epigastric pain are indicative of bile duct obstruction. Small bowel obstruction is characterized by crampy pain, vomiting, constipation, and distention.

Reference: Luckmann, J., and Sorensen, K.C.: Medical-Surgical Nursing: A Psychophysiologic Approach, 3rd ed. W.B. Saunders, Philadelphia, 1987.

3–163. (**B**) As peritonitis develops from ulcer perforation, the patient breathes shallowly to avoid the pain caused by diaphragm expansion and body movement. Hyperactive bowel sounds might develop in small bowel obstruction but not after perforated ulcer. Hyperglycemia is associated with pancreatitis. Jaundice is associated with bile duct obstruction.

Reference: Luckmann, J., and Sorensen, K.C.: Medical-Surgical Nursing: A Psychophysiologic Approach, 3rd. ed. W.B. Saunders, Philadelphia, 1987.

3–164. (**B**) The semi-Fowler's position, in which the patient sits up and draws the knees up to the abdomen, is the most comfortable position for severe abdominal pain. This position reduces the tension on the irritated abdominal muscles. It also promotes drainage of fluid to the pelvic region so that drainage or abscess treatment is more easily managed.

Reference: Luckmann, J., and Sorensen, K.C.: Medical-Surgical Nursing: A Psychophysiological Approach, 3rd ed. W.B. Saunders, Philadelphia, 1987.

3–165. (**D**) Laxatives are used in the treatment of cardiomyopathies to prevent Valsalva responses, which increase myocardial oxygen consumption and decrease cardiac output by altering ventricular filling time. Bedrest decreases myocardial oxygen consumption and limits sympathetic increases in heart rate and contractility that result from exercise.

Reference: Underhill, S., Woods, S., Froelicher, E., et al.: Cardiac Nursing, 2nd ed. J.B. Lippincott, Philadelphia, 1989.

3–166. (**A**) A key element that must be remembered with cerebral aneurysm patients is that they are often unaware of their condition until the aneurysm ruptures and they require immediate hospitalization and emergency surgery. The patient with cerebral aneurysm may or may not present with symptoms of actual neurologic deficit; however, that risk is always likely. Activity and visiting restrictions need to be explained carefully. Certainly, concerns regarding a lengthy hospitalization must be addressed.

Reference: Caine, R.M., and Bufalino, P.M.: Critically Ill Adults: Nursing Care Planning Guides. Williams & Wilkins, Baltimore, 1988.

3–167. (**D**) Heparin interrupts clotting by blocking the conversion of prothrombin to thrombin and by inhibiting thrombin-induced platelet aggregation. This serves to reduce clot formation and the subsequent consumption of clotting factors that is occurring intravascularly.

Reference: Mathewson, M.K.: Pharmacotherapeutics: A Nursing Process Approach. F.A. Davis, Philadelphia, 1986.

3–168. (**C**) The repeated unsuccessful weaning attempts indicate that the patient has become dependent upon the ventilator and is unable to cope with the withdrawal of ventilator support. The repeated attempts also tend to disprove the other options as the causes of her distress.

Reference: Belitz, J.: Minimizing the psychological complications of patients who require mechanical ventilation. Crit Care Nurs, 3:42–46, 1983.

3–169. (**C**) All but age cause the compliance to decrease because of stiffer lungs and thorax or reduced expansibility. As adults age, the rib cage becomes more distended, thereby increasing compliance.

Reference: West, J.B.: Respiratory Physiology: The Essentials, 4th ed. Williams & Wilkins, Baltimore, 1990.

3–170. (**A**) By administering any blood product to the patient, the nurse would have broken an implicit promise to act as his advocate and demonstrated that the nurse valued saving the patient's life above his right to self-determination. The nurse could be held legally liable for assault and battery for acting on the person against his wishes.

References: Creighton, H.: Law Every Nurse Should Know, 4th ed. W.B. Saunders, Philadelphia, 1981.
Dixon, J.L., and Smalley, M.G.: Jehovah's Witnesses, the surgical/ethical challenge. JAMA, 21:2471–2472, 1981.
Gardner, B., Bivona, J., Alfonso, A., et al.: Major surgery in Jehovah's Witnesses. NY State J Med, 5:765–767, 1976.

3–171. (**C**) Acting as a patient advocate is an ethical duty of a nurse, whether or not the nurse agrees with the values held by the patient. The supervisor should be notified at once to support the nurse and the patient. A nonblood plasma expander might be used to preserve the life of the individual.

References: Creighton, H.: Law Every Nurse Should Know, 4th ed. W.B. Saunders, Philadelphia, 1981.
Dixon, J.L., and Smalley, M.G.: Jehovah's Witnesses, the surgical/ethical challenge. JAMA, 21:2471–2472, 1981.
Gardner, B., Bivona, J., Alfonso, A., et al.: Major surgery in Jehovah's Witnesses. NY State J Med, 5:765–767, 1976.

3–172. **(B)** The complaint of stabbing chest pain in a patient with hypertension may signal a dissecting aortic aneurysm. Before any other measures are taken, this potential must be assessed. Because the patient complained of a "funny feeling" in his arms, his pulses in these extremities should be palpated and results compared with previous findings. Stabbing chest pain is the most common complaint of persons with aortic dissection.

Reference: Underhill, S., Woods, S., Froelicher, E., et al.: Cardiac Nursing, 2nd ed. J.B. Lippincott, Philadelphia, 1989.

3–173. **(C)** The nitroprusside reagent reacts with acetoacetate and acetone. It does not react with 3-hydroxybutyrate. During diabetic ketoacidosis, the 3-hydroxybutyrate level is usually two to three times greater than the acetoacetate level. In this patient the negative test result suggests an absence of acetoacetate and acetone. With insulin therapy, the nitroprusside test may more likely become positive as 3-hydroxybutyrate converts to acetoacetate.

Reference: Kohler, P.O., and Jordan, R.M. (eds.): Clinical Endocrinology. John Wiley and Sons, New York, 1986.

3–174. **(A)** Serum potassium may be elevated during untreated diabetic ketoacidosis secondary to hemoconcentration, decreased uptake by the cell, and a shift of potassium out of the cell and hydrogen ion into the cell. With hydration and insulin therapy the above phenomena are reversed, and the potassium level will fall. Potassium is lost during osmotic diuresis, and there may actually be a total body potassium deficit despite high serum levels. When serum potassium falls to 5 mEq/l, replacement therapy is warranted.

Reference: Hamburger, S., Rush, D.R., and Bosker, G.: Endocrine and Metabolic Emergencies. Robert J. Brady, Bowie, MD, 1984.

3–175. **(A)** The patient is acidotic and should be hyperventilating. Excess hydrogen ion (H^+) combines with bicarbonate buffer (HCO_3^-) to form carbonic acid (H_2CO_3). Carbonic acid readily dissociates into H_2O and CO_2. Elevated serum CO_2 stimulates the respiratory center in the medulla to increase respiratory rate and depth. As a result, the arterial CO_2 tension is lowered.

Reference: Holloway, N.M.: Nursing the Critically Ill Adult, 3rd ed. Addison-Wesley, Menlo Park, CA, 1988.

3–176. **(C)** Endocarditis associated with aortic regurgitation may be complicated by infarctions resulting from the embolization of valvular vegetation. As the site is located on the aortic valve, arterial embolization would be anticipated in the spleen, causing left upper quadrant pain; in the kidney, causing hematuria; or in the brain, causing paralysis. An embolization site originating from the right heart, such as from the tricuspid or pulmonic valve, would be associated with the development of hemoptysis. Tachycardia is present in endocarditis and is related to fever, congestive failure, and anemia.

Reference: Underhill, S., Woods, S., Froelicher, E., et al.: Cardiac Nursing, 2nd ed. J.B. Lippincott, Philadelphia, 1989.

3–177. **(B)** Symptoms associated with cocaine intoxication include hyperexcitability, anxiety, headache, hypertension, tachycardia, hyperpnea, tachypnea, fever, nausea, vomiting, abdominal pain, delirium, convulsions, and coma.

Reference: Alspach, J.G. (ed.): AACN Core Curriculum for Critical Care Nursing, 4th ed. W.B. Saunders, Philadelphia, 1991.

3–178. (**B**) An *aura* refers to a peculiar sensation that some patients with seizures experience immediately preceding the definite symptoms of a seizure. An aura may be visual, auditory, or gustatory, or it may be numbness or tingling of a body part. *Prodromal* is a term used to describe early symptoms of a disease. *Ictus* refers to an acute seizure. An *epileptic cry* is a sound sometimes produced during a seizure.

Reference: Hickey, J.V.: The Clinical Practice of Neurological and Neurosurgical Nursing, 2nd ed. J.B. Lippincott, Philadelphia, 1986.

3–179. (**C**) The patient has decreased WBCs and T cells as well as a reversed T4:T8, indicating decreased immune system function and increased risk for infection. The red cell count is normal, therefore eliminating anemia and polycythemia. The platelet count is also normal, eliminating an increased risk of bleeding.

Reference: Alspach, J.G. (ed.): AACN Core Curriculum for Critical Care Nursing, 4th ed. W.B. Saunders, Philadelphia, 1991.

3–180. (**A**) The decreased WBCs and T cells as well as the reversed T4:T8 are strong indicators of the presence of HIV infection. The western blot test would be done to confirm the presence of HIV infection. A Coombs test detects the presence of immune antibodies and is used to differentiate types of hemolytic anemias. A bleeding time is used to assess platelet function as well as capillary function. Since the platelet level is normal and there is no history of bleeding, there is no reason to perform a bleeding time.

Reference: Gee, G., and Moran, T.A.: AIDS—Concepts in Nursing Practice. Williams & Wilkins, Baltimore, 1988.

3–181. (**C**) The clinical picture presented suggests a tension pneumothorax. As air fills the pleural space, the intrathoracic pressure increases, which triggers the high pressure alarm on the ventilator and causes the affected side to become larger and the intercostal spaces to bulge.

Reference: Kersten, L.D.: Comprehensive Respiratory Nursing: A Decision Making Approach. W.B. Saunders, Philadelphia, 1989.

3–182. (**A**) Early ambulation is essential to maintain and improve muscle strength as well as to mobilize secretions. Smoking should be stopped at least 48 hours prior to surgery and not resumed until recovery is made. A change in smoking habits will not have much of an effect, unless the patient stops smoking. Prophylactic antibiotic therapy may promote growth of resistant bacteria or other organisms such as viruses and fungi.

Reference: Alspach, J.G. (ed.): AACN Core Curriculum for Critical Care Nursing, 4th Ed. W.B. Saunders, Philadelphia, 1991.

3–183. (**B**) After carotid endarterectomy, there may be transient impairment of carotid sinus reflexes causing inhibition of the vasomotor center, resulting in hypotension. Reflex vagal stimulation causes bradycardia. Increased intracranial pressure would cause an increase in blood pressure. Cerebral ischemia and blood loss would both cause an increase in the heart rate.

Reference: Fahey, V.: Vascular Nursing. W.B. Saunders, Philadelphia, 1988.

3–184. (**C**) Although dialysis may eliminate some uremic symptoms, the patient will not feel perfectly well. It is important that the nurse not convey to the patient that she can be restored to her previous state of health. The nurse needs to recognize the stressors the patient is experiencing. Even though the patient will be able to perform activities of daily living, her lifestyle will have to be adjusted to the dialysis treatments, and she needs time to accept this.

References: Eccard, M: Adjustments and psychosocial impact of end stage renal disease: Nursing intervention. In Lancaster, L.E. (ed.): The Patient with End Stage Renal Disease, 2nd ed. John Wiley and Sons, New York, 1984.
Thompson, J., McFarland, G.K., Hirsch, J.E., et al. (eds.): Mosby's Manual of Clinical Nursing, 2nd ed. C.V. Mosby, St. Louis, 1989.
Ulrich, B.T.: Psychological aspects of nephrology nursing. In Ulrich, B.T. (ed.): Nephrology Nursing: Concepts and Strategies. Appleton and Lange, Norwalk, CT, 1989.

3–185. (**D**) All are possible nursing diagnoses, but this patient is expressing a problem in coping with her disease, its treatment, and her inability to return to a "normal" state of health.

References: Jett, M., Lancaster, L., and Small, S.: Renal Disorders. In Renal and Urologic Disorders. Springhouse, Springhouse, PA, 1984.
Thompson, J., McFarland, G.K., Hirsch, J.E., et al. (eds.): Mosby's Manual of Clinical Nursing, 2nd ed. C.V. Mosby, St. Louis, 1989.

3–186. (**A**) The patient's low blood pressure and wedge pressure together with a hematocrit less than 30% indicate the need for a transfusion. A fluid bolus may improve the blood pressure and filling pressures temporarily, but would not improve the oxygen-carrying capacity or hematocrit. Dopamine in this situation would increase the myocardial work and oxygen demand. Verapamil would decrease the heart rate, which for this patient is the compensatory mechanism for his hypovolemic state.

Reference: Daily, E., and Schroeder, J.: Techniques in Bedside Hemodynamic Monitoring, 3rd ed. C.V. Mosby, St. Louis, 1985.

3–187. (**D**) Excessive chest tube drainage that abruptly stops may signify a pericardial tamponade or hemothorax. Chest x-ray and laboratory studies may be ordered to confirm blood losses and to rule out the presence of tamponade or hemothorax.

Reference: Millar, S., Sampson, L., and Soukup, M.: AACN Procedure Manual for Critical Care. W.B. Saunders, Philadelphia, 1985.

3–188. (**B**) Mineralocorticoids, primarily aldosterone, enhance sodium reabsorption from the renal filtrate across the distal tubular epithelial cells. The rise in serum electrolyte concentration results in an additional renal reabsorption of water to maintain normal serum osmolality. This preserves intravascular volume. In the absence of aldosterone, intravascular fluid volume becomes contracted, as manifested by orthostatic hypotension.

Reference: Kohler, P.O., and Jordan, R.M. (eds.): Clinical Endocrinology. John Wiley and Sons, New York, 1986.

3–189. (**B**) A bracelet identifying a risk for adrenal insufficiency should be worn by the patient to protect him in the event of injury or unconsciousness. It is also desirable for the patient to carry an emergency kit containing hydrocortisone and instructions for injection. The patient should contact a physician to adjust the steroid dosage.

Reference: Muthe, N.C.: Endocrinology, A Nursing Approach. Little, Brown, Boston, 1981.

3–190. (**A**) Complete transsection of the spinal cord causes irreversible loss of sensory and motor function below the level of the lesion. A spinal cord injury between T1 and L2 causes varying degrees of intercostal and abdominal muscle loss. In the acute phase, cardiac output is diminished owing to the loss of sympathetic outflow caused by the transsection; vasodilatation, decreased venous return, and hypotension result. Bradycardia is also seen a result of the sympathetic blockade. Typically, vital capacity is diminished as a result of hypoventilation in injuries below C4. Intracranial pressure is not usually affected.

Reference: Alspach, J.G. (ed.): AACN Core Curriculum for Critical Care Nursing, 4th ed. W.B. Saunders, Philadelphia, 1991.

3–191. (**D**) The nurse should first ascertain whether the patient is in stable or unstable supraventricular tachycardia by assessing blood pressure and level of consciousness. The patient who has just had his AICD removed may need adjustment of his antidysrhythmic medications.

Reference: American Heart Association: Textbook of Advanced Cardiac Life Support. Dallas, 1987.

3–192. (**D**) The cause of DIC is not clearly understood. However, many conditions have been identified as possible triggers for developing DIC. These include infections, including gram-negative infections; oncologic problems, including leukemias and prostate cancer; and trauma, such as crush injuries and near-drowning.

Reference: Shoemaker, W.C., Ayers, S., Grenvik, A., et al.: Textbook of Critical Care Medicine, 2nd ed. W.B. Saunders, Philadelphia, 1989.

3–193. (**B**) This patient's sensory-perceptual alteration is mostly likely related to ammonia retention associated with her hepatic failure. Retained ammonia is very toxic to nerve cells. As ammonia intoxication progresses, patients proceed from irritability to confusion, coma, and asterixis (liver flapping).

References: Ganong, W.F.: Review of Medical Physiology, 13th ed. Appleton and Lange, Norwalk, CT, 1987.
Holloway, N.M.: Nursing the Critically Ill Adult, 3rd ed. Addison-Wesley, New York, 1988.

3–194. (**C**) 1:4 augmentation is utilized in intra-aortic balloon pump weaning protocols to determine the ability of the heart to compensate for increased afterload. Generally, the patient is weaned from 1:1 to 1:2 augmentation before being placed on 1:4 augmentation. Although the pulmonary capillary wedge pressure is 12 mm Hg, this is considered to be in the high range of normal. The patient is therefore demonstrating neither continued failure nor intra-aortic balloon pump dependence. Early sepsis would cause lower blood pressure and increased heart rate, which are not present in the example given.

Reference: Weeks, L.: Advanced Cardiovascular Nursing. Blackwell, Boston, 1986.

3–195. (**C**) The main inspiratory muscles are the diaphragm and the external intercostals, with the accessory muscles being the scalene and sternocleidomastoids. The diaphragm is supplied by the phrenic nerves from C3 to C5. The external intercostals are supplied by the intercostal nerves, which come off the spinal cord at the same level of the rib they innervate.

Reference: West, J.B.: Respiratory Physiology: The Essentials, 4th ed. Williams & Wilkins, Baltimore, 1990.

3–196. (**C**) Compression (TED) hose do not prevent pulmonary emboli. They provide support for the vascular system.

Reference: Braunwald, E., Isselbacher, K.J., Petersdorf, R.G., et al. (eds.): Harrison's Principles of Internal Medicine, 11th ed. McGraw-Hill, New York, 1987.

3–197. (**C**) Stiff neck, or nuchal rigidity, photophobia, blurred vision, and positive Kernig's and Brudzinski's signs are indicative of subarachnoid hemorrhage. Kernig's sign is assessed by flexing the patient's hip and knee while the patient is in the dorsal recumbent position. The examiner flexes the patient's hip at 90° and attempts to slowly extend the knee. The patient experiencing resistance or pain has a positive Kernig's sign.

Reference: Hickey, J.V.: The Clinical Practice of Neurological and Neurosurgical Nursing, 2nd ed. J.B. Lippincott, Philadelphia, 1986.

3–198. (**B**) Epidural hematomas usually form quickly, within 6 hours of injury, as a result of arterial bleeding. They usually cause periods of lucidity and may or may not cause loss of consciousness. Whereas epidural hematomas, if left untreated, are fatal, subdural hematomas actually have the highest mortality of all head injuries (60% to 90%).

Reference: Cardona, V.D., Hurn, P.D., Mason, P.J.B., et al. (eds.): Trauma Nursing: From Resuscitation Through Rehabilitation. W.B. Saunders, Philadelphia, 1988.

3–199. (**A**) Finding out how the patient behaved with life changes prior to this crisis will identify the patient's usual coping mechanisms and encourage their use at this time.

Reference: Thompson, J., McFarland, G.K., Hirsch, J.E., et al.: Mosby's Manual of Clinical Nursing, 2nd ed. C.V. Mosby, St. Louis, 1989.

3–200. (**C**) Since there is no correlation between the P waves and the QRS complexes, this rhythm is due to third degree heart block. The P waves are regularly occurring at a rate of 100 per minute. Some P waves are identifiable on the S waves of the QRS complexes. The QRS complexes are wide, indicating ventricular origin, and cannot be attributed to conduction from the preceding P waves.

Reference: Andreoli, K., Fowkes, V., Zipes, D., et al.: Comprehensive Cardiac Care, 6th ed. C.V. Mosby, St. Louis, 1987.

Annotated Bibliography

PULMONARY

Alspach, J.G. (ed.): AACN Core Curriculum for Critical Care Nursing, 4th ed. W.B. Saunders, Philadelphia, 1991.
Updated edition presented in nursing process format with nursing diagnosis and interventions. Excellent reference for both beginning and advanced critical care nurses.

Bordow, R.A., and Moser, K.M.: Manual of Clinical Problems in Pulmonary Medicine, 2nd ed. Little, Brown, Boston, 1985.
Excellent handbook reference for pulmonary problems and therapy. Physiologic basis of disease is limited, but the text covers many diseases and most therapy.

Braunwald, E., Isselbacher, K.J., Petersdorf, R.G., et al. (eds.): Harrison's Principles of Internal Medicine, 11th ed. McGraw-Hill, New York, 1987.
Extensive reference for pathophysiology and medical treatment. Normal physiology is not generally reviewed, but the text covers a wide scope of medical conditions in a concise manner.

Civetta, J.M., Taylor, R.W., and Kirby, R.R.: Critical Care. J.B. Lippincott, Philadelphia, 1988.
Reference on critical care that is conceptual in nature. Discusses the team approach to critical care, physician-nurse relationships, and ethical issues such as termination of life-support, as well as disease processes. A must for any nurse in critical care.

Kersten, L.D.: Comprehensive Respiratory Nursing: A Decision Making Approach. W.B. Saunders, Philadelphia, 1989.
An invaluable resource for nurses. Covers respiratory nursing care exhaustively with graphs and tables that concisely and simply describe physiology, signs, and symptoms. Provides interventions and information on psychosocial and rehabilitation aspects. A must for any nurse in pulmonary nursing.

Kinney, M.R., Packa, D.R., and Dunbar, S.B.: AACN's Clinical Reference for Critical Care Nursing, 2nd ed. McGraw-Hill, New York, 1988.
Comprehensive text for all critical care nurses. Excellent reference of physiology and pathophysiology integrated with nursing care.

Millar, S.: Procedure Manual for Critical Care, 2nd ed. W.B. Saunders, Philadelphia, 1985.
Reference manual for critical care procedures. Procedures based on research. Standards listed for all critical care patients.

Shapiro, B.A., Harrison, R.A., Cane, R.D., et al.: Clinical Application of Blood Gases, 4th ed. Year Book Medical Publishers, Chicago, 1989.
Excellent reference for reviewing blood gases and physiology associated with oxygen transport. Bedside and noninvasive measurements of blood gases are also reviewed and case studies of different pathologies are presented at the end for illustration of physiologic principles.

Shoemaker, W.C., Ayres, S., Grenvik, A., et al.: Textbook of Critical Care, 2nd ed. W.B. Saunders, Philadelphia, 1989.
An excellent resource on many areas of critical care. This text is more physiologically based and technical. Discusses pathology as well as monitoring techniques.

Snyder, J.V., and Pinsky, M.R.: Oxygen Transport in the Critically Ill. Year Book Medical Publishers, Chicago, 1987.
Excellent resource on all aspects of oxygenation and oxygen transport.

West, J.B.: Respiratory Physiology: The Essentials, 4th ed. Williams & Wilkins, Baltimore, 1990.
Classic text for pulmonary physiology. Easy to read and understand, yet comprehensive.

West, J.B.: Pulmonary Pathophysiology: The Essentials, 3rd ed. Williams & Wilkins, Baltimore, 1987.
Companion text for the physiology text. Discusses disease states and pathophysiology associated with the diseases. Some therapy is discussed, but not in depth.

CARDIOVASCULAR

Alspach, J.G. (ed.): AACN Core Curriculum for Critical Care Nursing, 4th ed. W.B. Saunders, Philadelphia, 1991.
Primary text upon which the content for the CCRN examination is based. It includes much of the relevant physiology, clinical symptomatology, nursing diagnoses, and nursing interventions upon which critical care nursing practice is founded.

American Heart Association: Textbook of Advanced Cardiac Life Support. Dallas, 1987.
Excellent review of current standards of practice in advanced life support. This text also reviews cardiac dysrhythmias, physiology, cardiac medications, and risk factors.

Andreoli, K., Fowkes, V., Zipes, D., et al.: Comprehensive Cardiac Care, 6th ed. C.V. Mosby, St. Louis, 1987.
Superb review of ECG interpretation, dysrhythmias, coronary care, and physical assessment of the patient with cardiovascular disease.

Bustin, D.: Hemodynamic Monitoring in Critical Care. Appleton-Century-Crofts, Norwalk, CT, 1986.
A simplified approach to hemodynamic monitoring with multiple choice questions for practice after each chapter.

Daily, E., and Schroeder, J.: Techniques in Bedside Hemodynamic Monitoring, 3rd ed. C.V. Mosby, St. Louis, 1985.
Principles and practice of hemodynamic monitoring are explained concisely in this text, which also gives case studies of selected cardiovascular and pulmonary conditions affecting the critically ill patient population. Interventional strategies in relation to hemodynamic monitoring are provided.

Fahey, V.: Vascular Nursing. W.B. Saunders, Philadelphia, 1988.
Describes pathology, physiology, and surgical processes in vascular surgery. Postoperative care of the patient is described well.

Hurst, C.: Dysrhythmia Interpretation Based on Cardiac Suppression and Irritability. J.B. Lippincott, Philadelphia, 1986.
Text is an excellent reference on dysrhythmia interpretation. Utilizes the concepts of suppression and irritability to define the ECG and discusses the hemodynamic effects of both dysrhythmias and

189

their therapies. Contains also a well-organized, excellent discussion of action potentials and pacemakers.

Kenner, C., Guzzetta, C., and Dossey, B.: Critical Care Nursing: Body—Mind—Spirit. Little, Brown, Boston, 1985.

Holistic approach to critical care nursing. Text first describes assessment findings and then discusses clinical disease states for each body system. Provides nursing diagnoses and interventions as well as directions for future research and alternative approaches to nursing care.

Kinney, M., Packa, D., and Dunbar, S.: AACN's Clinical Reference for Critical Care Nursing, 2nd ed. McGraw-Hill, New York, 1988.

Excellent text for nurses who have been involved in critical care for a number of years. Gives extensive information on complex conditions and practice in critical care.

Millar, S., Sampson, L., and Soukup, M.: AACN Procedure Manual for Critical Care. W.B. Saunders, Philadelphia, 1985.

Excellent AACN text is a good review for discussion and rationale of critical care nursing procedures.

Reuther, M., and Hansen, C.: Cardiovascular Nursing. Medical Examination Publishing, New York, 1985.

Straightforward text utilizing the nursing process approach to cardiovascular nursing. Gives a holistic view with simplified explanations and suggestions for patient teaching. Many case studies are offered, and although the nursing diagnoses are not standard, they are useful in nursing care planning.

Underhill, S., Woods, S., Froelicher, E., et al.: Cardiac Nursing, 2nd ed. J.B. Lippincott, Philadelphia, 1989.

An expensive book but well worth the price. Contains everything the critical care nurse needs to know about the cardiovascular system and how to assess and care for patients with cardiovascular problems.

Weeks, L.: Advanced Cardiovascular Nursing. Blackwell, Boston, 1986.

Excellent text for advanced practitioners, containing a chapter on cardiac assist devices. Text is divided into sections including pathophysiology, assessment, interventions, and professional issues.

NEUROLOGIC

Alspach, J.G. (ed.): AACN Core Curriculum for Critical Care Nursing, 4th ed. W.B. Saunders, Philadelphia, 1991.

Excellent, comprehensive review of critical care nursing presenting content in detail. Provides an appropriate synthesis of essential knowledge of the critical care patient experiencing neurologic and neurosurgical disorders. Presented in nursing process format, the text is organized in outline form to facilitate understanding.

Caine, R.M., and Bufalino, P.M.: Nursing Care Planning Guides for Adults. Williams & Wilkins, Baltimore, 1987.

A valuable resource for nurses who provide care in a variety of acute and rehabilitative settings for the patient with neurologic and neurosurgical disorders. The text provides a thorough discussion of the nursing process as it relates to patients with specific medical-surgical problems. The patient as an individual with social and family roles is emphasized throughout.

Caine, R.M., and Bufalino, P.M.: Critically Ill Adults: Nursing Care Planning Guides. Williams & Wilkins, Baltimore, 1988.

An excellent resource for nurses who provide nursing care to neurologic and neurosurgical patients in a variety of acute care settings. The nursing process is the format utilized. Nursing diagnoses are presented along with rationale and expected outcomes. Nurses can utilize various aspects of the content to facilitate care, apply information as it pertains to specific patients, and individualize care for the critically ill adult. The chapters on neurologic disorders are excellent.

Caine, R., Molla, K., and Reynolds, R.: Malignant hyperthermia: A critical care challenge. Dimen Crit Care Nurs, 5(3):144–154, 1986.

Review article that is an outstanding reference on the pathophysiology and nursing care of the patient with malignant hyperthermia, a pharmacogenetic disorder. Includes a case study and excellent tables to facilitate understanding.

Cardona, V.D., Hurn, P.D., Mason, P.J.B., et al. (eds.): Trauma Nursing: From Resuscitation Through Rehabilitation. W.B. Saunders, Philadelphia, 1988.

Comprehensive and well-written text that discusses trauma along the continuum from time of injury through rehabilitation. A conceptual framework of trauma is utilized throughout. The neurologic chapter is excellent, presenting comprehensive pathophysiology, interventions, and rehabilitation concepts.

Hickey, J.V.: The Clinical Practice of Neurological and Neurosurgical Nursing, 2nd ed. J.B. Lippincott, Philadelphia, 1986.

Comprehensive text on neurologic and neurosurgical conditions. Excellent tables and illustrations. Presents complex material in an understandable manner.

Hartshorn, J., and Hartshorn, E.: Pharmacology update: Vasopressin in the treatment of diabetes insipidus. J Neurosci Nurs, 20(1):58–59, 1988.

Good review article dealing with diabetes insipidus and vasopressin administration. Easy to read and understand.

Holloway, N.M.: Nursing the Critically Ill Adult, 3rd ed. Addison-Wesley, Menlo Park, CA, 1988.

Good review text for understanding multiple critical care disorders. Text uses a FANCAS model for presentation of material. Neurologic chapters include an easy-to-understand review of pathophysiology related to various disorders. Nursing diagnoses are used throughout.

Kinney, M.R., Packa, D.R., and Dunbar, S.B. (eds.): AACN's Clinical Reference for Critical Care Nursing. McGraw-Hill, New York, 1988.

An excellent comprehensive text for critical care nurses. Pathophysiology is presented thoroughly as it relates to basic neurologic function and various neurologic disorders. Numerous tables and illustrations are used to enhance understanding. This book is directed at the advanced clinician desiring detailed information related to critical care nursing.

Larson, E.L., and Vazquez, M.: Critical Care Nursing. W.B. Saunders, Philadelphia, 1983.

A reference text for critical care reviewing pertinent assessment, diagnostic, and nursing management information. Sections related to the neurologic and neurosurgical patient are good refreshers for the nurse desiring a quick review of applicable information.

Nikas, D.: The Critically Ill Neurosurgical Patient. Churchill Livingstone, New York, 1982.

Valuable advanced text on neurosurgical nursing. Provides a good understanding of the pathophysiologic basis for various neurologic conditions requiring surgery. Appropriate treatment and rationale for interventions are provided.

Rudy, E.: Advanced Neurological and Neurosurgical Nursing. C.V. Mosby, St. Louis, 1984.

Advanced text detailing neurologic and neurosurgical information in a readable format. Physiologic presentations are directed at both the beginning and the advanced clinician.

RENAL

Alspach, J.G. (ed.): AACN Core Curriculum for Critical Care Nursing, 4th ed. W.B. Saunders, Philadelphia, 1991.

Utilizing outline format, text covers all areas of the nursing process for body systems. Information is concise and serves as a refresher or as a basis for further study of renal dysfunctions in critical care. An excellent reference for critical care nurses preparing for the CCRN certification examination.

Cardona, V.D., Hurn, P.D., Mason, P.J.B., et al. (eds.): Trauma Nursing: From Resuscitation Through Rehabilitation. W.B. Saunders, Philadelphia, 1988.

An excellent reference for any nurse managing care of trauma patients. Included are chapters on single system injuries, as well as ethical and legal aspects, infection control, and unique patient populations, such as trauma in the elderly. The chapter on genitourinary injuries and renal management gives useful information on the types of injuries that may result in renal failure, complications, and rehabilitation.

Fincke, M., and Lanros, N.: Emergency Nursing: A Comprehensive Review. Aspen, Rockville, MD, 1986.

Good reference for nurses, covering major conditions patients present in the emergency department. Includes a chapter on fluids, electrolytes, and hemodynamics.

Gilman, A.G., Goodman, L.S., Rall, T.W., et al. (eds.): Goodman & Gilman's The Pharmacologic Basis of Therapeutics, 7th ed. Macmillan, New York, 1985.

Comprehensive drug reference dealing with all aspects of pathophysiology, medication usage, indications, and actions.

Hamilton, H., and Rose, M.B.: Renal and Urological Disorders. Springhouse, Springhouse, PA, 1984.

A good basic book for renal disorders. Presented in an easy-to-understand format and accompanied by illustrations and tables that are very useful.

Lancaster, L. (ed.): The Patient with End Stage Renal Disease, 2nd ed. John Wiley and Sons, New York, 1984.

Deals with all aspects of caring for the patient with end stage renal disease (ESRD). Written for nurses interested in nephrology, this book covers areas from pathophysiology and psychosocial aspects to modes of treatment and public policy. Provides a good basis for care of these patients.

Massry, S.G., and Glassock, R.J.: Textbook of Nephrology. Williams & Wilkins, Baltimore, 1983.

Two-volume medical text covering topics of anatomy and physiology, endocrine function of the kidney, altered water and electrolyte balances, and analysis of disease states and their treatments. Difficult for beginning practitioner in nursing, but a good reference.

Roberts, S.L.: Physiological Concepts and the Critically Ill Patient. Prentice-Hall, Englewood Cliffs, NJ, 1985.

Various categories of critically ill patients receive a detailed discussion in this text. Focus is on the physiologic concepts. Each chapter contains a definition of terms. Renal assessment, diagnosis, and interventions are covered in detail.

Thompson, J., McFarland, G.K., Hirsch, J.E., et al.: Mosby's Manual of Clinical Nursing, 2nd ed. C.V. Mosby, St. Louis, 1989.

Comprehensive nursing text covering all areas of nursing practice. Each system is covered in a separate chapter. In addition to the system review and related diseases, chapters cover nursing diagnosis in great detail.

Ulrich, T. (ed.): Nephrology Nursing: Concepts and Strategies. Appleton and Lange, Norwalk, CT, 1989.

Very good text for nurses interested in any aspect of renal failure, either acute or chronic. Covers topics from anatomy and physiology through quality assurance and research. Also includes a chapter on the pediatric renal patient. Well written and easy to understand.

ENDOCRINE

Alspach, J.G. (ed.): AACN Core Curriculum for Critical Care Nursing, 4th ed. W.B. Saunders, Philadelphia, 1991.

Content organized in outline format. Includes an overview of endocrine anatomy, physiology, and pathophysiology. Also featured are a general nursing assessment database and commonly encountered nursing diagnoses relevant to endocrine problems.

Brenner, Z.R.: Diagnostic Tests and Procedures, Applying the Nursing Process. Appleton and Lange, Norwalk, CT, 1987.

Laboratory tests, their purpose, normal values, and applicable nursing actions are organized according to the nursing diagnoses to which they apply. Descriptions of diagnostic procedures include relevant nursing diagnoses, assessment parameters, and nursing interventions.

Hadley, M.E.: Endocrinology, 2nd ed. Prentice-Hall, Englewood Cliffs, NJ, 1988.

Comprehensive and complex description of neuroendocrine physiology at the chemical and molecular level versus the clinical level. Molecular structure of hormones and hormonal regulation is emphasized. Pathophysiology is briefly addressed.

Hamburger, S., Rush, D.R., and Bosker, G.: Endocrine and Metabolic Emergencies. Robert J. Brady, Bowie, MD, 1984.

Clinical medical reference that briefly addresses common endocrine and metabolic states that warrant emergency treatment. Information such as signs and symptoms, laboratory diagnostics and abnormalities, and complications and treatments are highlighted for rapid reference. Included is a "diagnostic syllabus appendix" geared for the emergency room or critical care practitioner.

Holloway, N.M.: Nursing the Critically Ill Adult, 3rd ed. Addison-Wesley, Menlo Park, CA, 1988.
Emphasizes assessment parameters of pathophysiologic states and highlights nursing diagnoses that are applicable. Nursing care content is organized according to nursing diagnosis. Numerous illustrations and sample nursing care plans enhance content.

Kohler, P.O., and Jordan, R.M. (eds.): Clinical Endocrinology. John Wiley and Sons, New York, 1986.
Comprehensive clinical text featuring molecular, cellular, and clinical aspects of endocrine physiology and pathophysiology. Clinical manifestations, medical diagnostics, and treatment are emphasized. Numerous illustrations and diagrams enhance content.

McLane, A.M. (ed.): Classification of Nursing Diagnoses. Proceedings of the Seventh Conference. C.V. Mosby, St. Louis, 1987.
Includes a current list of nursing diagnoses and their definitions, risk factors, and major and minor defining characteristics. An essential reference for nursing diagnosis.

Mountcastle, V.B. (ed.): Medical Physiology, 14th ed. C.V. Mosby, St. Louis, 1980.
Provides detailed endocrine physiology, including hormone biosynthesis, secretion, and regulation. Diagrams of chemical and molecular structures and biochemical processes simplify content.

Muthe, N.C.: Endocrinology, A Nursing Approach. Little, Brown, Boston, 1981.
Organized overview of endocrine physiology and pathophysiology. Diagnostics, medical interventions, and nursing care are addressed in textbook format.

Wills, S.L., and Tremblay, S.F.: Critical Care Review for Nurses. Wadsworth, Belmont, CA, 1984.
Includes a basic and brief overview of endocrine anatomy and physiology, assessment guidelines, and endocrine disease states. Nursing interventions are listed. Important concepts are summarized as "key concepts," and self-assessment tests are offered throughout the text.

HEMATOLOGY

Alspach, J.G. (ed.): AACN Core Curriculum for Critical Care Nursing, 4th ed. W.B. Saunders, Philadelphia, 1991.
Comprehensive overview of basic information required by critical care nurses. Presented in an outline format, the hematology chapter covers most essential material for today's practitioner.

Bonato, J.: Blood transfusions: Are they safe? Crit Care Nurs, 9:40–46, 1989
Article explores the issues surrounding the safety of blood transfusions. Presents basic points related to managing the transfusion of major blood components.

Cox, H.C., Hinz, M.D., Lubno, M.A., et al.: Clinical Applications of Nursing Diagnosis. Williams & Wilkins, Baltimore, 1989.
Text provides a summary of current nursing diagnoses, defining characteristics, nursing orders, and patient evaluation.

Crow, S.: Asepsis as a part of the patient care plan. Crit Care Nurs Q, 11:11–16, 1989.
Author provides a straightforward overview of the principles of asepsis and applies them to basic patient care planning.

Dickerson, M.A.: Anaphylaxis and anaphylactic shock. Crit Care Nurs Q, 11:68–74, 1988.
Article presents a comprehensive overview of the mechanism for the development of anaphylaxis and anaphylactic reactions. In addition, the rationale for signs and symptoms and treatment is fully covered.

Dickerson, M.A.: Protecting yourself from AIDS: Infection control measures for the critical care practitioner. Crit Care Nurs, 9:26–28, 1989.
Article explores concern about protecting the individual health care provider from infectious diseases such as HIV infection and AIDS. Development of infection control practices and appropriate implementation of those practices are also discussed.

Doenges, M., and Moorhouse, M.: Nursing Diagnosis with Interventions. F.A. Davis, Philadelphia, 1988.
Excellent book that provides definitions of the nursing diagnosis as well as various etiologies, defining characteristics, and treatments. Useful in planning care for the critically ill patient.

Gee, G., and Moran, T.A.: AIDS—Concepts in Nursing Practice. Williams & Wilkins, Baltimore, 1988.
Comprehensive text explores the various aspects of AIDS and HIV infection.

Griffin, J.P.: Hematology and Immunology. Appleton-Century-Crofts, Norwalk, CT, 1986.
Author discusses various types of disease and treatment modalities for patients who have hematologic disorders.

Littleton, M.T.: Pathophysiology and assessment of sepsis and septic shock. Crit Care Nurs Q, 11:30–47, 1988.
Article describes the pathophysiology, etiology, assessment, and treatment parameters for septic shock. Excellent summary article.

Mathewson, M.K.: Pharmacotherapeutics: A Nursing Process Approach. F.A. Davis, Philadelphia, 1986.
Author explores the various medications, including anticoagulants, given today to patients. Has an excellent emphasis on patient teaching, side effects, and care planning.

Shoemaker, W.C., Ayers, S., Grenvik, A., et al.: Textbook of Critical Care Medicine. W.B. Saunders, Philadelphia, 1989.
Textbook provides a definitive description of common critical care problems. Excellent chapters on physiology, DIC, transfusions, and septic shock.

Smith, S.: The Immune System: Physiologic Considerations in Critical Care. In American Association of Critical-Care Nurses. Proceedings of the Sixteenth Annual National Teaching Institute. American Association of Critical-Care Nurses, Newport Beach, CA, 1989.
This article provides an overview of the physiology of the immune system and its application to critical care.

Von Rueden, K.T., and Walleck, C.A.: Advanced Critical Care Nursing. Aspen, Rockville, MD, 1989.
A case study approach to provide insight into primary problems encountered by nurses in critical care, including patients with DIC, AIDS, and immunosuppression.

Wall, S.C.: Septic shock. Nursing '89, 19:52–60, 1989.
Article provides an overview of the stages of septic shock, the changes in hemodynamic parameters, and nursing care for the patient.

193

GASTROINTESTINAL

DeGroot, K.D., and Damato, M.B. (eds.): Critical Care Skills. Appleton and Lange, Norwalk, CT, 1987.
Discussion of beginning to advanced critical care skills. Easy-to-follow outline format with emphasis on what to do and how to do it. Excellent diagrams, charts, and photographs of critical care skills. Strengths of the chapter on the gastrointestinal system include assessment methods and practical procedure guides.

Drossman, D.A.: Manual of Gastroenterologic Procedures, 2nd ed. Raven Press, New York, 1987.
Concise presentation of current gastroenterologic diagnostic procedures. Also describes nonsurgical treatment procedures. Written for the physician but very useful for the nurse who wants to know the steps of a procedure and appropriate postprocedure follow-up.

Ganong, W.F.: Review of Medical Physiology, 13th ed. Appleton and Lange, Norwalk, CT, 1987.
One of two essential physiology reference books that includes up-to-date human physiology based on research. Content is written in straightforward, narrative style.

Gitnick, G. (ed.): Handbook of Gastrointestinal Emergencies, 2nd ed. Medical Examination Publishing, New York, 1987.
Systematic review of appropriate rapid response to gastrointestinal emergencies seen in the emergency room and hospital. Content is confined to essential emergency care. Very useful in emphasis on critical responses to gastrointestinal patient crises. Written as a study text for physician board exams.

Guyton, A.C.: Textbook of Medical Physiology, 7th ed. W.B. Saunders, Philadelphia, 1986.
One of two essential physiology reference books that includes current, research-based physiology. Content is comprehensive but clear and straightforward.

Holloway, N.M.: Nursing the Critically Ill Adult, 3rd ed. Addison-Wesley, New York, 1988.
Successful integration of the art and science of critical care nursing. Strong psychosocial emphasis but not at the expense of the more traditional critical care content such as disease process and treatment. Organized from a nursing framework and cross-indexed to disease process.

Johanson, B.C., Wells, S.J., Hoffmeister, D., et al. (eds.): Standards for Critical Care, 3rd ed. C.V. Mosby, St. Louis, 1988.
Presentation of critical care nursing practice standards for interdependent and independent practice. Straightforward outline format includes brief discussions of disease processes followed by specific patient problems with nursing diagnoses, expected outcomes, and interventions. Excellent teaching plans.

Kinney, M.R., Packa, D.R., and Dunbar, S.B. (eds.): AACN's Clinical Reference for Critical Care Nursing, 2nd ed. McGraw-Hill, New York, 1988.
Comprehensive critical care nursing reference that exemplifies a collaborative approach to critical illness. Sound discussion of issues in critical care and phenomena of concern to critical care nurses is followed by a systematic review of patient care problems. Gastrointestinal patient care problems are reviewed for data acquisition, pathophysiology, diagnosis, medical/surgical therapies, and nursing

interventions. An essential critical care nursing reference book.

Luckmann, J., and Sorensen, K.C.: Medical-Surgical Nursing: A Psychophysiologic Approach, 3rd ed. W.B. Saunders, Philadelphia, 1987.
Comprehensive medical-surgical nursing reference that integrates pathophysiology and disease process with nursing process and practice. Well-referenced content is presented in clear narrative format. Excellent illustrations and photographs support a well-written text. Critical illness is covered in more depth than many critical care texts with a follow-through for patients after critical illness. An essential nursing reference book.

Myers, A.R. (ed.): Medicine. John Wiley and Sons, New York, 1986.
Review of disease processes presented in a succinct outline format. The gastrointestinal chapter is clear and comprehensive. Includes the etiology, clinical features, diagnostics, and appropriate medical therapy for each disease presented.

Sleisenger, M.H., and Fordtran, J.S. (eds.): Gastrointestinal Disease: Pathophysiology, Diagnosis, Management, 4th ed. W.B. Saunders, Philadelphia, 1989.
Classic gastrointestinal textbook for physicians. Presents state-of-the-art gastrointestinal pathophysiology, diagnosis, and treatment. Appropriate for careful study, but content exceeds that generally needed by the critical care nurse.

Swearingen, P.L., Sommers, M.S., and Miller, K.: Manual of Critical Care: Applying Nursing Diagnoses to Adult Critical Illness. C.V. Mosby, St. Louis, 1988.
Discussion of 70 critical patient conditions presented in a combination narrative/outline format. Indexed by system and disease process, discussed by pathophysiology, diagnosis, medical/surgical intervention, and nursing diagnosis. Very thorough cross-index. Outstanding presentation of interdependent and independent nursing interventions. Good highlighting of specific areas of concern in intervention sections. Primary gastrointestinal dysfunctions are clearly presented, as are those gastrointestinal patient care issues secondary to other etiologies.

ETHICAL/LEGAL

American Heart Association: Textbook of Advanced Cardiac Life Support. American Heart Association, Dallas, 1987.
Excellent reference on care of the acutely unstable patient who may have or has suffered cardiac arrest. Includes post-resuscitation management and ethical/legal and psychosocial information.

Armiger, Sr. B.: Ethics of nursing research: Profile, principles, and perspective. Nurs Res, 5:330–336, 1977.
Complete discussion of the personal and social issues involved in the research process. Remains relevant.

Beresford, H.R.: Legal aspects of terminating care. Sem Neurol, 1:23–29, 1984.
Discusses the legal constraints on the care providers in the decision whether to continue care. Includes the patient who can speak on his or her behalf, and substituted judgement.

Corbett, K., and Lynch, L.: Professional nursing issues in the administration of investigational antiarrhythmic medications. Heart Lung, 4:395–399, 1984.
Describes the process of FDA approval for drug trials and the legal and ethical obligations of the research

team. Also discusses psychosocial needs of the patient participating in an investigational drug trial.

Creighton, H.: Law Every Nurse Should Know, 4th ed. W.B. Saunders, Philadelphia, 1981.
Clear, concise general text on the legal system as it affects the practice of nursing.

Creighton, H.: Legal implications of the impaired nurse—Part I. Nurs Manag, 1:21–23, 1988.
Legal advice for the supervisor and colleagues of the impaired nurse. Discusses identifying and preparing to confront the impaired professional, and appropriate actions to be taken to assist the impaired nurse to enter a treatment program.

Creighton, H.: Legal implications of the impaired nurse—Part II. Nurs Manag, 2:20–21, 1988.
Includes assisting the person in rehabilitation and appropriate licensure constraints imposed upon the impaired individual.

Douglas, S., and Larson, E.: There's more to informed consent than information. Focus Crit Care, 2:43–47, 1986.
Clear discussion of the ethical problems of obtaining truly informed consent, both for treatment and for research.

Gaines, C., and Carter, D.: Overtime: A professional responsibility? Focus Crit Care, 4:270–273, 1989.
Analysis of the ethical/legal dilemmas in the problem of working overtime. A decision-making process is outlined to help the nurse clarify his or her position when faced with the conflict of the obligation to work versus the obligation to refrain from working.

Meisel, A., Grenvik, A., Pinkus, R.L., et al.: Hospital guidelines for deciding about life-sustaining treatment: Dealing with health "limbo." Crit Care Med, 3:239–246, 1986.
Includes discussion of ethics committees, patient autonomy, collaborative decision-making, incompetent patients, advance directives, and appropriate documentation.

Rahn, J.G.: General theories of hospital liability for negligence. Focus Crit Care, 2:48–49, 1986.
Outlines the responsibility borne by an agency for the negligent acts of its employees and the individual liability of the negligent person. The concept of the "deep pocket" is covered.

Smith, D.H., and Veatch, R.M. (eds.): Hastings Center Guidelines on the Termination of Life-Sustaining Treatment and Care of the Dying. Indiana University Press, Indianapolis, 1987.
Analysis of the many ramifications of ceasing life-sustaining care.

Thompson, J.B., and Thompson, H.O.: Ethics in Nursing. Macmillan, New York, 1981.
Complete text on the ethical issues in health care from a nursing perspective. Includes case studies.

Veatch, R.M.: Medical Ethics. Jones and Bartlett, Boston, 1989.
Especially good discussion of current ethical issues brought about by recent technological advances.

Wlody, G.S., and Smith, S.: Ethical dilemmas in critical care, a proposal for hospital ethics advisory committees. Focus Crit Care, 5:41–46, 1985.
Excellent discussion of the ethical frameworks underlying hospital ethics committees and the appropriate application of each model.

Yob, M.O.: Communication issues: a potential source of liability for nurses. Focus Crit Care, 2:78–79, 1988.
Describes the legal pitfalls of the interdependent relationship between nursing and medicine.

Younger, S.J.: Do-Not-Resuscitate orders: No longer a secret, but still a problem. Hastings Center Report, 1:24–33, 1987.
Although commonplace, DNR orders are not always easy to write or to follow. This article discusses some of the difficulties.